*f***P**

Menopause and the Mind

The Complete Guide to Coping with Memory Loss,
Foggy Thinking, Verbal Slips, and Other
Cognitive Effects of Perimenopause
and Menopause

CLAIRE L. WARGA, Ph.D

The Free Press

THE FREE PRESS
A Division of Simon & Schuster Inc.
1230 Avenue of the Americas
New York, NY 10020

THE FREE PRESS and colophon are trademarks
of Simon & Schuster Inc.

Designed by Carla Bolte

Manufactured in the United States of America

10   9   8   7   6   5   4   3   2   1

Library of Congress Cataloging-in-Publication Data
Warga, Claire.
    Menopause and the mind: the complete guide to coping with memory
    loss, foggy thinking, verbal slips, and other cognitive effects of
    perimenopause and menopause/by Claire Warga.
        p.   cm.
    Includes bibliographical references and index.
    1. Menopause—Psychological aspects.   2. Cognition disorders—
Endocrine aspects.   3. Estrogen—Therapeutic use.
4. Perimenopause—Psychological aspects.   I. Title
RG186.W34   1999
618.1'75'0019—dc21   99-11244
                                                    CIP

ISBN 0–684–85456–2

Note to Readers

This work is based on research by the author, and the ideas, procedures and suggestions in this book are not intended as a substitute for the individualized medical evaluation and advice of a qualified, licensed health professional. The author and publisher do not recommend changing medication, adding hormones or implementing dietary regimes without consulting your personal physician. Individual differences in health and family history require individualized health assessments. You should consult your health professional before adopting any of the suggestions in this book or drawing inferences from it. The author and publisher disclaim any liability arising directly or indirectly from the use of the book, or any of the products or treatments mentioned in it. In addition, the statements made by the author regarding certain products and treatments represent the views and opinions of the author, and do not constitute a recommendation or endorsement of any product or treatment by the publisher.

Dedication

This book is dedicated with love to
My wonderful husband, Jerry Landsberg, who values learning, books,
and the freedom to be, more than material possessions,
My clever gentle-hearted little boy, Joshua, whose existence lights my
life daily and who on summer nights loved brainstorming with me for
this book,
To my mother, Raia, for so many years of love, devotion, and
inspiration,
And the memory of my father, Gedaliah, who taught me to feel free
to step up and ask the world some questions.

Contents

Acknowledgments

I t has been a pleasure writing this book because of the help of so many people. My wonderful agent, Katinka Matson; my incisive, soothing, and highly constructive editor, Elizabeth Maguire; Chad Conway for his ever-readiness to help and delightful manner; Celia Knight and David Frost for their willingness to help so graciously.

My sincere thanks to the many scientists and physicians who gave freely of their time, often on numerous occasions: Dr. William Andrews, who has been listening well these many years; Dr. Maurice Cohen for our many talks, research articles, and news updates; Dr. Bruce McEwen for giving precious time and help amongst so many competing demands; Dr. Victoria Liune for being so open-minded early on and later; Dr. Dominique Toran-Allerand for talk, tolerated intrusions and her offers of help; to Dr. Barbara Sherwin for conversations and for laying the groundwork for this book with great skill and dedication to a field of research; to Dr. Robert Greene; to Dr. John Arpels, Dr. Roberta Diaz Brinton, Dr. Jim Simpkins, Dr. Stanley Birge, Dr. Victor Henderson, Dr. William Greenough, Dr. Claudia Kawas, Dr. Richard Mayeux, Pam Boggs, Dr. Paul Shaghrue, Dr. Paul Gold, Dr. Howard Fillet, Dr. Lila Nachtigall, Dr. Carol Shively, Jed Diamond, Dr. Nancy Desmond, Dr. Jill Einstein, Dr. Tina Williams, Dr. Sheryl Smith, Dr. Mary Lou Voytko, Dr. Janice Juraska, Dr. Annlia Paganini-Hill, Dr. Donna Korol, Dr. Doreen Kimura, Dr. Diane Jacobs, Dr. Jim Morrison, Dr. Susan Resnick, Dr. Jerri Janowsky, Dr. Sonia Lupien, Dr. Tom Foster, Dr. Claude Hughes, Dr. Frederick Naftolin, Dr. Allan Kluger, Dr. Elkanon Goldberg, Dr. Jamie Golumb, and the many others who graciously gave of themselves.

ACKNOWLEDGMENTS

My profound thanks go to the many women who entrusted me with their stories and taught me. To Letty Cottin Pogrebin, whose courage to "tell it like it is" confirmed a piece of this puzzle for me through her excellent book, her curiosity, and her openness—she continues to be a feminist leader; to Sherry Strumph, Polly Van Benthusen, Cheryl Calhoun and all the many alias women who shared with me this adventure in living; to the women in my reading groups who shared with me their private stories and the excitement of tracking this discovery during its varied stages.

Lastly to the firemen of Battalion 31 and the firemen of Middagh Street, without whom this book truly would not exist.

Introduction

This book is intended for women in their thirties, forties, fifties, and beyond who may be experiencing unusual come and go memory, speech, attention, behavior, thinking, and time-tracking symptoms no expert ever prepared them for and who want help in understanding and possibly treating such symptoms. It is for all women who may in the future experience such symptoms and prefer to be forewarned and forearmed rather than be caught helpless. It is for women who want to know the latest research news on the estrogen and Alzheimer's disease evolving frontier.

This book is also for women's physicians who want to understand the plausible basis for cognitive, speech, and behavioral symptoms women experiencing perimenopause, menopause, or estrogen loss for any reason may be reporting to them.

Lastly, this book is for neuroscientists eager to mine not merely a good but a "great" research topic rife with the potential for yielding not only major pure science discoveries about the mind and brain but discoveries that will have life altering applications for millions and millions of women now and in the future.

In this book I make a rather dramatic revelation. I report that there is something new under the sun about women's *biology* that has been missed before: a set of *interior,* sometimes visible symptoms that frequently occur in association with menopause and perimenopause in many but not all women that are as common, normal, similar in cause, and variable in pattern as hot flashes are. These symptoms have been previously overlooked because no one asked women the right questions. Most of the health and mental experts women see today, I maintain, now know virtually nothing about the symptoms, yet neuroscientists studying the brains of different species have been wondering expectantly how their findings would manifest in women. They have been looking for these symptoms. Here they are.

I link these symptoms to very recent but as yet little-known brain and clinical research evidence in the neurosciences that I argue explains why the symptoms occur, indicates that the symptoms can largely be reversed, and reveals how this may be done.

I present for the first time anywhere in symptomatic detail the lives of many women who have experienced these symptoms in great perplexity, isolation, and often fear and describe how they coped with and around them. I offer women multiple tools for assessing, speaking about, and getting competent help for treating their symptoms, if they need to—and many don't—and for assessing whether any proposed treatment is actually helping. For many women simply understanding what is happening may be all the help they need.

I also propose that I have detected the "larger meaning" of these symptoms within the framework of evolutionary biology. I believe these symptoms lead us to important clues about how our human psychology has been adaptively shaped, honed, buffed, and polished by evolution. I contend that the cognitive/behavioral/speech symptoms that commonly show up in women during perimenopause and menopause, when fertility sequentially declines and then ceases, are the opposite or flip side of the very traits of mind and behavior that "nature" most highly values and typically keeps tightly regulated, controlled, or "girdled" during women's reproductive years because they confer unique survival advantages to those who have them. When the stakes of reproducing the species, i.e., species survival, are no longer an issue, "nature," I contend, pragmatically draws an exhaling breath of relaxation and says in effect, "You no longer need to be as tightly tuned for hypervigilance as before. It's OK to just 'be' during this time." The subtle symptoms of what I have named the WHM Syndrome (WHMS), for Warga's Hormonal Misconnection Syndrome, I contend, are the outward signs of that relaxation, of that altered biological agenda.

For modern women who intend to live long and well beyond the end of their fertility and whose quality of life is affected by these symptoms, biology need not be destiny I say. I point to plausible ways for living longer well, presenting the input of neuroscientists, menopause, and memory experts, who offer scientific rationales for treatments. I offer self-help behaviors that can have neurological/physiological consequences, along with practical little-known self-help aids and tools.

I argue that these symptoms are now epidemic among women because the first waves of the baby boom generation have reached the maturational landmarks of perimenopause and menopause and will continue to hit those markers in great numbers for some two decades to come. Ignoring women who suffer most with this syndrome, I suggest may have important public health consequences now and quite possibly for the future of our nation.

My goals in this book are:

- First and foremost to help women with these symptoms understand what they are experiencing now
- To educate the medical and mental health professionals women see so *they* can help women now
- To put this syndrome on the scientific map so that researchers can investigate all facets of its basis and devise multiple safe strategies for helping women now
- To offer researchers a testable scientific rationale for the syndrome that has heuristic value, that can be aimed at and validated, or if need be, shot down
- To draw attention to an as yet unrecognized major public health epidemic affecting the lives of millions of women now that may have important long-term consequences.

BACKGROUND

In this book I report on a discovery I made in the fall of 1996—the WHM Syndrome—after several years of initially detecting "glitches" in speech and behavior in women I knew very well in diverse settings.

Some of the women I knew well from my work as a New York state-licensed psychologist treating patients with health and stress-related problems with the tools of health psychology and behavioral medicine. They told me things, which at first I didn't understand, but which I mentally tucked away somewhere.

Some of the women I knew well from belonging to two reading groups that met monthly for over a decade—that still meet—and that included, on average, eighteen to twenty women, some my age, some older, and some younger, spanning in recent years ages from about thirty-eight to sixty-two. I knew these women to be highly bright and verbal. And the monthly spacing of our meetings provided sufficient distance to "see" changes in some of them over time. The intimate familiar nature of these groups also made it possible for me during my initial inklings of discovery to get individual confirmation from more than a few women in private about the reality of the symptoms I was detecting. I received more of the same confirmation from interviews with women I had come to know while living outside of New York City for a number of years, who were, on average, four to seven years older than me. The women I collectively observed in these settings were all either perimenopausal or menopausal. Considerable trust I believe is essential for discussing these symptoms, though sometimes need alone will suffice.

Confirmation of what I was detecting fueled my later drives to obtain interviews with many women I did not know about what cognitive or behavioral or speech symptoms they associated with perimenopause and menopause. I solicited interviews with these women through advertisements and referrals made by ob/gyns. I also interviewed women I did not know who responded to an article I wrote in *New York* magazine in 1997. But I am getting ahead of myself.

At some point in the fall/winter of 1996 I could stand it no longer and set off one evening to find out if science knew anything about the symptoms I was detecting in women. I went to do a computer search at the medical library of New York University Medical Center, where for three years I had done research on Alzheimer's disease years before, as a clinical research psychologist testing Alzheimer's patients on a neuropsychological test battery before and after experimental treatment with hyperbaric oxygen.

I loved the medical library and knew it well. Fishing to see what would turn up, I typed into the computer such paired terms as "menopause" and "mind" and came up with very little if anything. I persisted typing in different terms until I suddenly hit gold. I had typed in "estrogen" and the "brain" and out poured a wealth of references and abstracts mainly from the 1990s from leading research laboratories that represented a virtual revolution in prior thinking about both the brain and the roles of estrogen.

Estrogen loss, some of the studies noted, could produce detectable changes in parts of the brain having to do with memory and attention and could affect multiple neurotransmitter systems involved in thinking and memory. Other clinical studies found small but consistent (reliable) evidence of changes in verbal memory and learning in women with estrogen loss. I'll let you read about these discoveries in chapters 3, 4, and 5.

I didn't initially understand the overall significance of many of these studies, but what I did understand was that they could easily dovetail with the observations about unusual symptoms I had made in women—they dealt with overlapping areas of function. In my readings later I discovered that neuroscientists had actually been wondering how their basic-science discoveries in animals about the potential effects of estrogen loss on the brain would show up in women.

After reading through these studies, facilitated by my earlier study of the neurophysiology of sleep and wakefulness with the eminent scientist Dr. Raul Hernandez-Peon, and later research on the psychophysiology of sleep, dreams, and sexual arousal, I next started calling for interviews with the experts who had published the research I had discovered in the medical library. I had learned that I could pretty much call any expert for an interview, when I had adventitiously stumbled into a side career as a medical/science broadcast and print journalist, during a return to graduate school for a doctorate in psychology at New York University, after a near decade engaged in exciting research as an experimental psychologist. (I had a master's degree in experimental psychology and additional graduate courses.)

My interviews with these experts convinced me that the symptoms I thought I had detected were not merely a figment of my imagination and that there was a plausible scientific basis for them. Dr. Bruce

McEwen, an eminent research psychologist and neuroscientist who had done much of the important research in this area with students and colleagues at Rockefeller University and was president of the Neuroscience Society that year, in particular, surprised me by being aware that women were having these difficulties. He urged me on in my efforts.

I wanted to find out if women were being told by anyone about these possible symptoms, since the research evidence supporting their existence was "out there." And so I next called officers of the American College of Obstetrics and Gynecology and the North American Menopause Society to see if their organizations formally recognized any speech, memory, attention, or cognitive/behavioral symptoms in women, in the educational materials they made available to women patients in doctor's offices. They didn't, I soon learned. I decided to find out why. So I called the presidents or scientific directors of these organizations to find out if they were aware of the estrogen/mind/brain research. They were, I discovered. Why then, I asked, weren't they informing women that cognitive changes could be associated with the hormonal changes of perimenopause and menopause. "It was too soon," the leader of one group said. They were waiting "to develop consensus," a leader of the other group said. Meanwhile, as I saw it, millions of perimenopausal and menopausal baby boomer women in the midst of high-demand lives were floundering in the dark, silently wondering what was happening to them. I felt I had to act in some way.

I contacted the director of the New York City branch of the Women's Health Initiative, the huge government-sponsored national study assessing among other things the effects of estrogen on women, and met with her, presenting a list of the symptoms I had by then enumerated. She was very interested in what I had to say, appeared to recognize the merits of what I was describing, and suggested I write up an "ancillary study" for her to submit for review to the national head of the Women's Health Initiative Study at their upcoming meeting in two weeks. The ancillary study was submitted and ultimately rejected.

I decided to use my sideline skills as a published medical/science journalist to get word out to women about these possible symptoms, which I had discovered could vary in intensity and inconvenience in different women in much the same way that hot flashes did. On August

11, 1997, I succeeded in having published a cover article in *New York* magazine titled within the magazine "Estrogen and the Brain" and "Can Estrogen Make You Smart?" on the cover. The focus of the article was the little-known new research on estrogen and the brain and a conference titled "Estrogen and the Brain" that had been held recently at Mount Sinai Medical Center to present the new research. At that conference the president of the Mount Sinai School of Medicine and the Mount Sinai Hospital, Dr. John Rowe, himself a leading researcher on aging, had opened the proceedings by saying that on the basis of the new research "The equation for taking estrogen has now changed. . . . We know now that women taking estrogen after menopause reduce their chances of getting cognitive impairments"—not a wishy-washy statement.

My article alluded briefly to the symptoms perimenopausal and menopausal women were experiencing and that I describe in detail for the first time in this book. After the article was published, I received countless phone calls from friends and friends of friends—total strangers—who said they were so relieved that there was a basis for their symptoms and that they didn't, as feared, have Alzheimer's disease or a brain tumor. For months after the article came out, at parties and meetings, women with the symptoms came up and told me conspiratorially what had happened to them. The president of the Ms. Foundation, Marie Wilson, who had experienced some of the symptoms I described, reported that friends of hers too feared they were developing early Alzheimer's disease or a brain tumor, in a letter to the editor at *New York* magazine published September 9, 1997, in response to my article. (In my article, the president of the National Organization for Women, Patricia Ireland, also had acknowledged experience with word loss and uncharacteristic scheduling errors—WHMS symptoms—before treatment reversed her symptoms.) Shortly after the article came out, when I attended a meeting of the North American Menopause Society in early September in Boston that year, I was amazed to discover how many people there were suddenly familiar with the article. At a party at the New York Academy of Sciences I discovered that copies of the article had been distributed by the academy at a fall meeting on estrogen and the brain. I was delighted that the message I had sent out was finding an audience. That message is presented in much greater detail in this book.

———

Looking back it seems to me now that virtually everything I have ever done professionally as a basic sciences researcher, and as a clinician interested in seeing how "adaptation to stress" really works in people from the "laboratory" vantage point of a private practice (in health psychology), has been relevant to my detecting these symptoms and what I suspect they mean. Even many of the readings I did as a science journalist in preparation for radio interviews with leading scientists, while working toward my doctorate in psychology were interviews in the fields of sociobiology, evolutionary psychology, anthropology, and physiology: interviews with Edward O. Wilson, Donald Symons, Niles Eldredge, Donald Johanson, Mary and Richard Leakey, Tim White, Rene Dubos, Sir John Carew Eccles, and others. Even the many articles I wrote for medical and popular magazines on women's reproductive lives, infertility treatments, and other aspects of women's health have proven relevant.

Reviewing the work I have been engaged in most of my adult life has revealed to me that unwittingly I have been virtually "tap dancing" around topic areas that border on the study of the science of perimenopausal and menopausal women in virtually a connect-the-dot fashion that leads to the present picture. In the study of adult life development my life would make an interesting case example of something, I'm not certain what, since not only self-direction but factors I had no control over—the deaths of two relatively young people I worked for—shaped the course of my work.

My earliest research was at Bar Harbor's Jackson Laboratory for Mammalian Genetics Research. There under a National Science Foundation fellowship I independently studied what pregnancy, over its course, does to the self-regulation skills of the body—its bounce-back ability (homeostasis). I examined the effects of different stages of pregnancy on the ability of mice to get their body temperature back to normal after exposure to cold, a stressor. For this research I studied reproductive endocrinology and the physiology of temperature regulation, both areas that prefigured my present interest in the effects of hormonal changes in women (hot flashes). I later did research on the psychophysiology of sleep, dreams, sexual arousal during sleep, insomnia, and the effects of different emotions on the body at the Psychophysiology Laboratory of what was then Downstate Medical Center and is now known as SUNY Health Sciences Center in Brooklyn.

After the fifty-three-year-old leader of our research group unexpectedly died, I studied sleep and dreams again in research at New York University's Research Center for Mental Health. Both research positions again entailed study of topics that bear directly on the many mysteries that still surround the experience of perimenopause and menopause for many women: potential sleep disruptions, potential changes in sexual arousal, potential changes in emotional lability and baseline mood.

When yet again the relatively young leader of our research team died unexpectedly at fifty-four, I became involved in research on an experimental treatment for Alzheimer's disease and studied the research literature on memory, aging, and Alzheimer's at NYU Medical Center's Rusk Institute for Rehabilitation Medicine. I observed "up close and personal" all the cognitive/behavioral/speech "glitches" of patients in different stages of decline during lengthy hours of testing and of interviewing them and their relatives, before and after treatment with hyperbaric oxygen.

Familiarity with these patients primed me for "thinking about thinking" and for detecting WHM Syndrome symptoms. Familiarity with Alzheimer's patients also prepared me for noting the distinctions between Alzheimer's disease and WHMS symptoms even when they appear related.

A return to graduate school for a doctorate after this research led to my doing a doctoral dissertation in the field of neuropsychology on the role of the two hemispheres of the brain in the expression of positive and negative emotions and how these can show up in subtle differences between the two sides of the face during the expression of emotions. The topics of brain-control-over-emotion and neuropsychology again bear upon issues central to my interests in understanding perimenopausal and menopausal women.

After receiving my doctorate from NYU in 1982 I became director of research programs at the new Institute for the Advancement of Health, then in New York City. It was devoted to funding and giving prominence to the then-emerging interdisciplinary mind/body/health field of psychoneuroimmunology. I began to fund research, organize and attend conferences, and write about developments in different facets of psychoneuroimmunology. At that time psychologists/psychiatrists didn't know or read much about immunology, and immunologists didn't know or read much about the mind and brain. I loved my work and in relation to it even studied immunology at Mount Sinai's School of Medicine. I was immersed daily in research findings that described the negative compromising effects of stress on different aspects of the body, brain, and mind. But while the research was highly credible and intriguing intellectually, the fact was that it didn't mesh with my personal experience in living. I had long thrived on stress. Stress made me feel intensely alive, and I enjoyed rising to the occasion of it, having "Mission Impossible" tasks to accomplish in "x" number of minutes or hours. I enjoyed the "rush" of skiing and even liked to play the piano and type fast, even if I did both badly. I had long enjoyed the excitement of working on multiple projects at once, e.g., the science journalism while in graduate school.

Intrigued by conferences I had been part of, and experts I had heard, to make sense of it all, I decided to become retrained in the "applied" end of psychoneuroimmunology, the then also emerging fields of health psychology and behavioral medicine, and see how life really played itself out in relation to stress. My prior research in psychophysiology related directly to this new work. Over the course of three years I received training in biofeedback; cognitive therapy; hypnosis; pain management; and the self-regulation tools of progressive relaxation training, imagery, breathing and meditation techniques (initially being as much of a skeptic and an unrelaxed person as one could be). Before starting my own private practice I trained in the offices of a neurologist who had many car accident patients suffering profound headaches, backaches, and post-traumatic stress reactions. My main interest was in wanting to hear and understand what happened to people with life stresses—acute and chronic illnesses, pain states, panic attacks, headaches, irritable bowel problems, upcoming surgery—how they managed, what they said to themselves, what made things better, what made them worse.

I was very interested in what happened to patients' lives around their symptoms, and over time, I became adept at teaching and applying the tools of health psychology and behavioral medicine and looking for patterns. You could say I became a sick person's delight. I didn't easily tire hearing the details of symptoms. I wanted to understand their subtleties, detect their sequence in relation to other events, understand what thoughts and feelings they triggered. I enjoyed demonstrating how even a fast-talking, hyper child of wound-up Holocaust survivors could relax in an instant, becoming a puppeteer over my nerves and muscles and mind when I needed to. I enjoyed teaching patients how they could make use of a "medicine shelf" of behavioral tools that could be "popped" in an instant, anywhere, once learned, that could adjust and "tune down" their physiology and mind efficiently and with multiple levels of "payoff."

The relevance of this work to the present is that I became a fairly good listener and observer tuned into observing people and trying to understand the subtleties of their symptoms from their perspective. Biofeedback, for example, taught me not to trust my first impressions. From working with it I learned that people who could look outwardly cool and calm could be highly tense when measured with muscle-tension and temperature-monitoring devices.

So here I am.

It is my hope that this book helps many women now and over the long run. In the course of researching it I have also come to the suspicion that for similarly hormonal reasons, having to do with estrogen's newly discovered roles in both men's brains and bodies, that some men at similar ages also experience at least some WHMS symptoms. In chapter 14 of this book I explain what I have uncovered in this regard.

I also believe that WHMS symptoms are "normal" in the way that hot flashes are "normal" and use new evidence I present of WHMS symptoms existing in estrogen-deprived breast-feeding women in chapter 6 to frame the claim of "normality." I also propose that the experience of women with WHMS symptoms may offer us a novel perspective on one possible basis for the symptoms of attention deficit disorder in children. So stay tuned. This is an evolving story that will have many ramifications.

———————

The postwar population boom we commonly refer to as the baby boom generation lasted for an amazing length of time—twenty years according to some sources, eighteen according to others. In 1997 the first wave of baby boomer women reached the average age of menopause. For the next eighteen years millions of baby boomer women will be hitting that marker if they haven't already. Many of these women during years of perimenopause have already been experiencing in great perplexity the on-and-off array of intermittently flashing symptoms I have named the WHM Syndrome, without knowing what was happening to them or who they could turn to for help.

These women need to understand *now* what is happening to them. Before they give up careers and jobs they have often spent long years training for and striving at. Before they start sidelining themselves out of dreams and plans and hopes from a sense of despair and hopelessness. Before others needlessly sideline them out of a salary they and their families may be depending on for survival.

At present, as I see it, the world of science knows virtually nothing about the many kinds of WHMS symptoms that are possible with estrogen loss. The research "pipeline" of science could take years to investigate and credit this syndrome with the gold-standard imprimatur of double-blind, placebo-controlled trials. The results of the Women's Health Initiative Study will not be out until the year 2008. And at present in this study the effects of estrogen on some aspects of cognitive functioning are only being examined in women sixty-five years and older. While interest in women of menopausal age is growing at the research level, it will take a long long time, I fear, before researchers in turn discover that some proportion of women, even in their thirties, can be affected cognitively by hormonal loss (as you will see in this book).

It is my belief that the converging evidence on what estrogen does, in different animal models, in women deprived of estrogen for different reasons and given replacement hormones, in women at different hormonal tides in their menstrual cycle, in cell culture, from epidemiological studies of the effects of estrogen therapy on the risk of developing Alzheimer's, collectively offers a sufficient basis for alerting women now to what may be happening to them and to their options, particularly since estrogen replacement therapy is already an available treatment with many other proven benefits to women.

In view of the epidemic number of women potentially affected by WHMS symptoms today and in the near future, in view of the evidence of the potential reversibility of the symptoms by estrogen and in the future likely with yet-to-be designed estrogen substitutes, in view of the fact that knowledge alone can relieve the suffering of women fearful about the meaning of WHMS, and in view of the potential personal and public health costs of not doing so, I believe *women need to be informed of their options now* so that they can become health research advocates acting to secure the research they need now. So they can educate each other and, if necessary, their doctors. To do otherwise, to not inform women in light of what I know, for me would constitute neglect.

Lastly, as you read this book I ask you to ponder, as I often have, the question "How could this syndrome have been kept a secret for so long?"

Claire L. Warga, Ph.D.

I

IDENTIFYING THE PROBLEM

1

What Are These Strange Symptoms I'm Experiencing in the Middle of My Life?

Mrs. Malaprop: a character in Richard Brinsley Sheridan's 1775 play *The Rivals.* "A . . . woman of *almost fifty* [emphasis added] who . . . is famous for misusing . . . long words that sound similar to the correct words."

—*Larousse Dictionary of Literary Characters*

Malapropisms: the type of verbal errors made by the character Mrs. Malaprop.

There are some topics almost no one talks about till you do first. The stampede for the male impotence drug Viagra unveiled one such topic. This book is about another one: the previously unrecognized cognitive symptoms that are caused by the effects of perimenopause and menopause on the mind.

Sometimes it begins out of the blue with occasional slips of the tongue, meaning to say one word and unexpectedly hearing another pop out. Or when you realize that you, once a champion speller, aren't so sure

3

anymore how to spell "potato" or "forty." Sometimes it begins with uncharacteristically forgetting important appointments or drawing unexpected momentary blanks—total blanks—when it comes to remembering your only child's or best friend's name, or how to turn on the computer you've been using for years. Sometimes with feeling mentally "hazy," "foggy," or "spacey" and not being able to clear things up though you need to be "sharp" at that moment. "What's happening to me?" you wonder. "Could this be early, early, early Alzheimer's disease or a brain tumor?"

But it is usually not early Alzheimer's disease or a brain tumor. It is something else, a particular set of symptoms—a syndrome—that can occur in women beginning in their mid to late thirties or in their forties or fifties that more than likely can be halted and even largely reversed according to the best evidence available today. It is a syndrome associated with estrogen loss that is mainly experienced from within, and that until now, amazingly, no one has recognized as common among women or has linked to the wealth of post-1990s research evidence revealing the many important newly discovered roles estrogen plays in the remembering, naming, and attending parts of the brain. This is research that helps explain why the symptoms occur and why they can often be reversed.

———————

"I'm losing it," women say. "I'm going out of my mind," "I'm falling apart at the seams." "I'm flipping out." "I'm cracking up." "I'm having a nervous breakdown," "I'm just not myself." "I don't know what's wrong with me." "I do the strangest things." "I think I'm getting early Alzheimer's."

These are *not* the hysterical rantings of women with vague psychosomatic complaints but rather the blanket descriptions frequently used by perimenopausal (women experiencing or undergoing changes associated with the shifting hormonal functioning of the ovaries that precedes the last period. Symptoms can begin four to fifteen years before menopause.) and menopausal (women who have had their last period twelve months ago) women to describe the dislocating experience of confronting an assortment of unpredictable mind, speech, and behavioral "flash" symptoms. These are surprising symptoms no one has ever prepared them for.

Physicians hearing these dramatic statements over the years have simply had no basis in training for understanding what they were hearing and as a result have been able to offer no, or minimally constructive, help to women who dared to mention them.

THE SYMPTOMS OF PERIMENOPAUSE AND MENOPAUSE CAN BE VERY STRANGE BUT NORMAL

Before describing the specific symptoms I am referring to it makes sense first to agree about certain realities of a perimenopausal/menopausal symptom you already *do* know something about. Hot flashes. Consider this: If we on earth had never heard of hot flashes as a "normal" midlife symptom associated with ovarian and hormonal changes, and a returning astronaut-discoverer of a twin planet to ours reported drenching, unpredictable, overheating episodes as normal in otherwise healthy midlife-and-older women, we would likely say in quick dismissal, "Go away! You must have gotten something wrong there. The women were probably fooling with you in some way. You couldn't be right. That symptom is just too weird to be true of normal people."

And yet the reality is hot flashes are definitely normal but strange symptoms for healthy women to have. The fact that they are so common makes them seem normal to us. What makes them believable apart from their strangeness is the fact that they are also sometimes observable to others, leaving "tracks" of the internal experience visible to those who don't have them* and who might otherwise be inclined to dismiss them as "too crazy" to credit as real.

PERIMENOPAUSAL AND MENOPAUSAL SYMPTOMS CAN OFTEN BE CURED EVEN WHEN NOT FULLY UNDERSTOOD

It's also useful to point out that though science does not yet have a clear consensus on what specific sequence of events produces hot flashes in

---

*In Japan though, hot flashes are not common "normal" symptoms cited by menopausal women. "Tight shoulders" are much more commonly cited as symptomatic of this period in a woman's life.

women—beyond the bigger picture of changing ovary and estrogen function during perimenopause and menopause—nevertheless medicine has developed at least one quite effective empirical treatment for hot flashes based on trial-and-error experience, even in the absence of a clear scientific understanding of their basis. Namely, estrogen replacement.*(Other remedies that apparently work for some proportion of women have been considerably less tested and proven.) Successful treatment therefore of a symptom associated with ovarian/hormonal changes can precede biological understanding of the full complexity of the symptom.

The broad array of symptoms I have named the WHM Syndrome—for Warga's Hormonal Misconnection Syndrome—may at first, I suspect, appear as strange and bizarre as hot flashes do to those unfamiliar with them. But in the years to come, I believe, it will seem one of the great mysteries of our time that such a common, unusual, but apparently typical set of biologically based symptoms could have been overlooked for so long. Cultural and medical historians of the future, I predict, will long ponder the great divide of female patient/doctor noncommunication that is implicit in physicians not having "heard" and detected this set of symptoms and its cause in women for so many years.

What WHMS Is Like

The list of possible symptoms I am specifically referring to is presented in Table 1 to help you better understand the cases you will shortly be reading about. (A fuller description of possible WHMS symptoms with examples of how they actually occur in women's lives follows in chapter 7.) In Table 1, however, I list only the mind/speech/attention/behavioral symptoms to which I have given the name "WHM Syndrome," or "WHMS." This table does not include any of the *mood* or *physical* symptoms that are also frequently but not inevitably associated with menopause and the years preceding menopause. (These are more fully described in Appendix I.)

*The progesterone that is typically given with estrogen is essentially to counter the cell-proliferation effects of estrogen.

TABLE 1

The WHM Syndrome: Warga's Hormonal Misconnection Syndrome

As you examine the following chart keep in mind that the symptoms below typically occur as brief come-and-go episodes within the context of a functional ongoing nondisabled life, not unlike the manner of hot flashes. Women who experience *some* of the symptoms need not experience *all* of the symptoms or even *many* of the symptoms. Some symptoms may appear similar but are experienced by women as different from each other and are thus listed as distinct, pending additional research. Implied in each symptom is the sense that it occurs with a greater frequency than it did in the past. The symptoms most typically do not occur continuously but in erratic on-and-off intermittent episodes, in the pattern of occurrence of "hot flashes," so each symptom should be read preceded by the phrase "Flash episodes of." The headings over the symptoms are provisional pending further research, i.e., whether a specific symptom belongs under a speech, memory, or attention category may ultimately change as more is discovered about the symptom's biological basis.

Symptoms of Warga's Hormonal Misconnection Syndrome

THINKING CHANGES

- Losing your train of thought more often than in the past
- Forgetting what you came into a room to get more than in the past
- Not being able to concentrate as well upon demand
- Feeling foggy, hazy, and cotton-headed and not being able to clear it up at will
- Experiencing a thought blockade: an inability to pull ideas out at will
- Fluctuating agility in prioritizing as well as in the past

SPEECH CHANGES

- Naming difficulties for long-known names: children, best friends, things, places
- Finding yourself at a loss for words in how to express something while speaking

continued

TABLE 1 *continued*

- Experiencing "It's on the tip of my tongue but I can't get it out" sensation
- Making malapropisms: saying wrong words that are related somehow to the intended one
- Reversing whole words while speaking
- Reversing the first letters of words while speaking
- Experiencing "echo" words as unintentional intrusions into present speech
- Relying on "filler" words more often: "whatchamacallit," "that thing," "you know what I mean"
- Organizing sentences and ideas less efficiently while speaking

CHANGES IN THE "BEAM" OF ATTENTION
- Blinking social attention when interested and interacting: listening but not always attending
- Blanking-out amnesia for what you just did
- Experiencing increased distractability

MEMORY CHANGES: SHORT- AND LONG-TERM
- Forgetting what you just did, or past occurrences, with no threads of association to getting back to what's missing: missing links
- Changing certainty in how words should be spelled in once good or great spellers
- Fluctuating agility in calculating and in "counting with a quick scanning look"
- Experiencing changes in the speed and accuracy of memory retrieval
- Forgetting the *content* of a movie right after seeing it but remembering your *emotional* reaction to it

BEHAVIORAL CHANGES
- Making behavioral "malapropisms": unintended slips in behavior that are related to the intended behavior somehow, such as putting shampoo in the refrigerator

- Forgetting briefly how to do things long known, such as where to turn on the computer
- Feeling that automatic skills such as driving for a few moments are not "automatic" in the same way as usual
- Dropping things more often that require fine finger/hand coordination
- Absentmindedly, leaving out or reversing letters in words while writing
- Forgetting how to write a word in the middle of writing and having to leave blanks
- Experiencing "translating" hesitations in converting what's heard into writing
- Not handling the same amount of stress in the same way

SPATIAL SKILLS CHANGES

- Changing skill in remembering and/or recognizing faces (*not* well-known faces)
- "Looking at but not seeing" what you are looking for when it's right there ultimately, more than in the past
- Changing reading skill in visually "seeing" and comprehending reading material
- Spending less time reading, without difficulties above (for formerly heavy-duty readers)
- Forgetting briefly how to get to long-known landmarks in your life
- Experiencing familiar locales in one's experience as momentarily unfamiliar

ALTERED SENSE OF TIME

- Forgetting appointments more or not anticipating events of personal importance with the same accuracy as in the past
- Forgetting important events in your personal history timeline, i.e., which breast you had biopsied
- "Living more in the moment" out of necessity: a "spliced-film-frames" sense of personal time

WHY IT'S CALLED THE WHM SYNDROME

I have named this set of symptoms the WHM Syndrome, or WHMS, because women who experience the symptoms often feel subjectively as if they are observing their own "bad show," watching their mind behaving whimsically, unexpectedly taking off on a whim with seeming intentions of its own while violating *their* intent.

In my mind WHM originally stood for the Women's Hormonal Misconnection Syndrome. I felt the acronym in good measure characterized the subjective experience of women who had the symptoms without stigmatizing them. And the words behind the letters described what I believe is going on at the neurophysiological level—namely, cognitive*/behavioral/speech episodes that are mis-hits. Episodes that are off the mark misconnections, in which the mind's intentions are not producing the right physiological connections that they used to in the preexisting circuitry and/or chemical flow patterns of the brain. The reason for the misconnections? A body/brain retooling or "retuning" brought on by the effects of declining ovarian function and declining estrogen hormone supplies on a thinking, remembering, attention-creating brain that science has recently learned (see chapter 4) depends heavily on estrogen as a brain "transmission" fluid of sorts, as a fortifying performance-enhancing steroid or multivitamin. (Estrogen is after all a steroid hormone even though it isn't the kind typically used by athletes. I'll explain this more later in chapter 4.)

However, as I continued interviewing women and experts and reviewing the research literature in this area over the span of several years, I came to the conclusion that calling this the *Women's* Hormonal Misconnection Syndrome would not be prudent. (You'll have to read chapter 14 to find out exactly why.) But for the moment suffice it to say that I learned that science had very recently discovered that male thinking/remembering brains and sex organs *also* depend on estrogen supplies for their normal function. So for reasons of faltering estrogen hormonal lev-

---

*By cognitive I am referring collectively to thinking, attention, memory, time-estimation-and-flow sense, and perceptual/spatial/navigational skills.

els in their brains I began to suspect that at least some men too may have similar WHM symptoms at possibly similar ages. What to do?

To preserve the acronym WHM and prevent the syndrome from being called the rather farcical HM(mmm) Syndrome, I have renamed the set of symptoms Warga's Hormonal Misconnection Syndrome. It turns out that naming new medical syndromes and hormonal/behavioral phenomena after their discoverer has a long history, respectively, in both medicine and behavioral neuroendocrinology (the hormones and behavior branch of science), according to the eminent sociobiologist Edward O. Wilson. Describing a series of known behavior-and-hormones effects in the animal kingdom—i.e., the Bruce Effect, the Lee-Boot Effect, the Ropartz Effect, and the Whitten Effect—Wilson in his landmark 1975 book *Sociobiology,* writes: "In the manner of the medical sciences, the different kinds of physiological change are often called after their discoverers."

Why have I called this set of symptoms a *syndrome?* Because the set of symptoms occur frequently in association with each other, as a constellation, or sets of subconstellations. Certainly not all women who have some of the symptoms have all of the symptoms, but sufficient cumulative experience interviewing women has persuaded me that the symptoms represent a possible set that are part of the same causative agent.

WHMS SYMPTOMS HAVE TYPICALLY BEEN IGNORED OR WALLPAPERED OVER

Till now in the relatively few instances when popular writers have referred to the above symptoms they have usually used seemingly mild, and nonspecific terms such as "concentration problems," or "forgetfulness," or "memory problems" to refer to women's experiences during these years, without an appreciation of the range of possible "glitches" in speech, behavior, and cognition that women in actuality have been experiencing. Broad-spectrum terms such as "forgetfulness" or "concentration problems," in effect, "wallpapered" or plastered over the variety and the bizarreness of the symptoms women have encountered. The casual, familiar terms masked or obscured the specific reasons why otherwise seemingly normal and healthy women might be inclined to say such phrases as "I think I'm losing it" or "I think I'm flipping out" or "I think I'm cracking up."

If you had occasion to go into major bookstores at the time I am writing this to look in the indexes of the many books now on the shelves currently addressing menopause or perimenopause for such terms as "memory" or "concentration" or "forgetfulness," you would find that in the vast majority there is either no mention of even these broad-spectrum terms or at most a one- or two-line reference to their possibility at this time of life but without much in the way of elaboration. There is virtually no reference in most of these books to the unusual behavioral symptoms listed in Table 1.

HOW DO WHMS SYMPTOMS PLAY OUT IN WOMEN'S LIVES

But how do these symptoms actually play out in the lives of real women? Let's look at three very different women:

Case 1: Katherine Kennedy

Katherine Kennedy (alias) is a thirty-eight-year-old professor of English at an Eastern university who also hosts a weekly talk-radio show. She is married to a scholar, has no children yet, but hopes to have them in the future.

Reproductive state: still gets her period regularly. Appears to be perimenopausal, though she does not yet realize it.

When I was younger I had the most retentive memory for everything, especially names and faces. Friends in college would say, "Your mind is like a Rolodex." When I entered my thirties I started having these strange symptoms. I would meet people and the next day felt as though I had never seen them before. They'd know me but I had no clue as to who they were. Their faces were just not registering. It so happens that I had begun to menstruate copiously around that time, more than before but I did nothing about it. Not recognizing faces still happens. I find that slightly scary because my grandmother was demented; and I sometimes wonder if it's hitting me very early.

What drives me mad is that I now forget the precise names of things, objects, and will end up saying "that thing" instead of "diploma" for example. It's the same with verbs. I will use the word "doing" instead of the verb I actually want to use. I also have the sense that sometimes I'm grasping for a word and I can't get to it. It feels like mental clutter, like I'm shuffling around inside not finding what I want. I find it hard to retrieve things. I'll have a sense of what I want—it's not even the sense of being on the tip of my tongue but rather I can't get it to my tongue. I'll want to say "chair" and will think "something about sitting" but can't fill in what I want. It's like mental miasma. This happens not all the time but intermittently enough so that it concerns me.

I find it [these symptoms] enormously frustrating. One of the ways it affects me is when I'm having a disagreement with my husband. I'll know there's a point I want to make but I can't make my point. Either that or I lose it midstream.

The difficulty in retrieving, to some degree, also overlaps with what I call fog or haziness. My mind sometimes feels foggy, hazy, or cloudy. If it's fog I'm feeling it's more confused, more grasping than when I'm trying to retrieve something. With fog I don't know what I'm looking for—that's the worst—being lost in the fog. When this happens I think I'll end up like my grandmother, not knowing the names of my family and having lost decades. Or like my friend who got ECT [electroconvulsive therapy] and lost decades of her life, big chunks of her brain. At times like this I feel like I'm losing it. And I'll think to myself "I didn't even drink or take drugs and I'm losing it."

In the classroom and when I'm on radio I want to be sharp and alert, and it hasn't happened terribly much, these blunders, when I'm working. In fact when I'm in front of a class or microphone I'm somehow sharper. I have to be really alert and thinking and focused. And when I'm working I'm better than in my private life.

I find now that often when I walk into a room and want to get something, I'm apt not to recall what I went to find. I think it's a little early for this to be happening to me. My mom and grandmother do this. I never did this as much as now.

In my late twenties if I was writing fast I noticed that I started to reverse letters on words. I also used to be a great speller. Now if I see something that's wrong I won't realize what the correct thing should be. Strangely though, I started doing crossword puzzles only recently as a way to reassure myself of my verbal skills, and I can finish *The New York Times* crossword puzzle pretty easily writing in ink. But at the same time I just feel really stupid. I used to be and probably still am pretty smart. I always did very well in school. Verbal things were very easy for me. Now I'm still strong verbally but I hate any slippage. It might be analogous to being really gorgeous when you're young and now not feeling as radiant.

I don't think others have noticed the verbal changes because I'm still better than most at noticing names. I'm always the first person who knows the name of a writer or actor. At the same time though I will mispronounce words and can't get back to recalling the correct word. Recently, for example, I was trying to say the plural of roof and couldn't recall if it was "roofs" or "rooves." Both sounded wrong. It's this confusion over basics that I find scary. In the past once I learned something I would have remembered it always. I seem to need a lot more reinforcement than I used to, to learn new commands on the computer.

In the last couple of months I've also begun to lose things and I never ever did that before. My wallet, for example. I lost it and I couldn't think at all where I might have lost it. I had absolutely no associations the way I normally would as to where it might have happened. Fortunately a Good Samaritan returned it. I have a special telephone message pad that's been by the phone forever that's got important numbers on it. I just couldn't remember what happened to it in my home office. It's the lack of associative threads that seems so strange.

I'm the treasurer in my family who does all the practical things. My husband is incredibly brilliant but doesn't really live on this planet. He always loses things and people return them. Recently, I thought I had cash in the bank and when I looked I had appreciably less than I recalled. I couldn't think at all where I spent it. Nothing came to mind in the way of any associations. It's as though I had no links to the past when this happens.

I think I tend to compensate for all of this fairly well. I keep lists and write things down and use the mnemonic devices from childhood that I was always great at. But at the same time all these things affect my whole identity. I've always thought of myself as verbally skilled and these episodes affect my sense of self. I met a woman at the radio station a few weeks ago. Then I met her again two nights later and didn't recall her at all.

Another night I asked the same couple twice if I gave them passes to something and they got annoyed with me. I had already given them the passes.

The ironic part is that as a teenager I had unbearable contempt because my mother couldn't recall the names of people. But she could recall other things really well—what she paid for something.

All this makes me feel diminished. I now feel not as sharp as I used to be. I'm not depressed but feel like I'm getting dim, with the foggy, hazy, cloudy episodes.

At the same time I'm probably happier in my life than I've ever been. I'm in a great marriage that's working well. My husband and I have a wonderful relationship. Over the years I have had depressions on and off but things are going well now both in my private and professional life. I love the work I do.

I don't go to doctors unless I'm dying and I wouldn't know who to go to with these symptoms anyway. I just keep hoping they'll go away on their own.

Katherine Kennedy's case is an example of pure WHM cognitive/speech/behavioral symptoms occurring at a rather early age—what I think of as a "one-ring circus" of symptoms—with no body symptoms (i.e., hot flashes or vaginal dryness) or associated mood/emotional symptoms except for her diminished sense of self in reaction to having the symptoms. Her symptoms can't be said to be occurring in reaction to sleeplessness, or hot flash disruptions, or depression because she does not report these. Like many women her age she isn't thinking about hormone changes in relation to these symptoms, but her mention of greater bleeding in her early thirties when her WHM symptoms appeared to her to begin, likely reflects the increased variability of periods (more, less, longer, shorter) that typically characterizes perimenopause. I view her case as being linked to hormone changes because, as you will see with later cases, it echoes in its pattern of specific symptoms so many of the other women whose symptoms *did* begin in association with hot flashes or vaginal dryness—indicators of hormonal changes. Like many women Katherine Kennedy has not seen a doctor about these symptoms. She has been coping with them in multiple ways. As with many women the symptoms are occurring within the context of a fully lived functional life. They are mainly invisible to others though very noticeable to her.

Case 2: Sherry Strumph

Sherry Strumph (actual name) is the forty-nine-year-old president of a highly successful major office-services company in New York City that now employs over thirty-five people. She has built this company from a one-person venture over a twenty-year period through great initiative, ability, creativity, and sustained directed effort. She owns another unrelated business as well. Sherry is married and the mother of a grown daughter.

Reproductive state: "I'm perimenopausal now. I'm still regular but my periods come for ten minutes. The last one was over before I knew it."

I remember this beginning about two to three years ago when I caught myself saying something wrong to myself. I said to myself, "You used to have a 'photogenic' memory" and then said, "You fool, you mean 'photographic'" and now you can't even remember what your husband told you ten minutes ago." This was in response to my husband reminding me that he would be out that evening and my not remembering it at all. He said we spoke about it several times. For me it was the first time. I laughed it off thinking "OK here comes old age." I thought memory problems began around age seventy-five, not in your forties. Another time a friend asked me something and I said I didn't remember; and she said, "But you always remember everything. I can't accept that you say you can't remember." She was so taken aback because my memory had always been phenomenal—everybody relied on it. My husband started saying things like "You used to be so reliable and I used to be able to count on you. Now I never know when you'll do whatever you say you'll do." I realized myself that I wasn't the same as before but I said to myself, "It's the way I am now." I was very accepting. Maybe because I had been so responsible all these years. I used to be so driven to be right. It's kind of refreshing for me not to have to do that.

When this began I had been away from the office for two years. I had excellent management there. I was free as a bird so it wasn't job burnout or stress. My memory lapses created havoc for some of the people around me, but not me. I just accepted it. But then too I didn't know what to do about it and it's not my style to complain to people.

Before I started using estrogen cream nine months ago, I'd say that my worst memory issues were one to two years ago [ages forty-seven to forty-eight]. When I'd forget something I would joke with people and say "Mind-like-a-sieve strikes again."

When this began I had no idea this could even be related to hormonal changes. I learned this from the experience of my friends. I thought menopause was about going through hot flashes. I didn't associate hormonal changes with what I was experiencing. I didn't have any mood swings during this time the way some women do. In fact I was the calmest, most unflappable I'd ever been. Things I had feared doing before I could do now, like driving at night. But my memory was a mess. I'd write things down and forget where I'd put the list.

I thought about going to a doctor but I'm not one to go running to them very readily. I thought maybe I was pre-Alzheimer's but then I said to myself, "No one in my family has ever had it." I did stop using my deodorant, however, because I had read that something in deodorant—aluminum—caused Alzheimer's. I also stopped using aluminum foil and switched to shrink-wrap for that reason.

My concentration also changed. I would start to read a book and pick it up two weeks later and have absolutely no memory of any of it. As though not a trace had stayed with me. However, when I tested myself, by pulling cards from a deck and reading them to myself, to see how many I could remember, I could do it if I tried. This forgetting happens more when I'm on automatic pilot. I need to really pay attention to "get" some things now, more than I used to. And I can but I need to make a conscious effort to do so.

I finally broke down and bought a date book and I'm pretty religious about writing in it but not at all religious about looking at it.

I started to make the connection that the things happening to me were related to hormones when friends started telling me what they were going through. My friend A. said to me one day that she was much more forgetful than I was. She was diagnosed as needing estrogen for her bones and started being treated with it, and she said it was working for *all* her symptoms. Then another friend said that she'd been put on estrogen and could think like a young girl, meaning that things came easily again. I was percolating on this information and then my friend A. said she was switching to an estrogen cream. She used to be a chemist. After she went on the hormone cream she said she stopped being hot all the time (the way I am too all day without any hot flashes), her memory got better, and amazingly she was able to successfully lose weight.

I started using the [estrogen] cream in August (nine months ago) and they say to give it three months. I've noticed a difference in some things but not a great difference in everything. But I also haven't used it consistently—probably about 50 percent of the time. I forget to. But I'm also afraid of hormones because of my family history. I'm the only one in my family who hasn't had cancer. So I've got a love/hate relationship to taking estrogen. Now at least I know I have a choice in whether I want to stay this way if it lasts.

After I went on estrogen my attention got better. I'm more focused. It might also be because I'm back at work full-time. It kind of forces me to be focused. The result is I appear more focused than I am in my personal life. Besides my husband and good friend, I don't think others noticed any difference in me. The changes weren't blatantly observable.

Did I go to a doctor about this? Yes and no. At regular intervals I would go to my internist and when I told her what I was experiencing she said, "Well, welcome to the club honey." She's only a bit older than me. She didn't offer me anything. She knows better. I'm normally unwilling to take even aspirin. I mentioned the heat thing to my gynecologist. He felt that since it was constant it wasn't likely related to menopause. He did take blood level tests and told me I'm peri-menopausal.

I'll do these strange things every now and then. The vice president of my company and I take turns picking each other up on alternate days to drive in to work. One day I left the house, got into the passenger seat, and sat there waiting. When I realized what I'd done I started laughing. Even more recently I unpacked groceries. I put canned tomatoes into the fridge and put fresh lettuce and spinach in the pantry closet where I found them a week later. Other times I'll be cooking and go into the pantry and say, "Now why am I here?" and then realize I meant to go to the freezer or spice shelf. This now happens all the time.

Spelling too is strange. I used to be a great speller. I didn't have to think about it. Now I have to think about it. The other day I couldn't remember if the word "comrade" had an *e* at the end. Working with language has been my business so this is not like me. I'll also now substitute short words for the ones I can't think of. I also have more difficulty prioritizing things than before. I'm still very good at it but I feel there's a change in the directness with which I organized a task before.

I used to be able to compute things mentally and now I have to write them down. I sometimes have someone check it for me. I now blank out on phone numbers and names that I've known forever. I never needed a phone book but I think now I should start writing them down. I've also blanked out on mail I received at home that I acted on. I wouldn't remember having talked to anyone about what was involved but then they would tell me I *had* already.

I'll also catch myself now half focusing on things. People will be speaking and I'll have no idea what we just spoke of. My friend M. was speaking the other day and I realized I had no idea what the conversation was about. I've also stopped carrying keys. Keys no longer exist in my consciousness. I have given new meaning to the phrase "living in the moment." I own a house and two businesses but I no longer carry *any* keys. They were gone all the time. I had a garage opener built into my car for that reason. It's funny because my husband always relied on me for locking everything up. Now he does it all. I used to be obsessive about it. Now I'm cavalier about it, nonchalant. I'm also not as suspicious as I used to be. I'm more trusting of people. In the past if I got on a train I used to automatically size people up and think "Do I want to be caught in an alley with this person?" Now I don't look for traits in that way anymore. I'm less mistrusting of the looks of someone.

Would I rather go back to the way I was? I don't seem to feel as much need to control everything. To me I think estrogen is like the fuel that wants me to try to get big bites out of life and my appetite has diminished somewhat with the diminishing of the estrogen.

Sherry is an old friend who was unaware of what I had been doing the last several years. When she read the *New York* magazine article I had written in the summer of 1997 and my allusions to WHM symptoms in the article, we spoke. She said, "That's me," and proceeded to tell me her story.

Like many women Sherry did not connect the symptoms she was experiencing with hormonal factors, but instead attributed them vaguely to aging or the possibility of developing early Alzheimer's disease and went so far as to make changes in her life. Like many women with WHMS she did not run to a doctor after experiencing the symptoms or get much specific help from doctors in response to describing some of them. What stands out about her case to me is the atypical equanimity with which she accepted the cognitive/behavioral symptoms she watched herself exhibit, the attributions she ascribes speculatively to her reproductive hormones, the motivational drives she suspects they impelled her to, and the diminished vigilance around safety she describes in herself, i.e., less suspiciousness, diminished fears around driving at night, less compulsiveness around keys, locking up, etc. Are these new traits unique to her? Is there something here to follow up? I'm not sure. Sherry was experiencing what I think of as a "two-ring circus" of symptoms associated with hormonal changes. She experienced the cognitive/speech/behavioral changes—the mind changes, and one physical change—she was hot all the time.

Like many perimenopausal or menopausal women with erratic memory who take hormones, Sherry's symptoms lead her to sometimes forget to take medications consistently (although in her case, ambivalence due to fears of cancer related to her family history may partially account as well for her forgetting). Product manufacturers need be mindful of memory as a basis for noncompliance with prescribed and nonprescribed treatments.

Case 3: Quiana Mortier

Quiana Mortier (an alias) was referred to me by one of the menopause experts I had come across in my research. He had recently started to treat her at the time of our interview. Ms. Mortier is widowed, the mother of a daughter now twenty-one, and supports herself in a position she has long held, working in the billing department of a physician.
Reproductive state: now fifty-two and in menopause.

I'm now fifty-two but my symptoms started when I was forty. I was perimenopausal then. I went to the doctor because I wasn't feeling right. Weird words were popping out of my mouth that I hadn't intended to say, and I'd cry constantly. I thought I was cracking up. This had been going on for a couple of months and my husband and I went to our internist. I told him about the wrong words that would come out. And I told him it felt like I was seeing things. I'd go to take something that I was sure was there before. And then it wasn't there when I went to look for it again. He diagnosed me as having paranoid schizophrenia. He told my husband that in private and my husband was very upset. He told me that night what the doctor had said. I was very upset and called the doctor and said, "Did you really say that?" He denied he told my husband that. But I believe my husband more than I believe him.

I was so upset with what he said that I went to another doctor, a psychiatrist, to check it out. After telling him the same things, he said it wasn't schizophrenia or paranoia. He didn't know what it was.

Then I started getting hot flashes. My body started to change. My periods came real heavy. Then they didn't come. I never knew what was going to happen from month to month. When I was forty-three or forty-four my memory started to get even worse. I thought it might be due to stress. Frustrating things would happen. I was going into the bank to pay my bank mortgage one day and parked my car and saw the meter maid behind me. I had the coin in my hand and intended to put it in the meter, but I forgot in a second what I was going to do and went into the bank holding it. When I came out the meter maid was writing the ticket. I was so mad. Things that frustrated me like that kept on happening. In a second I'd forget what I was going to do. I'd misplace things I'd kept in the same place forever. This happens with keys, money, earrings. I'll look in the refrigerator and think "Who ate this?" You know you brought it in and you can't find the food. At one point there was a reason for this happening—my daughter had a girlfriend living here, and she was hiding her. But this happened before and after that too.

But you become paranoid. You suspect people because you are missing things, misplacing things. At times I'd say to myself, "This must be Alzheimer's."

I did speak to another doctor about this. He said it was probably related to stress and never related it to menopause.

This has gotten better though—the misplacing things. I just take Rejuvex and I think it's helped me. It relaxes me. But even now I still come into a room and don't remember what for. I have trouble with speaking. It's as if you don't remember any words in a sentence. If the sentence I wanted to say was "The cow jumped over the moon," I couldn't remember the word for cow. Even now, I have difficulty repeating a sentence back. It's like the recall button takes longer to bring things to the mental screen. Names escape me the minute I hear them. I still have difficulty with my memory. If I don't write things down, forget it—which is usually what I do. But I forget to write things down. I have only short-term memory now. I thought it was just aging.

I didn't know this could possibly be related to menopause until Dr. D. told me that it could. Before him I went to an Italian gynecologist about all of this, and he just didn't believe in taking hormones. The speech difficulties he said were due to stress! He said to relax, which didn't help much.

For the last seven to ten years I've felt like I was in a bubble. I've only recently come out of that bubble. I felt like I was in a vacuum and certain things weren't important to me, like the silver candelabra my mother left me when she died. My family thought I was crazy. "Leave her alone," they would say. My daughter would say this too. My sister even tried to take advantage of my memory problems. She thought I had forgotten that she had the candelabra and acted surprised when I asked about it a year later.

But other times if something wasn't directly in front of me it was out of my mind, as if I had amnesia or something. At different times I've forgotten my ATM code, my social security number, my family's birthdays, which I've had in my mind forever. They just flew out and later just flew back in. That's what it feels like. It feels like you are going crazy. You don't know what's going to happen next.

How did I manage at work? My husband is dead now and I work in a doctor's office on billing. The computer has a format for what I do so I can handle it. I have to focus in on it but I do OK. I've been at it a long time. At home I studied to become a travel agent a couple of years ago when it was really bad and things would just go out of my head. I have to read something over and over and over to retain it and within a week it's gone. I'll forget it like I never read it before. It all feels brand new if I read it again.

Now it's a lot easier. Whatever was going on with me the last ten or so years has leveled off. It was a really bad time. I just recently went to Dr. D. He wants me to take estrogen. He's for it but I went to two other gynecologists who were against my taking estrogen. They still don't relate any of this to menopause. Dr. D. knew what I was talking about and said it's related to menopause, but nobody else ever said that. I'm still not sure of taking it [estrogen-progesterone hormone replacement therapy (HRT)], even though nobody in my family ever had breast cancer. The other doctors said not to. So I'm not sure yet what I'll do.

What is revealing about Quiana Mortier's case is the many years that this syndrome can apparently persist and that it can become better with time; also, that verbal and perceptual (cognitive) errors together with reduced control over her emotions were Ms. Mortier's earliest symptoms, preceding hot flashes and menstrual irregularity. What stands out too is the misdiagnosis of her symptoms as "paranoid schizophrenia" by an internist, and complete unawareness of the basis for her symptoms by other physicians, except for Dr. D., a male ob/gyn who specializes in treating perimenopausal and menopausal women and has been correctly sensing what women have been trying to communicate to him about their experiences over the years.

WOMEN, WHMS, AND DOCTORS: WHAT HAPPENS NOW WHEN WOMEN REPORT THEIR SYMPTOMS TO DOCTORS

The bigger picture at present is that most physicians know very little if anything about the specific mind/speech/behavioral symptoms I have named the WHM Syndrome. They haven't been taught of their possibility during medical training. They may have learned something about these symptoms if they have been carefully listening to some of their patients over the years. However, some women, as we've seen, don't go to physicians about these symptoms for multiple reasons, but some women do speak up about their symptoms.

At present when women go to their ob/gyns or other physicians with their symptoms here is what may happen:

1. Women are told to relax more, or to take a vacation, that the symptoms are probably stress-related. The cost of following this seemingly innocuous advice, however, can sometimes be high. A woman with multiple WHM symptoms, for example, was led by her doctor to believe her symptoms were due to stress. She quit an exciting, demanding job she loved, only to discover her symptoms did not improve at all with a less stressful job, but got worse. They did improve significantly after she was put on a three-month diagnostic test-trial of estrogen alone to see if estrogen decline was the basis for them.* When she had determined that her symptoms *were* related to estrogen loss, wary of estrogen for family history reasons, she then went off the pharmaceutical estrogen her doctor had prescribed and turned instead to weaker plant-based estrogens, phytoestrogens. And it worked in her case. The three months

*My thanks to Dr. Maurice Cohen for elaboration of this type of diagnostic use of estrogen in assessing the basis for symptoms associated with perimenopause and menopause.

of estrogen was used as a diagnostic tool, to identify the cause of her symptoms. (See chapter 10 on treatments.)

2. Women are told the symptoms are the result of aging and to "accept it" as inevitable.

3. Doctors, like many other human beings, tend to deny or dismiss what they don't understand. And their training to date hasn't included any grounded scientific rationale that would logically explain the basis for the symptoms. So women are given "It's probably nothing" admonitions, or quizzical looks that imply *they* don't know what they're talking about. The tone of these encounters is "if the doctor hasn't heard about it, it is probably nothing too important, or it doesn't exist."

4. Women who show up in doctors' offices with WHMS can be misdiagnosed as having a psychotic condition. You saw that this is what happened to Quiana Mortier. Describing her WHM symptoms as best she could, "strange words popping out" and "things being there and then not being there," Mrs. Mortier's internist attributed her strange unfamiliar symptoms to a psychotic condition, paranoid schizophrenia, and gave this diagnosis to her husband but not to her directly. But what if her job had depended on this diagnosis? What if this diagnosis unbeknownst to her became part of a permanent HMO medical record made available to others? Mrs. Mortier's prudent decision to see a psychiatrist for a second opinion paid off in her case, when the psychiatrist was forthright enough to say he didn't know what disorder she had. But do all psychiatrists exercise this option? How often can they say "I don't know" to those who refer patients to them for a diagnosis? *I* don't know.

5. Sometimes women with WHMS symptoms are diagnosed as having Attention Deficit Disorder (ADD). Two women with WHMS symptoms I interviewed were given this diagnosis, one by a psychologist, the other by a psychopharmacologist she was referred to. Both were advised to take Ritalin, the stimulant drug used to help focus attention in youngsters with ADD. Taking Ritalin helped one of the two women with WHMS symptoms. (Might this be a potential form of treatment for some women with WHMS attention changes?) Both women had no prior history of attention, reading, or word-reversal difficulties.

After interviewing these women I decided to interview several experts on ADD. I asked if ADD ever manifested with adult onset—if the disorder could show up initially in adulthood without a prior history in childhood. I was told that in instances where ADD is first detected in adulthood, the assumption commonly made is that it was likely present in childhood but not detected or diagnosed at that time! It is my suspicion that in some women with WHMS an intermittent ADD-like disorder can show up in adulthood for the first time as one possible subset of WHMS symptoms in association with estrogen loss. It's important to be aware, however, that not all women with WHMS symptoms have ADD-like symptoms.

6. Sometimes women with WHMS who insistently pursue their quests for diagnosis at memory or Alzheimer's disease research centers within major medical centers are suspected of having early Alzheimer's disease and given this tentative diagnosis. Though they test normal on the battery of cognitive tests they are given, the symptoms these women describe lead clinicians to suspect a diagnosis of Alzheimer's disease, since the symptoms outwardly can sometimes appear to overlap. The women are then asked to return at regular intervals for follow-up testing and evaluations, to see what happens to their symptoms—if they progress with time, stay stable, or disappear. What happens over time helps the experts clarify the diagnosis. Imagine, however, being told by experts that your WHMS symptoms might indeed be Alzheimer's disease! You might very well redirect the whole course of your life or live in a bubble of suspended anxiety if you thought your remaining cogent time on earth was likely very limited.

The reality is that Alzheimer's disease researchers know very little as yet about how true instances of Alzheimer's disease begin in very specific detail—how they play out in everyday life. As a former Alzheimer's disease researcher, I know. I would often ask the relatives of patients I was evaluating what were the earliest signs *they* saw. Typically the first signs were only recognized in retrospect, after the full-blown picture of Alzheimer's had later emerged. "So that's why he acted so funny back then two years ago," they would say.

Alzheimer's disease researchers aren't yet aware of WHMS as a distinct set of symptoms among perimenopausal and menopausal women, even though they may be aware overall of the neuroscience research showing a connection between estrogen loss and changes in the structure and chemistry of the brain, and recent research on Alzheimer's disease and estrogen (see chapter 7). Alzheimer's disease experts are reading about the existence and details of the WHM Syndrome at the same time you are reading this. They aren't yet prepared to diagnose WHMS. They can't diagnose what they don't yet know. But they might mistakenly diagnose WHMS symptoms in relation to what they are familiar with and unintentionally derail the course of a life. I have nothing against the clinicians who diagnose memory disorders or Alzheimer's disease. I am merely cautioning women with WHMS symptoms about what could theoretically happen. Hopefully WHMS will be given the attention it deserves in research efforts so that memory and Alzheimer's diagnostic centers will be aware of it soon. Without intending to add to the fears of women with WHMS, I feel it would be negligent of me not to add that some true cases of Alzheimer's disease can occur within the age range of the forties and fifties. The youngest presumed* Alzheimer's patient I ever tested was a forty-two-year-old male. It is my belief, however, that the preponderance of cases of WHMS in women are not manifestations of early Alzheimer's disease cases. As anchoring points for this view, I use as evidence the absence of droves of sixty-year-old Alzheimer's-like women wandering the streets of major cities. (If WHM symptoms are present to one degree or another in a significant proportion of fifty-year-old women, then if it truly represented the beginning of Alzheimer's disease, ten years should be sufficient time for the condition to "bloom" into Alzheimer's disease.) Also in my experiences as a health psychologist treating patients with chronic disease sometimes in rehabilitation and nursing home settings, I found few sixty-year-old women or men with Alzheimer's disease. For very specific reasons that will become clearer in a later chapter, I believe that WHMS in most women represents a "normal," though until now undetected, series of changes.

---

*Alzheimer's disease can't be diagnosed with certainty till after death.

More Encounters with Doctors

Here are two more experiences of women with self-described WHMS symptoms and encounters with their doctors. They are letters to the editor that arrived in response to publication of my August 1997 article on "Estrogen and the Brain" in *New York* magazine.

Thank you for validating the absolute nightmare I lived for at least four years. I make a living as a salesperson on the wholesale level. I have always thought on my feet and counted on doing several things at one time. Words cannot express the sheer terror I lived through, losing my quick thinking and my memory, being depressed, and going to doctor after doctor who had no idea what was wrong—and I was already taking estrogen.

Fortunately, I found a new gynecologist and she picked up my symptoms. My body was not absorbing enough [estrogen] to get me back on track mentally. [Women can differ biologically in their reaction to the same drugs.] Everything is now pretty much back to the way it was—except that I lost a job that I loved and was working at for fourteen years. (Name listed in the article, Manhattan)

Here is another:

How good to read [my article]. In my early thirties, I went into premature menopause. With it came what I call "teflon brain" and aberrant bouts of halting speech. Pieces of simple information would fly through my brain, skipping over a slick surface. . . . No small problem for a television-news producer. Of course, when I would tell this to my doctors—and then add that it had to be because my brain was malnourished from lack of estrogen—they determined that lack of estrogen had rendered me daft, not forgetful. Now, it seems medicine is wiser. . . .
(Name, Manhattan)

THE WHM SYNDROME PARALLELS HYPOTHYROIDISM

In many ways the WHM Syndrome parallels, in its effects on thinking and behavior, an established hormone-deficiency syndrome that is also known for having cognitive/behavioral consequences—hypothyroidism.

In those with hypothyroidism, the very basic hormonal "fuel" that "drives" the body's metabolism efficiently—thyroid hormone—becomes deficient for one of several reasons. People with insufficient supplies of the hormone can experience not just mood and physical symptoms such as bone-wearying fatigue and a persistent cloud of depression (as do some women with WHMS), but also well-established cognitive-deficit symptoms ranging from subtle to very serious, in memory, attention, and the fine-tuning of thinking and speaking. The precedent thus exists for a known hormone-deficiency state producing cognitive symptoms in the manner of WHMS. It is even possible that hypothyroidism and WHMS may be related, i.e., that estrogen loss may trigger changes in thyroid function. While little is known about the relationship of estrogen changes on thyroid changes, it is known that changes in thyroid functioning often increase significantly in frequency among women during intervals of rapid hormonal shifts—e.g., following the birth of a child and around perimenopause and menopause. Some clinicians who treat menopausal women have observed that in association with menopausal symptoms often thyroid disregulation of one kind or another is not an uncommon finding. Moreover it has been discovered in recent years that the respective receptors that bind thyroid hormones and estrogens are part of the same superfamily of steroid receptors and may have evolved in tandem and work in tandem. Both are hormonal systems in charge of major, basic life-sustaining functions— thyroid hormones for driving the metabolism of cells for daily living and estrogen for underwriting and "fueling" the survival of the species and directly or indirectly affecting many brain, bone, heart, and other body-system functions. Just as the symptoms of hypothyroidism are now known to be readily correctable with thyroid hormone replacement therapy, in the years to come, the cognitive and behavioral symptoms of the WHM Syndrome, I believe, will be formally recognized as a comparably correctable hormone-deficiency state reversible with estrogen hormone replacement or custom-designed drugs or products mimicking estrogen's effects in the brain.

WE DON'T CREDIT HOW MUCH NORMAL WOMEN CAN DIFFER FROM EACH OTHER BIOLOGICALLY AROUND REPRODUCTIVE HALLMARKS

It is my goal in this book to communicate what the WHM Syndrome is and what it feels like, but it is also my express goal not to do harm, not to paint all women broadly with the same brush since WHMS symptoms affect some women not at all, some only mildly, and some seriously. I believe that central to any woman's or health expert's understanding of WHMS symptoms, perimenopause, menopause, research on menopause, and the treatment of menopausal symptoms is a considerably heightened appreciation of how much normal women can differ from each other with respect to any of the stages on the time line of women's reproductive events.

Consider for the moment what you already know about otherwise healthy normal women. Some have a monthly momentary twinge that announces their period is coming, whereas some go through days of premenstrual syndrome (PMS) agony with intense and disruptive mood and physical symptoms hammered in often by grueling migraine headaches. I have treated such women. Some women during pregnancy are sick to their stomachs practically every day while others fall in love with the psychological state pregnancy induces and keep wanting to repeat it over and over. Some women suffer postpartum effects that lead to thoughts of suicide and infanticide while others experience postpartum euphoria and bliss.

When I first heard about PMS and later postpartum depression as states that could induce dire mood alterations in women the truth is I suspected that some poor male psychiatrists had had the wool pulled over their eyes by females who were malingering for some unknown reason. I doubted that women could experience such intense reactions since *I* was a woman, after all, and assumed *I knew* what the universal experience of having a period was like. It was a "nothing" experience for me. Nothing to balk about. Only with time have I come to truly appreciate how diverse and divergent the experiences of women in this regard normally can be.

Let me share with you one moment of insight when this appreciation forcefully embedded itself in my psyche. Since graduate school I have used medical/science journalism as a means for extracurricular graduate study, for developing expertise by getting paid access to experts I wanted to interview in relation to my work as a research psychologist and later as a clinical health psychologist. I could ask the experts "up close and personal" what I wanted to know. When I was working with patients with chronic pain I proposed to the editors of *Psychology Today* doing a profile of one of the leading research psychologists of our day, Dr. Ronald Melzack. Melzack and a colleague, Patrick Wall, had put forth an important theory on pain—the gate control theory—that ultimately stimulated generations of research and progress in the field of pain. Melzack had studied the experience of pain in women during childbirth and had earlier developed a novel pain questionnaire that helped in the communication of a difficult topic—how much and what kind of pain a person had. When I interviewed him at McGill University in Montreal, Canada, he told me that the pain of giving birth could be compared to the acute pain of having a finger cut off. On the other hand he said there were some women who gave birth with no pain whatsoever. "No pain whatsoever?" I asked in amazement. "No pain whatsoever," Melzack said. I just couldn't believe such a thing was true so I asked the same question again in an even higher-pitched tone: "No pain whatsoever?" "No pain whatsoever," he said. Melzack indulged me this back-and-forth dance several times till I finally desisted and decided to store the information away, uncredited, in the back of my mind for some other day. It just seemed too amazing to be true.

Then one day into my office walked a woman who came to see me in my role as a health psychologist. In taking a history somehow the fact emerged that she had given birth with no pain whatsoever. "No pain whatsoever?" I again asked incredulously. "No pain whatsoever," she answered. I asked if this had ever occurred to anyone else in her family and she said, "Yes, to my grandmother. Maybe it skips a generation." At that pivotal moment of confirmation I "got it"—the bigger picture about the variability among normal women. I accepted as true what Melzack had told me and what this woman had told me. More important I "got" the message that a rose is not a rose is not a rose. Menstruation is not menstruation is not menstruation in the same way for every woman; pregnancy is not pregnancy is not pregnancy for all women; delivery is not delivery is not delivery for every woman; that menopause and perimenopause are often far from the same experiences from woman to woman to woman. I realized that these reproductive biological hallmarks can and often do vary enormously among women so that, to overstate the case somewhat, there are virtually different species of women when it comes to the "fine-tuning" of their brain and body's reproductive infrastructure.

The morals: (1) You can't know the interior experience of the woman sitting next to you by knowing your own. (2) You shouldn't be intolerant of women whose experiences in this regard differ from your own. (3) You can't characterize the experiences of all women by knowing the individual experiences of some women. Some women first experience WHMS symptoms in their thirties, some in their sixties. Some never do.

The existence of many distinct biological subgroups of women means in terms of research on perimenopausal and menopausal women that very large-size samples are needed to get accurate findings that detect accurately what is true in nature about women. Small-size sample studies may obscure and find insignificant what may be very true in nature. What this means in terms of treatments for perimenopausal and menopausal women is that possibly very different forms or intensities of treatment may be needed to help women with different biological natures.

I became familiar with the research literature on menopausal women only after first detecting the symptoms of the WHM Syndrome via interviews with women. What I discovered in my interviews with ultimately some 160 perimenopausal and menopausal women did not correspond with what I later read in the professional "menopause research literature." I had interviewed women who reported being hot all the time, like Sherry Strumph and her friend. The menopause literature made no mention of such women—though they might be in there somewhere I haven't yet read. Menopause experts I interviewed about such symptoms didn't know what I was talking about. Some even told me that women only developed hot flashes during menopause, not during perimenopause, which entirely defied what informants had told me.

I discovered there were more than a few women who were now menopausal who had *never* had a hot flash or only one to date, but who had lots of WHMS symptoms to one degree of intensity or another. These women didn't have physical symptoms to speak of. Their memory wasn't blinking from nighttime awakenings. Their relationships, their diet, and their exercise were essentially the same. Their ability to recall where they had just put something down wasn't. The menopause field said women with lots of complaints around the time of menopause who went to menopause clinics for help were having secondary reactions to their body symptoms and tended to overuse the mental health and health systems altogether, i.e., they were crackpots, so to speak, and couldn't be assumed to be representative of most menopausal women who didn't go to doctors. To the contrary, I discovered that quite a few women with many WHMS symptoms and other mood complaints *rarely or never went to doctors* for help and that women who did seek out help were not typically crazy, but likely resourceful or desperately bothered by biological systems, which weren't doing what they expected them to.

This insufficiently recognized biological variability among women with regard to perimenopause and menopause, together with the lack of awareness of the biological effects of estrogen loss on behavior, thinking, and physiology, has rendered invalid, to my mind, many of the present "findings" produced to date by the professional menopause survey research literature. Researchers haven't asked the right questions of women so they haven't learned sufficiently what is happening to them and what is affecting them. Though this may sound like criticism my intention is not to be carping. It *is* my intention to spotlight what needs to be added to future research. Anyone involved in science long enough knows from personal experience that most knowledge in science is provisional, that etched-in-stone dogmas diligently learned in graduate school or medical school can be overturned in a night. Future research in this field, I hope, will routinely acknowledge women's evident biological diversity and work toward finding markers that predict that diversity. The field of menopause research needs to first observe women better and describe women's perceptions of change no matter the political fallout from either those who don't want menopause "medicalized" or from women fearful of finding biological differences among women or between women and men. It is time to acknowledge that not only do the sexes differ from each other in some important ways but that women can differ from each other in important ways. Understanding those differences, and in medical terms learning how to accommodate individual needs dependent on such differences, is where we should be heading.

2

Why the Syndrome Has Been Overlooked for So Long

Katherine, Sherry, and Quiana had no idea what was happening to them initially. And the physicians Sherry and Quiana discussed their symptoms with also had no awareness that memory and related symptoms could be associated with changing supplies of ovarian hormones, with the exception of Dr. D. (Katherine never sought a doctor's help for what she was experiencing.)

How could the medical establishment have failed to detect what was happening to so many women over such a long period of time? This is an intriguing and important question. Certainly, as we've seen, some women do keep their WHMS symptoms to themselves and away from the purview of doctors. But over a lifetime of practice undoubtedly many doctors have had patients like Sherry and Quiana at similar ages inquire about changing memory, speech, and mind symptoms year after year after year. How did they and society at large miss what was going on? Here are some answers:

1. RESEARCHERS HAVEN'T STUDIED HEALTHY MIDLIFE WOMEN ALTOGETHER.

Interviews with experts on aging and women's health indicate that there has not been much formal study altogether of *healthy* midlife men and women in their thirties, forties, and fifties within medicine and science. Researchers are only now beginning to study healthy people in their forties and fifties. Thus physicians didn't have a realm of formal knowledge to study in medical school about normal women. Paradoxically, however, the great consumer interest in *in vitro* fertilization and similar assisted-reproduction technologies has spawned the unintended side benefit of researchers learning much about *normal* younger women and their fertility and ovarian function. This has come from practice and experience in the removal of viable "donor" eggs from healthy younger women in their twenties and early thirties to "egg-receiving" women of different ages with impaired fertility. This work has revealed that some women develop evidence of ovarian decline at young ages, often as early as their twenties (a condition known as premature ovarian failure), and that one relatively precipitous drop in ovarian robustness and fertility occurs earlier than was recently thought—around age thirty-five. In doing this work fertility experts in general have discovered more variability among younger women in ovarian competence than they had previously suspected. This may be why the existence of WHMS symptoms in younger women such as Katherine Kennedy, described in chapter 1, may not be so surprising.

The absence of study of *healthy* normal women in their thirties, forties, and fifties has had other consequences as well—presumed basic "facts" have sometimes been based on a very small number of cases. At present even the ob/gyn basic facts of what goes hormonally up or down and for how long, during the very normal midlife stage called perimenopause are today in dispute and undergoing revision according to leading textbook writer and menopause expert Dr. Leon Speroff, of the University of Oregon Health Sciences Center. According to Speroff, a long-standing "dogma" about hormone levels in the years before menopause that has been taught for years to ob/gyns since 1976 was based on a limited sample of only eight women!

2. WHMS SYMPTOMS HAVE BEEN MISATTRIBUTED WHEN DETECTED.

At present most gynecologists and menopause experts—not necessarily overlapping categories as I once glibly assumed—don't know about the existence of most of the specific symptoms of the WHM Syndrome. They have not detected or isolated the biologically based signals of the syndrome. Instead amidst the complex interacting events that constitute a normal life for women, either psychosocial factors or the effects of experiencing the physical symptoms associated with perimenopause and menopause have been misattributed as the likely causes of women's complaints about attention or memory problems in the years surrounding menopause. Women with such complaints are often assumed to be depressed over such psychosocial factors as children leaving home, or "maxing out" in their careers as the result of professional "ceilings," or awareness of age-related changes, or seeing death looming on the horizon. Depression over such life events is assumed to be the basis of their memory and attention problems. Moreover, women's voiced complaints about memory and attention problems are now frequently interpreted as the likely result of experiencing sleeplessness from perimenopause- or menopause-associated night awakenings with or without associated hot flashes—as the result of the physical symptoms that can accompany perimenopause and menopause. And it is plausible. Some memory and attention problems in midlife women probably are due to these factors. But not always all of them. Animal research not confounded by psychosocial factors suggests that in rats and monkeys estrogen loss can respectively produce memory and attention deficits. Other animal research shows that estrogen loss can lead to the brain chemistry associated with depression. Depression, memory and attention problems, may therefore be real and associated with estrogen loss rather than the inevitable result of only life-events and/or physical factors.

3. THERE'S BEEN A "DON'T TELL, DON'T ASK" POLICY IN PRACTICE.

According to menopause expert Dr. William Andrews, former president of the American College of Obstetrics and Gynecology and a clinician who has been aware that cognitive changes can occur in women during these years, "Women are embarrassed to express these symptoms directly to doctors. But if a doctor takes a good history he can uncover the symptoms." Many women have been reluctant to voice WHMS symptoms to physicians in part for fear of undercutting their effectiveness with doctors as health partners in making health decisions. Like Katherine Kennedy they often feel diminished by the symptoms and fear they'll be "written off" as incompetent in future doctor/patient interactions. And it may sometimes be the case. One woman who complained of memory symptoms to her doctor found that the next time she came for an office visit she was asked—she had never been asked this before—to pay her bill before leaving!

4. WOMEN'S COGNITIVE COMPLAINTS HAVE FALLEN BETWEEN THE CRACKS OF DIFFERENT DISCIPLINES.

Dr. Andrews also says, "Gynecologists are more comfortable measuring objective indicators for treatment, like bone density or blood lipids. They aren't trained to give psychological tests." Gynecologists haven't been trained to study the mind, to ask or answer "mind questions." And guess what? Psychiatrists, psychologists, and neurologists don't order blood tests assessing women's ovarian hormone levels as a standard operating procedure. Women's WHMS symptom complaints, when voiced, fall too often on deaf ears. Ideally, interpreting the symptoms of WHMS requires expertise across multiple disciplines—reproductive endocrinology, psychology/psychiatry, neuropsychology, behavioral neuroendocrinology, and neurology; expertise specifically on menopause beyond a knowledge of an obstetrics/gynecology curriculum; knowledge about normal aging and about Alzheimer's disease; and expertise in understanding the current neurosciences research literature. Few medical specialists, much less general practitioners, have mastery of this broad realm, particularly as disciplines grow more scientifically complex and specialized. Women's lifetime medical care needs are now unfortunately largely chopped up and dispersed among doctors who specialize in and know well different organ systems, but not how a whole woman can function and variously behave over the span of a lifetime. Just as the mind/body/brain/immunology/health field of psychoneuroimmunology involved a synthesis of once distinct disciplines and cross-fertilization of ideas and techniques across disciplines, so too will this area require a new synthesis of disciplines, methods, and realms of expertise.

5. MEDICINE WAS AN ALL-MALE PATERNALISTIC PATRIARCHAL SYSTEM.

WHMS was overlooked because for a very long time obstetrics/gynecology was virtually an all-male surgical club in which, strange though it seems now, men taught other men about the experiences of women; they didn't have a firsthand basis for knowing what they were talking about. This was particularly true with respect to the subtle interior symptoms characteristic of WHMS. These mostly male gynecologists "knew" medically taught facts and apparently weren't readily educable by patients, much less women patients. Since the onset of the women's movement, obstetrics/gynecology as a field has been responsive and has made adaptive changes to the charge of paternalism—talking down to women in an all-knowing manner—but men still can't know firsthand the inner experiences of women. And though many more women have entered the profession many women gynecologists trained in recent years are only now approaching their perimenopausal/menopausal years and haven't yet reached a critical mass for being aware of WHMS symptoms. Also many female gynecologists are likely not to experience WHMS symptoms because as a group they are preferentially informed about clinical research attesting to estrogen's growing list of benefits and are more likely to be taking estrogen themselves for preventive bone and cardiovascular reasons.

Also, as applied scientists, ob/gyns tend to apply what they have learned and vested in their skills and expertise, and are likely to hold in abeyance or dismiss what they don't comprehend. Many haven't yet formally or informally learned about the 1990s evidence revealing the many new roles of estrogen in the thinking, remembering parts of the brain and haven't had a scientific rationale for understanding what women may have voiced to them over the years. "Many gynecologists are not aware yet of any cognitive symptoms that might arise with estrogen loss," affirms Dr. Andrews, "nor of the scientific research on estrogen's roles in cognition. Efforts" by the profession, he says, "are being made now to make this information available to [them]. At present," he says, "primarily experts on aging, menopause, and Alzheimer's disease are aware of this new research."

However, making this information available to practicing gynecologists in journals and professional meetings may not do the trick. A leading menopause expert I interviewed at the 1997 North American Menopause Society annual meeting in Boston (who I shall spare from the consequences of "dissing" his colleagues in public by not quoting him for attribution) told me, "After they start practicing, [obstetricians/gynecologists] often aren't receptive to new input." Why, I asked? "Because they think they know it all already," he said to my surprise, not joking. The information may be being made available to gynecologists, this leader was saying, but would they read it and take it "in" was the more salient question. Seeking explication and validation of the latter statement, at the same meeting I sidled up to another ob/gyn who was standing next to his poster-board presentation. I stated what I had been told. Was this how he saw it? I asked. He affirmed the same view. "What then would force already practicing gynecologists to absorb this new mind/brain/estrogen research?" I asked. "Being confronted by their patients with articles and books in the popular press and asked 'How come you haven't told me about this?'" he said. Namely, the fear of losing patients or losing status with their patients would be motivating. To help themselves and help disseminate knowledge of this research, therefore, women need to go and ask their doctors "Could you tell me what you know about the possible effects of estrogen on the mind and brain during perimenopause and menopause?" and "Are you familiar with that new book about the WHM Syndrome, *Menopause and the Mind*?" Even better I suggest you offer this book to your doctor as an educational present.

6. WOMEN'S SYMPTOMS WERE SUSPECT, OVERANALYZED, AND VIEWED THROUGH FREUDIAN AND PSYCHOSOMATIC LENSES.

For too many years women's female complaints were often viewed and "interpreted" through colored, sometimes distorting cultural lenses: from a "Freudian" perspective or a "psychosomatic" perspective. Women's stated complaints weren't trusted for what they were but were often seen as representing something other than what they ostensibly were about. A cigar was rarely only a cigar. Women were infantilized as credible informants and weren't much listened to as knowing about themselves. Male doctors—and until the seventies doctors were disproportionately males—assumed they knew "better" about women's bodies because they had studied what medicine had taught them; and it hadn't taught them about these strange WHMS symptoms. Even stand-up comedians in the prefeminist era routinely mocked dismissively women's professed physical woes. While psychosomatic and some Freudian interpretations *can* have validity they were overapplied and undercut women's credibility about what was happening to them.

7. WOMEN'S CHANGING AND VAGUE COMPLAINTS DUE TO THE SUBTLE REMODELING EFFECTS OF ESTROGEN LOSS ON THE BODY AND MIND WERE VIEWED SKEPTICALLY.

Because the effects of estrogen loss during perimenopause and menopause can be gradual, ongoing, diffuse, and pervasive in their effects on the bones, vascular system, the heart, the bladder, metabolism, skin, collagen-supported structures, and as we now know the brain and mind, the result can be a range of come-and-go symptoms that plausibly are numerous, subtle, and changing. (This isn't commonly appreciated even now as a possible correlate of hormonal loss.) However, women who may have accurately reported "many" and/or "vague" and/or an ever-changing parade of body symptoms or WHMS symptoms likely lost credibility as accurate reporters of their internal states and had their symptoms interpreted as "unhappy psychosomatic complaining" reflecting dissatisfactions over such things as their children leaving home (empty nests), not being needed, dissatisfaction with aging, and the like. Women weren't believed when they did complain about WHMS symptoms.

8. WHMS SYMPTOMS TEND TO BE INTERMITTENT AND DISAPPEAR WITH DIRECTED EFFORT.

Like hot flashes, WHMS symptoms tend to be erratic and intermittent, not continual. They tend to occur more when women are on "automatic pilot" behavior and are just "being" or coasting rather than "trying" or actively monitoring themselves. Women "try" for their doctors. Thus, WHMS symptoms were more likely to occur in the doctor's waiting room than in his or her office. Physicians didn't see the symptoms. Also, when women see doctors they tend to be focused in addressing their concerns and effortfully attuned to what the doctor is saying. They are also rarely "just being" before or during naked encounters in stirrups. Awareness of the time constraints often imposed on medical visits also tends to focus their efforts. Moreover, the intermittent nature of WHMS symptoms offers women respite and makes the symptoms tolerable even though they may be overall self-distressing. Reinforced by the symptoms going away—their intermittent nature—women with WHMS symptoms keep hoping theirs will, *for good,* and often don't go running to doctors with them or know who to "run" to.

9. PATIENTS WITH WHMS SYMPTOMS TESTED NORMAL.

Many of the standard neuropsychological tests used today to assess memory, attention, and thinking in all likelihood aren't sufficiently sensitive for detecting the subtle-but-present WHMS changes. Many tests in use today were developed to evaluate those with severe brain damage. The WHM Syndrome represents often intermittent, hide-and-seek, sometimes there/sometimes not symptoms that may fail to be present at the moment of testing, even if more sensitive tests were to be used. Furthermore, as noted, many of the symptoms can be overcome by directed effort, the kind of "trying" usually present when a person takes a test. So with WHMS symptoms the standard process of test administration may defeat its diagnostic intent. According to leading brain researcher Dr. Robert Sapolsky, Associate Professor of Neuroscience at the Stanford University School of Medicine, with whom I discussed some of WHMS' symptoms, tests that catch "testees" unaware, such as being asked to recall information about a scene casually walked through five minutes before, without advance warning that such follow-up questioning would occur, are the kinds of tests more likely to detect subtle attention or memory deficits, such as those present in the WHM Syndrome.

When I interviewed a leading estrogen-and-cognition researcher at a 1997 meeting of the Society for Behavioral Neuroendocrinology in Baltimore, her comments reinforced my suspicion of the likely insensitivity of standard neuropsychological tests for detecting WHMS symptoms in at least some of those with WHMS-like complaints. I asked the researcher, who is also affiliated with a menopause treatment center, why in her published reports she often minimized earlier research describing estrogen's effects on memory, which relied on menopausal women's self-report measures of improvement in memory after estrogen administration. She said because the research relied not on *objective* indicators of improvement but *subjective* "self-report" measures—women's own assessments. Such self-report measures she said could be unreliable from the standpoint of research. In partial explanation she added that when women came to the menopause clinic with which she was associated saying things like "I think I'm losing my mind," a WHMS kind of description, "and we send them out to be tested on neuropsychological test batteries, they [the tests] usually come back indicating [the women] are normal." That is, the tests are not "picking up" or detecting what the women are actively complaining about.

10. WHMS SYMPTOMS CAN REMAIN HIDDEN UNLESS WOMEN OPENLY TALK ABOUT THEM AND THEY OFTEN DON'T.

Though it's finally socially acceptable in the 1990s to talk about perimenopause and menopause, women no longer have the intimate forums for sharing and unmasking what is common to them, for making the personal public and political, for collectively informing physicians about personal realities. They are otherwise engaged in fitting careers, family needs, and fitness routines into "superwoman" expectations.

In the era of consciousness-raising groups in the 1970s, mainly younger premenopausal women broke the competitive barriers that divided them and often shared their most intimate experiences week after week in a programmatic down-the-list fashion. They did this as a way of learning about the varieties of experience of being a woman, of overcoming negative attitudes toward women's bodies, or as a way of examining and challenging negative stereotypes about women. Today those groups no longer exist and venues for intimately sharing subtle interior experiences about being a woman communally are limited. The political power of those groups collectively to inform physicians and alter medical practices is also limited now. Though books on menopause in the early 1990s by Gail Sheehy, Germaine Greer, and others helped make the topic culturally acceptable, ironically today's overcommitted, work-dominated, me-and-my-computer-isolated lifestyle makes it possible for WHMS symptoms to remain undiscussed and culturally invisible so that women can imagine their symptoms are an individual rather than a communal problem.

Even when some WHMS symptoms can be observed by others, the outward signs can easily be overlooked or viewed as isolated events in time and casually attributed to such factors as fatigue, or sleep deprivation, or an uncharacteristic "stumble" in the context of normal behavior.

Were women's consciousness-raising groups in existence today and attended by perimenopausal and menopausal women, not only would WHMS symptoms have been likely discovered communally but in the drive to make the personal political and public, women's physicians would have felt the pressure to attend to what large numbers of women would be telling them.

In many ways the hemispheric deconnection syndrome, which can result from surgery used to treat intractable epileptic seizures, provides a model of a similarly *subtle* cognitive/behavioral syndrome that was not detected for many years. In this form of treatment the cablelike structure linking the two brain hemispheres—the brain's corpus callosum—is sectioned or cut, to prevent the spread of seizures from one side of the brain to the other. As a result of this surgery one half of the brain often is unaware of what the other half knows. The symptoms of this syndrome are subtle and were only unmasked so that others could detect or infer the interior experience of those who had it, by devising very sensitive cognitive/behavioral tests that could reveal it.* Just as with the deconnection syndrome, WHMS may similarly require specially tailored tests, sufficiently sensitive, to fully reveal it or to assess changes in its symptoms over time.

The fascinating story of Polly Van Benthusen (a real person and not an alias) will reveal to you features that are common to many women in their encounter with and surprise at WHMS symptoms. Her case illustrates further why so many perimenopausal and menopausal women often don't "get" for a long time what is happening to them.

I heard about Polly Van Benthusen and her thirty-five-year-old gynecologist Dr. Robert Greene, a reproductive endocrinologist—a specialty of obstetrics and gynecology—through someone who knew what I was researching and had heard both her story and about her uniquely trained doctor.

Very atypically, Dr. Greene as a medical student knew he had a definite interest in studying menopause. After completing medical school he specifically sought out extensive training in menopause medicine (in contrast to some leading ob/gyn residency programs, where residents receive a scant two hours of training on the topic). He had become a researcher in the menopause field when he encountered Polly Van Benthusen as a patient. As you will see his training made a vital difference in the quality of Polly Van Benthusen's life.

Case 4: Polly Van Benthusen

Polly Van Benthusen is a bright, lively, fun-filled forty-eight-year-old field office assistant manager for a large branch of the Social Security Administration

---

*N. Geschwind and E. Kaplan, *A Human Cerebral Deconnection Syndrome,* Neur. 12, 1962, 675–85; Robert Ornstein, *The Right Mind, Making Sense of the Hemispheres* (Harcourt Brace & Co., 1997).

on the West Coast, where she has worked since she was twenty-three. In her professional life she engages in considerable public speaking and teaching in educational forums, informing people how the Social Security Administration works and how it can benefit them. Polly is married to her childhood sweetheart and is the devoted mother of a much-adored nineteen-year-old son born prematurely, whose developmental needs have been a loving focus of her life.

Reproductive State: was perimenopausal and may be menopausal now but can't tell since she is on hormones.

I think I'm menopausal now and when these symptoms began I was perimenopausal and had just started having hot flashes at forty. I thought that menopause began in your late fifties or early sixties. I didn't know anything about the topic. I thought it would take a few years. I'd be a little crazy and that would be it.

All this began at forty with my awareness of impatience. I remember always having a world of patience with my son who was then twelve and suddenly I realized I was getting short-tempered with him. I started to have these drenching night sweats that disrupted my sleep. Everything started going out of whack with my periods. I'd not have one period for a month and then have one for ten days. I wondered what in the world is going on. I went for a normal checkup and the doctor said at a certain time the cycles change and that it was not abnormal. He didn't mention menopause to me at age forty.

The first episode of what I call my memory changes came then with the apple juice incident. My son worships apple juice. We buy four to five gallons of apple juice at a time for him. It's a given. I'd gone to the refrigerator and put the juice on the counter and simply didn't remember in an instant that I put it there. It was apparently sitting there on the counter but I couldn't find it. I looked all over, the fridge, the counter, the kitchen, and just couldn't find it. So even though everything was set to go for dinner I ran to get some apple juice for my son. When I came back my husband said, "Honey are you alright?" He thought I'd lost a cog. There was the apple juice right on the counter. He said, "You set it out on the counter." I said, "No I didn't," and I was ready to do battle over this apple juice. He said, "You really are losing it now." I said, "I didn't put that apple juice there. I honestly don't recall doing that."

We then moved and my new gynecologist said, "You are pre-menopausal and we need to do some tests. I looked at him as though he had a chicken on his head and I didn't believe him. All I said was "Oh." At forty-one I felt I was too young to have this thing. I recall coming home and calling my mother and saying, "The doctor thinks I'm pre-menopausal." To my great surprise my mother told me that she had be-came *fully* menopausal when she was thirty and I said, "Mom, that doesn't sound normal. It sounds very early." She said, "I thought back then that I was losing my mind. I had trouble remembering where I put things. It was a very bad time for me."

My mother is a very southern lady and I said to her, "How come we never talked about this?"

You see I was known for remembering *everything*. I had a kind of photographic memory. I could very precisely see what I was recalling. Everyone would depend on me for it—at work, home, everywhere. That's why it was so frightening for me when my memory started to fail because I took it so much for granted.

At work I used to tell my secretary, "Put this in my appointment di-ary," and she would come in and I'd know by heart the meetings I was scheduled to go to for weeks. But between forty-two and forty-six I sud-denly became dependent on things being written down.

The weird thing is that I never linked what was happening to me to hormones. Even after the conversation with my mom I still didn't link the memory symptoms to menopause. I just didn't put them together. At the first meeting with my new gynecologist after we moved, I was alerted that hot flashes and irregular periods were problems of meno-pause. But he said my hormone levels were kind of in the normal ranges and he didn't recommend estrogen or anything.

Now, I'm pretty accepting of things. I said to myself, "If you get hot, turn on a fan." It was a little inconvenience but I just accepted it.

The next year my hormone tests were somewhat down but not in the low range. I wasn't told to do anything. Except more weird things kept on happening to me.

I didn't remember whole conversations I had with people. People would say "Don't you remember that?" and I didn't. That's when it be-gan to concern me. It would feel as though someone had kidnapped me from my life. Now, my husband's always been supportive and good-natured but he just couldn't believe what was happening to me. I'd begun to forget to show up at meetings, which is entirely not like me. I sat on a few boards in the community and I was absolutely aghast one evening when the blood center I was on the board of called and said, "You missed that meeting," a meeting that was on my calendar! I just hadn't checked it or recalled it. I apologized profusely and now knew I had to rely on writing things down. Before I never even used a shopping list.

I thought it was stress. I couldn't think of anything else. So I went to work problem solving and became what I call a "technoweenie." I got an electronic organizer that had alarms and it helped enormously. I had that and a written calendar, one at home and one at work. It worked. It was a lifesaver. I did really fine with this system. I became selective about what I kept in my head and relied on my organizers for everything else.

By age forty-six, however, things were really getting bad with my memory. I wondered if my asthma medication could be doing this and stopped taking it for a while. When I asked my internist about my memory all he said was, "We're all getting older and can't remember everything forever." He said, "You've just got to relax with all this." I love him and respected what he said.

But I thought memory problems started around sixty-five or seventy. I'd wake up in the dead of night and wonder had I locked the front door. And I'd think "Get it together." In those midnight walks to check, I'd think "Is this how it starts? Little things start and build and build and build?"

When my internist said it was about getting older I said to myself, "Well I've never been forty-six before so maybe this is what happens." I was afraid to reveal how much this was bothering me because I didn't really want to get involved with EEGs and brain scans. At the same time I was seriously going to get a blood test to see if I had that special apolipoprotein-E gene that's associated with a higher risk of Alzheimer's disease but I chickened out. I was afraid they would find it and afraid they wouldn't.

I didn't share what was happening to me with anyone besides my husband because I was a bit embarrassed and frightened. I don't think people had a sense of what was going on with me. I kept my work dead-lines pretty well and was managing fairly well.

One time though my boss, who I have a good relationship with and who had often depended on my memory, said in amazement, "Polly, I can't believe you can't remember this!" whatever it was. I said, "I honestly can't," and he said, "Are you alright?" Another time one of my staff members came in and said, "It's two o'clock. Time for the meeting!" I apparently had scheduled one and I didn't have a clue in the world what the meeting was about. So I said, "OK! Let's have a meeting!" I went with the flow. I said, "Refresh my memory on this." When they mentioned someone who was scheduled to meet with us and I had no idea who it might be, I said, "Can you spell their name for me?" and it turned out to be "Smith." We laughed hysterically.

During that time things were happening at home. My husband would say calmly things like, "Honey why is there a can of green beans in the refrigerator?" and I'd reflexively say, "Check and see if there's milk in the cupboard." And he'd say, "Yes, there's milk in the cupboard." And we laughed and laughed. It was as though my hands and mind didn't work together. They had separate lives. Whatever idea I last had in my head ruled my hands. I'd say, "This senility is really getting bad." Things like this happened over and over.

Also whatever I would have in my head would come out of my mouth. For example in making reservations instead of saying as I intended to, "One room with two beds," I heard the "two" echo in my words. I said, "Two rooms with one bed." "Good grief!" I thought. "If this wasn't so hilarious I'd be crying at what's happening to me." I'd switch the first letters of words around. One time I had to do a taped radio show for work and part of the line I had to say was "a fast buck." You can imagine what I said instead. We had to cut the tape. Sometimes in one-on-one conversations my mind would wander. It would be really embarrassing and I'd say, "Could you repeat that again?" In a big meeting I'd really be lost because I couldn't say that. Sometimes when it wasn't that crucial I would say, "I'm sorry, I was gone a minute but I'm back now." My husband at times like these would say to me, "Were we in ozone?"

During this time I also couldn't do simple math skills some of the time. I took a calculator with me everywhere when I used to be able to add things up in my head. In discussions I'd lose my train of thought when it came to making an argument. I'd be halfway through saying something and realize "I haven't got a clue where I'm going with this." It's like you're circling the field and your mind just refuses to land. I see this happening at work to both men and women.

I'd be standing in the kitchen and yell to my husband, "Why am I here at the cupboard?" and he'd yell back, "You needed oil for the skillet." Or I'd go into the bedroom and say, "Why am I coming through here?" and eventually realize it was to put some things in the closet. It's like your mind goes out of gear.

My mind at times would get hazy. It was like being drowsy. Almost like you want to shake your head to think. And then other times my mind would be clear but I couldn't come up with ideas. I've always been a great brainstormer, the ideas person. And I'd be in a meeting and for the moment feel as though I couldn't come up with an idea. People would be stunned that I didn't have an idea because I always had.

We have computers at work and I always turned them on and off. One day I couldn't recall where the "on and off" switch was. It was like getting lost. I walked up to the computer thinking "Now where is your switch?"

I'd go spell a word and drop a letter as I was writing. Because of this I now use an erasable pen. It becomes permanent after awhile.

Also my reading became so ponderous. I'd reverse words reading and lose the meaning by doing this. I was a big reader and halfway through a paragraph I'd think "That didn't make any sense." I'd make things into a question that weren't questions. My reading got so bad I had to read one word at a time. I had taken a speed-reading course and I couldn't skim anymore. I never had ADD [attention deficit disorder] and I had never had problems with this before. I'd think to myself "Here I am. This is like *The Exorcist*." I would read things wrong twice. It felt like I was dyslexic. And I'd say, "I really am losing it. It's pre-senile dementia."

One time I saw someone who turned out to be one of our neighbors from across the street from several years ago but I couldn't remember who she was and where she was from. It was most unusual. I had no recall of having ever met her. My husband had to tell me who she was. There have also been several instances of people at meetings knowing me and I wouldn't have a clue who they were.

A few times when I was driving things also seemed to be different somehow. I attributed it to my glasses. I would pull out into traffic and concentrate on one thing but not another. I didn't turn on my blinker the way I always do religiously. I misjudged the length of a car. Now, I've had exactly two tickets in my life. One at age eighteen and one at age thirty-six, so I have been and still am a good driver. And this hasn't happened since but it was strange when it happened. It had never happened before.

Then it became the time of the year when I make my ob/gyn appointments and they had a new doctor onboard. My older one had retired and they asked if I would see him. He had nice credentials and had done research in this area. He was young but real bright. We had good rapport. He did my physical and he asked if I had hot flashes or vaginal dryness. And I gave him my history of physical symptoms and then I said, "I can't remember a thing." To my complete amazement he said, "That's pretty common with menopause."

I was so taken aback I didn't say anything. I thought to myself, "Well where the heck have you been the last four years!" He took it as a matter of course, the association. I couldn't figure out why nobody else had said this to me before. He seemed to know it from the get-go. He said, "Your blood tests show that it's time for some hormones," and he gave me a sample of Prempro [a combination estrogen and progesterone] and said, "Take this." I said, "I don't think so. We have cancer in my father's family."

Then he discussed with me the latest evidence on breast cancer and endometrial cancer in relation to taking estrogen and progesterone, and he gave me some literature and suggested I read it. He also gave me a prescription, but I was fully *not* going to take it.

I didn't ask him about the memory problems because I was far more afraid of cancer than anything I was dealing with already. So I took the material home and read it and then read the warning on the medical insert of the Prempro and said "No" to myself.

Two months later I had to go to see him again for something. He asked if I was taking the pills. And I told him why not. I said I feared I would be the one person in a hundred who gets cancer. I was sharing with him the fact that I was beginning to have mood swings and that I would feel really, really depressed about not remembering things. I'd wake up in the middle of the night and think to myself "What in the world is happening!" He indicated that if I didn't take the estrogen and progesterone, life might be tough later. He feared osteoporosis for me because my mom had it. He said breast cancer is usually passed from the mother's side and that studies showed that for the first five years of estrogen usage breast cancer is not prevalent. He nonetheless said that there's always a risk with any medication. He said that the hot flashes would go away [with the estrogen] and I'd have no periods with the Prempro. And then he said, "I think you'll find your memory will improve."

I was so stunned by this again when he said it and he saw it. He said, "There exist studies that show it will improve your memory."

I took the Prempro, thinking "I'll soon find out if this will help." Afterward I just gradually had no more hot flashes. So many of the problems improved—the vaginal dryness, which had become so bad. A hair under my chin that I was so horrified by went away. I remember thinking when it arrived "This is just a bizarre rite of passage. I'm going to wake up one morning with some odd new thing on my face and it will be menopause."

There was no stroke-of-lightning moment but it must have been six to seven months [after I started to take the hormones] when I suddenly realized I wasn't making lists to go to the store. I was relying on my memory again. It felt good to remember things again. I began to take control of my life again and not have all those irritants. My memory, which had sunk to only 75 percent of what it had been—my husband would probably say that I couldn't remember anything then—is now probably at 90 percent of what it was. I feel so much more confident of my memory, that I won't forget a meeting, and things like that. Now I can come up with ideas all over the place and meet deadlines. It feels great to be able to do these things in the same way again. The reading improved too a great deal with the estrogen. I now get a lot of reading matter into my office and get on it and don't even have to take a break; I can focus so well.

Before the estrogen I found that unless I'd make lists I couldn't put things in order [in my head] unless I saw them. And I was always a great organizer. I found I couldn't always do that without more effort than I had been used to. This improved with the estrogen. I had a short deadline recently and I could think through the process and did it pretty well and met the deadline. I felt comfortable doing it. Just as a check on my skills I asked my boss to take a look at what I had done and to think if anything else was necessary and it wasn't. That was a good reinforcer for me.

I still will forget some things. My spelling, for example. During my forties it had gotten worse and it's not back 100 percent. I'd look at a word and it would not look right; and I'd have to get a dictionary out or use spell check [on the computer]. Even when I looked the words up they didn't look right. I couldn't explain the loss. It was just so absurd. I'd think "I have spelled this word nine hundred times!" Because I still forget some things I compensate by being more careful to use the tools I have. The electronic organizer is great for its alarm system. I find that a month-at-a-glance chart helps me remember the month visually and I find that writing things down in a calendar helps me remember them better. I can recall better in visual pictures.

I often think about women who might be going through this alone, or are working to support families alone, or with husbands who aren't supportive or funny the way mine has been, and I fear for them. I could see women going through these symptoms becoming realistically fearful if they'll make a faux pas that could cost them their job or going to drastic ends in fear over what's happening to them, and what it could lead to. It's also about not knowing what's happening and having nowhere to turn. Why didn't my other doctors know to tell me about this? It's very scary. The more people hear about this the better it will be for women. That's why I've decided to go public with this. Women have got to know what can happen so they don't slip into this abyss and feel so hopeless. I have a relative close in age to me. She's very shy and after I talked about this she said she's experiencing some of it too; but she had never been open or discussed it with me till I brought it up with her. I know that she would be reluctant to tell a supervisor what was going on. If we don't get educated about this and educate others many women will acquiesce and get fired for something than can be helped, for something they don't have to suffer through.

———————

Polly's case dramatizes the importance of finding a doctor who is up to date on menopause research and connecting estrogen to cognitive function. And Polly's own complex feelings toward the symptoms that were disrupting her life illustrate what happens frequently to many successful women experiencing WHMS—for many different reasons they often don't "get" what is happening to them.

WHY WOMEN WITH WHMS SYMPTOMS OFTEN DON'T "GET" WHAT'S HAPPENING TO THEM

- Unlike pregnancy, many women are not informed about peri-menopause or menopause before symptoms hit. There are no instructions in a box about these biological stages, in the way that many of us partially learned about menstruation from the insert in a box of Tampax. Like Polly many women don't know when menopause begins on average, at age 51.7, or which symptoms indicate that the functioning of the ovaries is beginning to *noticeably* wind down, the stage called by some perimenopause. Like Polly, few women know their mother's age of onset or experience with menopause. Few women sit around expectantly anticipating, thinking about, or planning for menopause, and even less so for the amorphously defined era called "perimenopause" (which even menopause researchers are still debating about), just as no one sits around saying, "I wonder when I'll begin noticeably aging." Women don't think about perimenopause or menopause till it's necessary. Former *New York Times* columnist and fiction writer Anna Quindlen, now in her mid-forties, recently gave testimony to this widespread ignorance (and a common WHMS symptom—forgetting *very* familiar names) when she wrote in *The New York Times* "I should know as much about menopause from talking and listening as I do about pregnancy. But I don't. That is why when I began to wake bolt upright in the middle of the night and started forgetting the names of my children, I initially thought I was losing my mind not simply my fertility. . . ."

• Women don't relate many of the WHMS changes to hormones or menopause because they are still menstruating and aren't "thinking hormones" or menopause yet, particularly in their thirties and early forties, just as Polly wasn't. They think of themselves as *young* and don't associate hormonal changes with "young." In the midst of busy lives they often haven't "tuned in to" or recognized subtle changes in their typical menstrual cycle pattern—greater variability—that can herald the onset of things like hot flashes and vaginal dryness and, as you've seen in the cases presented so far, can herald WHMS symptoms. Also, many women who have never had regular menstrual cycles but erratic patterns as the norm may particularly miss detecting greater variability in their periods as a trumpeting sign that more symptoms associated with perimenopause and menopause may soon follow.

• Many women don't realize cognitive symptoms can hit at all or so early, even in their thirties, and so don't connect them to changing hormone levels even when they start experiencing them in the vicinity of hot flashes, mood changes, or vaginal dryness as Polly did.

• Women often don't realize that the symptoms of hormonal change associated with declining ovarian function and estrogen availability can span such a broad *spectrum* of changes in multiple arenas: (1) WHMS cognitive/behavioral/speech changes, (2) mood and emotional changes, and (3) a wide array of possible physical changes and energy availability. Even Polly, who was aware that *some* of her "mind" and "behavior" symptoms were related to perimenopause and menopause because of what Dr. Greene ultimately told her, still during our interview had not connected *all* the dots between many of her other symptoms. She was surprised to learn when I probed at the end of our interview for the existence of other WHMS symptoms that she did indeed have other related symptoms but hadn't considered them before as connected to the others.

Even the professional menopause field hasn't yet connected many of these dots despite the fact that highly credible neuroscience research reports on the roles of estrogen in memory centers of the brain and in cognition in women have been published throughout the 1990s and some even in the mid-to-late eighties. For example, a 1996 review article of treatments for menopausal symptoms in the major professional menopause journal *Maturitas* states that "Recent cohort studies confirm that only flushes [hot flashes], night sweats and vaginal dryness are provenly associated with ovarian failure . . ." and that "Cognitive function is not related to menopause. . . ."

Reading through the menopause professional literature it can also seem as if menopause experts are telling physicians to look for a basis for women's complaints during this time in every other possible arena *but the biological one*. For example, in a 1997 Continuing Medical Education curriculum for ob/gyns, distributed at the exhibition area of the North American Menopause Society, titled *Postmenopausal Health Curriculum 101*, "produced in accordance with the Accreditation Council for Continuing Medical Education Essentials" by a company known as Pragmaton, "an accredited provider of continuing medical education," with a respectable Program Advisory Board that includes several key figures in the menopause field, the following statements appear in a table telling doctors what to do: "Clinicians [doctors treating perimenopausal women] should look beyond presenting symptoms [what women say is bothering them] into the patient's life for other factors (e.g., diet, exercise, history of depression, attitudes toward sexuality) and significant life changes (e.g., family relationships and function) that influence well-being." What this training material by menopause experts is telling doctors is don't take too seriously what women are really complaining about—poor memory, attention changes, etc. Look instead at what else might be going on in other parts of their lives as more plausible causes for the symptoms. And not *one* possible cause they cite, such as diet, family relationships, etc., hints that there might be any possible biological basis for the "presenting symptom."

In the same table it also says: "Vasomotor symptoms [e.g., hot flashes, night sweats] disrupt quality of life in perimenopausal and menopausal women and are significantly correlated with increased general complaints *not related to the climacteric* [menopause]." [Emphasis added.] Here again the menopause experts are denying that the complaints women present during perimenopause and menopause—things that Polly and Sherry or Katherine Kennedy or Quiana Mortier complained of, e.g., attention, memory, speech, and concentration difficulties—are categorically *not related to the climacteric* but *are* related to the disruptions in the quality of life caused by hot flashes and night sweats. Not all women during these years, however, experience vasomotor symptoms (hot flashes and night sweats—the physical symptoms) just as Katherine Kennedy didn't, but still show general complaints in phrases like "I think I'm losing it" that are referring to WHMS symptoms battering the normality of their lives.

- Women often don't know they are going through the WHM Syndrome till they look back later and realize they've just come out of a long bubble of a very difficult time period.
- It's often a language problem. Women are not trained neuropsychologists and are not used to dissecting, analyzing, and formally naming the subtle speech, behavior, thinking, attention, and perceptual "glitches" they experience on and off as WHMS symptoms. They don't know how to specifically characterize the many small unusual events they experience on and off and don't know how to accurately communicate them to a doctor. They are more likely to make summary statements that tally up in overview the impact of the different symptoms on their total awareness, with such statements as "I think I'm losing it."
- It's often hard for women with WHMS symptoms today to disentangle the causes of what is happening to them—what is due to physiological/biological/organic changes from what's psychological/stress/environmental/sociocultural. Women who are in their thirties, forties, fifties, and sixties today often lead packed, complex, time-pressured lives that are a reflection of the successful strivings of the women's movement. For many women it's easier to attribute their symptoms to things they can presumably control, such as stress, than to uncontrollable and more worrisome physiological causes they may not be able to control. Also stress is such a prevalent

factor in so many midlife women's lives that it can always serve as a "catchall garbage-pail diagnosis" and be plausibly pointed to as fitting the bill.

• Women with WHMS symptoms often deny what's happening. They hope that if they don't pay too much attention to the symptoms, they will just go away the way they came. They also use denial because to really focus on the symptoms evokes too much fear and the need for major medical follow through, i.e., EEGs and MRIs and deciding what kind of specialist to go to. And who in these organizationally shifting and fractured medical times wants to willingly undertake the task of trying to decipher the quality of the medical options available? It's easier to just deny or tune out on what you can't control or make sense of. Particularly since women find that by doing "double-time" in managing their symptoms with calendars and organizers, they can often carry on in their lives, despite the symptoms, very well, fairly well, or passably well. They function around the symptoms, but with an internal toll in stress considerably higher than in the past. As one forty-six-year-old woman told me who experienced waves of "fog" and forgetting-in-an-instant episodes of misplacing things while in the midst of using a newly minted master's degree for a new job, "I try to forget about them [the symptoms] as much as possible because if I didn't I'd get depressed. And there's no use getting myself upset. It won't help. So I try to stay calm and forget about them as much as I can. I've become very disciplined: I manage by writing everything down that I have to do for my job the next day and living by my daily diaries."

The reality is that in recent years, women have learned to accommodate stress in so many arenas in their lives: in tolerating messy homes, little downtime for themselves, and "winging it" meals in association with the benefits, enjoyment, and need for work. Many women also learn to accommodate peculiar—though often innocuous—symptoms. They work around them. What's a little more stress added to the pile, after all!

• Many women with WHMS symptoms suspect "It's probably just me." As a result of mainly keeping quiet about their frightening potentially status-diminishing symptoms, and with an absence of the consciousness-raising communal talkfests of the 1970s many women in their isolation have wrongly suspected that their WHMS symptoms are personally unique or due to bad-luck genes. As a result they have failed to appreciate how common the symptoms are among many but not all women experiencing *estrogen loss for any reason,* and they miss out on discovering that the symptoms can get better with estrogen replacement therapy. Polly, for example, didn't share what was happening to her over a span of years with anyone but her husband, who directly witnessed many of her "glitches." Polly also suspected she had "bad-luck genes" and debated whether to be tested for specific biological indicators associated with a higher risk of developing Alzheimer's. Sherry Strumph only realized what her WHMS symptoms were about when she heard her friends talk about their symptoms and realized the symptoms were potentially reversible. She didn't have a clue what they were due to before that. Like Polly she too thought she was developing Alzheimer's disease— a common suspicion as an explanation for the symptoms along with suspected fears of a brain tumor.

But not all women want to be open about these symptoms. When feminist writer Letty Cottin Pogrebin experienced WHMS symptoms at around age fifty and tried to discuss what was happening to her with friends the same age she found no one wanted to talk about the topic. "I was unable to ventilate on these issues. Nobody was talking about them [with me]" she told me after I read her description of WHMS symptoms in her wonderfully written 1996 book *Getting Over Getting Older.* "Whenever you would raise them, people either laughed them off or seemed embarrassed." That's why Pogrebin wrote her book. In it she describes making verbal "slips," specifically verbal malapropisms, and friends making what I refer to as "behavioral malapropisms" (see chapter 7) or "slips" among other symptoms and other topics. "Most low-birth-weight babies are born to women who had no prenuptial care," she told a group on one occasion, meaning to say "prenatal care." Another time she told a group, "We have lots of congressional singing at my synagogue," having meant to say "congregational singing." Pogrebin describes her friends' behavioral malapropism "slips": One friend threw her soiled underwear into the garbage pail instead of the proper receptacle—the hamper. Another insisted that the supermarket had not packed the shampoo she had bought, only to find it weeks later in the refrigerator—a storage center but not the exactly right one.

• Women and their doctors often wrongly assume that the symptoms are solely due to the effects of aging and have to be lived with, and that they are not reversible. Polly's internist made this attribution with the statement "We're all getting older, you can't remember everything forever," and she accepted it with the always valid and therefore not very discriminating explanation "Well I've never been this age before. Maybe this is what X age feels like." However, Polly's cognitive improvement after taking estrogen for some months suggests that her memory problems were predominantly estrogen-related and not inevitably the result of aging.

Pogrebin also made the assumption in her book that her WHMS-type changes were due to aging. Not until I interviewed her for my *New York* magazine article did she become aware there was brain research that made plausible an estrogen-loss basis for at least some of her symptoms.

It is ironic that within the field known as gerontology, "aging" is no longer thought of as a series of *inevitable* declines in physical function, but often the result of treatable or preventable diseases and conditions that can accompany aging. Certainly the many hardy eighty- and ninety-year-olds among us now give testimony to the validity of gerontology's revised view. It would be foolhardy to fall victim to outdated ideas in gerontology and to write off changes and erosions in youth or midlife as inevitable and due to inevitable aging when they might not be so. This is not to say that there may not be independent changes in memory, thinking, speech, and behavior that *are* the result of aging— whatever that is. But we should not be glib about the matter and toss off aging blithely as an answer without considerable investigation when it comes to defining the quality of what may be your life or mine for decades to come. Indeed some studies are now beginning to suggest that in comparisons of women of the same age who are and aren't menopausal, a change in the hormonal milieu that we term "menopause" appears to act as a trigger in orchestrating some or many of the changes that we now think of as aging: for example, the slowdown in metabolism; the changes in muscle versus fat proportions in body composition; and changes in spatial memory skills. The question then becomes, Are such changes amenable to compensatory or preventive treatments for those who want them? And can we do anything about these changes by means of safe behavioral, nutritional, or medicinal interventions that delay or postpone what may not be inevitable after all? Unless we ask and act on such exploratory questions we simply won't know.

What scientists have been asking, however, throughout the 1990s and in some instances since the mid-eighties is what happens to the brain in different regions—neurons, neurotransmitters, synapses, nerve growth factors, the mesh of nerve circuits that appear to underlie memory and more—when the seeming elixir of estrogen has been sequentially withdrawn from living systems and cells and then added back. It's been a dramatic story and one that is still unfolding in regular front-page headlines.

II

WHAT CAUSES THE SYNDROME?

3

Why Does WHMS Occur?
New Research on Estrogen's Roles in the Brain

What evidence do we have about the causes of WHMS? How widespread is it? In my view, and the view of some quite important others, it is considerable but dispersed across different disciplines or subspecialties of disciplines so that a bird's-eye view of the "whole" terrain is more impressive than a ground view of the discrete parts. But before getting immersed in this evidence let me begin with an anecdote.

While working as an experimental psychologist years ago at New York University Medical Center's Rusk Institute for Rehabilitation Medicine, I became for a time an uncharacteristically fearful person. I had occasion then to interview two men in their thirties who had been entirely paralyzed from the neck down for several years. In one instance the injury had followed what was described to me as a friendly tussle with another family member at a weekend gathering: The man had been caught off-guard and had fallen over a heavy piece of furniture, severing his spinal cord in an instant. In the second instance the man had become virtually immobilized after slipping while standing on the bathtub trying to change a light bulb.

After these interviews I became for a while inordinately cautious getting in and out of the shower, and particularly in crossing streets. My shield of invulnerability—the one most of us have—had been pierced by the facts of life. The possibilities for harm merely crossing the street suddenly seemed enormous to me in ways I hadn't given much thought to since childhood.

During those years too, outside my office in the waiting room area that linked our suite of offices, a children's clinic was held once a week. Children born with often multiple missing limbs were evaluated in their underwear for new prostheses or adjustments to old ones. Planning soon to have children myself, I became terribly fearful of the potential risks attendant upon having children. I had begun to write articles about infertility treatments at that time and it began to seem miraculous to me that things could go right as often as they did—i.e., normal children being born—given all the things that could conceivably go wrong.

I mention this now because the research I am about to present may have the sweeping effect of making you wonder how any sixty-year-old postmenopausal woman after years of relative estrogen deprivation could possibly still be cogent, intelligent, or sane; how anyone could possibly exist without practically bathing in estrogen replacement therapy. And yet as an observer it is clearly evident to me that countless sixty-year-old, and considerably older, women exist who continue to be exceptionally intelligent, verbal, and highly competent. I have had the good fortune to know more than a few in my life and they have not, to the best of my knowledge, been on estrogen replacement therapy. It is also the case that I don't see the streets, or the nursing homes I've sometimes seen patients in, swarming with inept, confused, lost women in their sixties. These too are anchoring observations for me.

So the "picture" regarding the role of estrogen loss on the mind and body need not be one of a marked inevitable downward slide in cognitive and behavioral function, just as the greater risks of developing osteoporosis and heart disease with estrogen loss do not inevitably portend these conditions for all women. While estrogen may indeed have many important roles to play in the thinking, remembering brain and the rest of the central nervous system, and while estrogen loss may offer potential explanations for WHMS-like glitches occurring, there are likely as well many individual differences among women, built-in biological failsafe "buffers," and reserve brain-capacity "cushions" that we as yet know little about that likely moderate the important estrogen/brain picture I am about to present. So, as you read the rest of this chapter do yourself the favor of keeping this broader perspective in mind.

OVERVIEW: THE ESTROGEN RESEARCH REVOLUTION AND HOW IT'S CHANGED OUR THINKING ABOUT THE BRAIN

Dr. Frederick Naftolin is an attractive man of once humble origins who has risen far in the world. In early 1997 as I was uncovering a part of this story a menopause expert said this to me about him: "Because of the position he holds, when Fred Naftolin speaks other ob/gyns listen. For that reason he can't readily afford to be rash in his statements. They carry considerable weight with the rest of his profession." Who is Frederick Naftolin? As professor and chairman of Yale Medical School's preeminent academic Department of Obstetrics and Gynecology he directs the training of successive generations of top-flight ob/gyn physicians, at the same time setting many of the standards for important policies for the ob/gyn field as a whole. As the clinical chief of the Ob/Gyn Department at Yale–New Haven Hospital and as a leading officer of the North American Menopause Society he also directly and indirectly affects the lives of women. Unlike most ob/gyns, however, Naftolin also happens to be a neuroscientist, one of the leading pure-science researchers who has been actively investigating the brain and the new roles of estrogen on its neuroanatomy and neurophysiology. It was therefore no throwaway comment when in the spring of 1997 Naftolin stood before his colleagues at the annual meeting of the American College of Obstetrics and Gynecology in Las Vegas and announced to the thousands of other ob/gyns present: "There is not a cell in the brain that is not directly or indirectly sensitive to estrogen."

"There are some four hundred intracellular actions of estrogen that have been identified to date," Dr. Naftolin's colleague at Yale Dr. Philip Sarrel told me, noting that many more estrogen paths of action were continually being discovered. A menopause researcher and a professor of both obstetrics/gynecology and psychiatry at the Yale University School of Medicine he said, "About a third of the menopausal women who took part in the Yale Mid-Life Study reported [having] memory problems that in intensity and frequency affected their *capacity to function*." [Emphasis added.]

If in the 1970s scientists first discovered the major roles that estrogen plays in maintaining the integrity of women's bones, and in the 1980s they discovered the major role the hormone plays in maintaining the integrity of the heart and its blood vessels in women, it has been in the 1990s, prophetically named the Decade of the Brain at its inception by former president George Bush, that scientists have been sequentially knocking over in haste what once seemed etched-in-stone commandments in the sciences. All to discover that estrogen plays, what appear now to be, leading roles in directly and/or indirectly modulating, "growing," and protecting the structure and chemistry and function of parts of the brain involved in learning, memory, verbal skills, emotions, and motor behaviors.

In the "dark ages" of only yesteryear scientists routinely believed in the "commandments" that estrogen was the "female" hormone, the hormone that only women had (and that only men had such androgens as testosterone). It was believed then that estrogen played a major role in the brain and body with respect to sex and reproduction but did virtually nothing else in the rest of the brain. It was thought that with development the adult brain became to a degree architecturally "set" and was no longer "moldable" or "plastic." (Studies of children with brain damage to their language-dominant brain hemisphere and related studies of injuries helped create this picture of limited plastic or "remodeling" potential in the brain past later childhood. The studies showed an ability for injury-lost speech capability to evolve again in undamaged parts of the brain before age eleven but not after that age.) The view was that in adulthood the brain at best could "hang on," staying the same, or begin to erode gradually with age, but *not* readily undergo organic structural interior renovations or improvements. To say the least, these views have now been rendered "old hat" by the new estrogen research and related research.

To fully grasp the "bigger picture" of what estrogen is now believed to do in the brain requires a composite sweep of informational "feeds" from many different arenas of research. It is a grasp few outside the neurosciences research community (and given the high level of specialization in today's sciences, even *inside* this community) at present have. Ideally, it spans a sweep of knowledge about different series of studies that have been done on:

(1) what estrogen does when it is added to nerve-cell tissue isolated from different brain regions and studied, in vitro, outside the body;

(2) what replacement estrogen does to the brain (its structure, chemistry, etc.) and to the behavior (attention, memory, speed, accu-

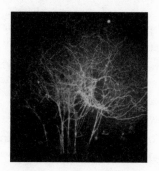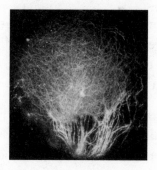

Figures 1 and 2
Two slices of brain tissue from the cerebral cortex. One grown with low-level exposure to estrogen (left) and one with greater exposure to estrogen (right). The one on the right reveals greater growth and complexity in neuronal structure: a denser mesh of axon and dendrite extensions potentially available for making connections—greater branching or arborization.

From the laboratory of Dr. Dominique Toran-Allerand at Columbia-Presbyterian Medical Center. Reprinted by permission.

racy, etc.) of mature female animals (rats, monkeys, birds, mice, etc.) who have had their estrogen-supplying ovaries removed (who have been "ovexed" as the researchers say) and been given add-back estrogen, compared to similarly surgically "modified" (I know some of you are thinking "abused") animals who have not been given replacement estrogen;

(3) how normally menstruating women perform during estrogen high phases versus estrogen low phases of their normal menstrual cycle on tests of verbal and spatial skills; (women consistently performed better on tests of spatial skill—more like men who, *on average*, tend to excel at tests of spatial skills—during phases in their cycle when estrogen was low; that is, estrogen may actually be a hindrance or impediment to spatial performance on tests);

(4) how adult women who have been deprived of estrogen because of either natural menopause or surgically produced menopause (having a hysterectomy with ovaries removed) perform on tests of cognitive function before surgery and before and after being given replacement estrogen treatment after surgery;

(5) how adult women given estrogen-suppressing drugs for the necessary treatment of medical conditions (such as fibroids, etc.) perform on tests of cognitive skills before, after, and with replacement estrogen while on treatment of this form;

(6) the degree of association in women between taking estrogen at some point in their lives and the risk of later developing Alzheimer's disease in epidemiological (observational) studies;

(7) how women with Alzheimer's disease perform on tests or are rated by others on cognitive/social skills, before and after treatments with estrogen, compared to control women with Alzheimer's given placebos;

(8) surveys on the frequency of complaints of memory and concentration problems of women who show up at menopause clinics;

(9) and still yet other studies observing the brain in physiological action noninvasively during different acts of thinking and being.

Those most familiar with these different streams of estrogen/brain/behavior research realize that while the entire picture puzzle on estrogen and its effects on the brain is far from complete, we have enough of the puzzle's outline and sufficient numbers of its interlocking pieces to discern what the puzzle depicts or conveys: two partners, estrogen and a cognitively functioning brain, engaging as an intertwining duo in an intense dance with as yet unspecifiable steps. Estrogen, it would seem, is a key partner in "cognition," which variously refers to one or all of the following: verbal memory, visual-spatial memory, perception, speech and language skills, problem solving, and higher-order intellectual functioning.

This "picture" is supported by the headline in the prestigious journal *Science,* in May of 1997, declaring ESTROGEN STAKES CLAIM TO COGNITION in a lengthy research news analysis article. It is also supported by the disarmingly simple words "Estrogen and the Brain" used to announce a conference at New York City's Mount Sinai Medical Center in the spring of 1997 at which leading researchers in the field reported on several of the content "streams" of the studies above. The same simple words were used to describe a four-article special supplement to the Journal of the Society of Obstetricians and Gynecologists of Canada, in October of 1997.

For some in the know, this research picture has lent a sense of urgency to the practical human implications they see in the new research. "Ample evidence has been accumulated in experimental animal models to clearly establish an effect of estrogen on the central nervous system [the brain and spinal cord]," writes a leading researcher on aging, neurologist/gerontologist Dr. Stanley Birge, Director of the Program on Aging, Jewish Hospital of St. Louis, Washington University School of Medicine, in a chapter titled "The Role of Estrogen Deficiency in the Aging Central Nervous System" in the medical textbook *Treatment of the Postmenopausal Woman.* "More recent observations," he writes, "indicate that these effects are not limited to only those regions of the brain involved in sexual [maturation] and function. Despite this evidence, *the role of estrogen in human [brain and spinal cord] function has largely been ignored by the scientific community* [emphasis added]," Birge adds.

"People—and I include doctors here—don't realize," says Dr. Dominique Toran-Allerand of Columbia University's College of Physicians and Surgeons, a highly regarded neurobiologist/researcher who has been studying the role of estrogen on fetal and postnatal rat-brain tissue in culture since the 1970s, "that the brain is a major target organ of estrogen, and if you deprive the brain of estrogen, whether in normal menopause or in an ovariectomy [ovary-removal, producing a surgical menopause] you will get the symptoms of estrogen deficiency in it. Fundamentally," she says, "menopause is a state of estrogen deficiency. It is an endocrinopathy [a disorder of hormonal failure], in the same way that diabetes and hypothyroidism are hormone deficiency states." Dr. Toran-Allerand says, "People worry about bone density and coronary artery disease in the postmenopausal state, but they should also be worrying about what's happening to the [brain's] neurons."

Whether ultimately proven right or wrong, this is not an uncommon view now held by more than a few of the leading *women* estrogen/brain/cognition researchers I interviewed for my article and this book. (When I described these successive views by female estrogen researchers to a leading male neuroscientist in this field, Dr. John Morrison, a researcher on aging and the brain at New York's Mount Sinai Medical Center, his initial reaction was laughter and the comment "A man could never get away with saying such things in public!") But Dr. Morrison too, discussing the many newly discovered functions of estrogen in a major 1997 review article, titled "Life and Death of Neurons in the Aging Brain" in the leading scientific journal *Science,* proposed with a colleague that the loss of estrogen's important functions might "lead to age-related impairment of memory and cognition. This effect," he writes, "is of obvious relevance to postmenopausal women. . . . Such multiple roles for estrogen would suggest that reproductive senescence [i.e., perimenopause and menopause] may have a multifaceted impact on memory loss and cognitive decline through decreased regulation of intact [memory] circuits as well as decreased protection of such circuits from degeneration."

Echoing sentiments I too had independently arrived at, and as probably many others will as well, Dr. Morrison and his colleague further write "It is perhaps not surprising that estrogen, a molecule that is so crucial to survival of the species through regulation of the female reproductive system, also plays a key role in the regulation of multiple neural [neuron/nerve] processes that confer significant survival value [i.e., survival advantages for oneself and one's offspring—one's genes—such as *remembering* where you last saw your children, where it's dangerous to go, what is dangerous to eat; being able to quickly name and find the words to shout to a child "Joshua, move, there's a rock about to fall on you!" while deftly holding on to another child and moving quickly to push your child out of harm's way while not dropping the day's bag of gathered foods]." Morrison and his coauthor write further: "As research in the neurobiology of aging moves forward . . . [progress can also be expected in the identification of clinically useful medical] interventions, such as estrogen, that will augment [boost] the continued protection and proper function of these [cognitive] circuits."*

What Has Been Learned About What Estrogen Does in the Brain

So what specifically does estrogen do in the brain? I will let one of the leading figures on the estrogen/brain research front, Dr. Bruce McEwen, variously describe this after first telling you something about his pivotal role in this emerging news picture. An engaging, muscular man, well liked by many—especially the many women researchers he has ably mentored and championed through the years—McEwen is a researcher's researcher who would not look at all out of place leading a squadron of bagpiper scientists down Fifth Avenue. Involved in estrogen/brain research for some thirty years, McEwen is director of the Laboratory of Neuroendocrinology at New York's Rockefeller University, a recent past president of the Society of Neurosciences, and was honored in the spring of 1997 with induction into the living scientist's hall of fame—the National Academy of Sciences—for his life accomplishments in estrogen/brain research and related scientific work. McEwen's lab has been a center for myth-shattering discoveries in the neurosciences for years now.

*John H. Morrison and Patrick R. Hof, "Life and Death of Neurons in the Aging Brain," *Science*, vol. 278, October 17, 1997, 412–419.

In the early eighties, for example, the estrogen/cognition revolution began in a sense when one of the researchers in McEwen's lab, Dr. Victoria Liune, now of Hunter College of the City University of New York, then studying the long-known *sexual* roles of estrogen, discovered in rats that in a special area of the brain known as the basal forebrain, estrogen boosted the activity of a specific enzyme known as choline acetyltransferase, which prompts special nerve cells to make the important memory-"ink" neurotransmitter, acetylcholine, a chemical that neurons use to communicate with other nerve cells. When Liune later read that in people with Alzheimer's disease there was characteristically an enormous loss in that same exact area of the brain, of the neurons that release acetylcholine, she had an insight: estrogen, acetylcholine, Alzheimer's disease, and cognitive function are linked. She realized that the loss of those acetylcholine-producing nerve cells *that were regulated one-step-removed by estrogen* were probably related to the cognitive decline in Alzheimer's disease and probably played a role in cognition. In later research she showed how the absence of acetylcholine in the basal forebrain negatively affected memory function in the learning-and-memory-important hippocampus of rats, helping to clarify how memory loss might evolve in Alzheimer's disease.

Liune also realized that estrogen might have treatment potential for Alzheimer's disease. And again in McEwen's lab one of the earliest studies of estrogen as a treatment for Alzheimer's was implemented by Dr. Howard Fillet together with Liune, McEwen, and others. They showed that in a small sample of women with Alzheimer's disease, some of the women improved in cognitive function to a clinically significant degree when given replacement estrogen.

In the early nineties working in McEwen's lab Catherine Wooley, and McEwen, made the discovery that contrary to all expectations estrogen given to *adult* female rats deprived of estrogen (they had had their estrogen-supplying ovaries removed) could reliably reshape the architecture of the brain in the memory-associated region known as the hippocampus within forty-eight hours. They discovered that the hormone, not unlike a revitalizing "watering" fluid, somehow prompted the sprouting of connection-hungry outgrowths known as dendritic "spines"—added potential docking sites for receiving and transmitting

incoming information to nerve cells via new synapses—on the projecting arms of nerve cell bodies in the brain. When estrogen was withdrawn the spines literally disappeared. When estrogen was added they
again grew. The *adult* brain was now seen as having synaptic and neuronal plasticity.

What seemed to be the case in the normal rats was that estrogen-
high phases, when the potential for conception and pregnancy were
high, appeared to be associated with a denser network of possible connections in a major memory and learning region of the brain—the
hippocampus. Perhaps the better to allow for pursuit of memorable potential mates navigationally over wider terrains than at other times of
their reproductive cycle, or related reasons. (In this regard estrogen researcher Dr. Sheryl Smith told me that in 1800 the name "estrus" cycle
in the rat was originally named for the frenzied motor activity that was
observed to occur in one out of the four days of the rat's estrus reproductive cycle when estrogen is high and when female rats run around
frantically.)

While many more studies remain to be done to make the practical
significance of this discovery clear, the study "opened up our thinking
about what hormones could do in the adult animal," says Dr. Victoria
Liune.

When I asked Dr. Bruce McEwen to summarize what estrogen has
been found to do in recent years he said: "Estrogen has been found to
have widespread effects in the brain through the nerve communication
systems that project messages throughout the cortex and other major areas of the brain, especially in the hippocampus, an area known to be
highly important for processing incoming information and for memory
and attention."

Estrogen has this widespread effect he says "in part by affecting the
availability of many of the chemical messengers in the brain we commonly call neurotransmitters, to the neuronal [message] projecting systems that depend on them. Estrogen has been shown specifically to
induce, to increase, the availability of the specific neurotransmitter serotonin, to increase the availability of acetylcholine which is an important
enabler of neural activity throughout the cortical areas that participate
strongly in memory. Estrogen increases the availability of the neuro-

transmitter noradrenaline, and enhances transmission of [the neuro-transmitter] dopamine. These are all systems of the brain that are very important in affect or emotion, in such things as depression and different forms of mental illness."

These systems—the cholinergic, the dopaminergic, the serotonergic, the noradrenergic—which estrogen affects, according to McEwen, all "have a utility role. They are important utility factors in everything from emotions to motor activity, in maintaining the capability of other systems of the brain to do specific things. So you could say that estrogen [by affecting these] affects *many* systems of the brain—not just one. It provides a general tone that maintains cells in the cortex and the ability of the hippocampus, to process and encode incoming information."

How relevant to humans overall, you may be wondering, are the animal studies that have been done in this area. I asked McEwen this question. "The organization of the brain of animals and humans is very similar," he said. "The differences of course are at the level of higher cortical functions, for things like language. But the human brain has evolved from a basic brain plan which was established in lower vertebrates—fish and reptiles—and has just been added onto over the eons. If you look at the consistency across mammals," he says, "with regard to, for example, the stress hormones, we know that the hippocampus of rats has receptors for stress hormones; we know that the hippocampus of rhesus monkeys have them; and that the hippocampus of humans have them. So we can point to many cases where there are very comparable anatomical structures, anatomical chemistries, and comparable functions.

"In neurobiology now," he says, "we are taking information from different sources [regarding the estrogen/brain/cognition picture] and putting it together into a coherent story.

"There is an interesting paradox regarding the data for humans in this area at the moment," McEwen says. "We have very good anatomical and mechanistic data for the genesis of synapses [in relation to estrogen] for rats. We don't have such a good idea what estrogens are doing to rat memory. We have a much better idea about what's happening to memory with estrogen loss from the multiple human studies of [experimental psychologist/behavioral neuroendocrinologist] Barbara Sherwin in which [estrogen-suppressing medical] treatment [produced] noticeable decline in verbal memory skills on tests in women which is reversed by replacement estrogen."[See chapter 5 for a review of this research.] "But we don't know as much about synapses in relation to estrogen in women," says McEwen. "We do however know from the field of neuropsychology and the study of brain injuries [in humans], and MRI scans [of the brains of such patients] and other studies of the human brain, that these memory processes are mainly the function of the hippocampus and the temporal lobe.

"We started putting two and two together," McEwen says, "saying 'Well this is what we see in the rat. It's very likely an explanation for the memory deficits that are evident in the women [in Sherwin's studies with estrogen deprivation].' It's like a big jigsaw puzzle and we have [been using] information from many different quarters in order to put together the whole puzzle—the information from human neuropsychology, from rats' brains, from infra-human primates together with the knowledge from all sorts of comparative aspects of brain function that has been accumulated over the last century. We know that we are talking about very similar processes going on in animal and human brains and therefore we assume that all these things fit together.

"Now ultimately," says McEwen, "we certainly will have to fill in all the dots in the animal and human research picture. But this will happen and is happening. Dr. Marylou Voytko, for example, presented a paper [not long ago] at a [Society for] Neurosciences meeting on cynomolgus monkeys. She looked at the effects of estrogen on behavior [in animals that had had their estrogen-producing ovaries removed] and found that [replacement] estrogen had a very positive effect on attention, a [function] also related to the hippocampus."

This kind of research McEwen said "is catching on all over the place which of course doesn't mean that we are guaranteed any particular outcome. We probably have a lot of surprises left to discover. The wonderful part of science," he says, "is the unexpected. Hypotheses are made to be refuted or changed. They are rarely ever true in their original way."

What do he and others suspect is happening to the nerve cells of the brains of perimenopausal and menopausal women losing estrogen? McEwen says, "Specifically in human menopause there are tremendous individual differences based upon things like body type. People with more body fat tend to have more estrogens. Their body fat converts [postmenopausal] androgens to estrogens and they tend to be protected against things like osteoporosis and heart disease perhaps more than very thin women. There is evidence that body type is very protective for dementia. It is the women who are very thin . . . with low body fat who are at increased risk. And so some women [with estrogen loss] may show impaired cognitive function, and changes in motor coordination, a slowing down of reaction times—Dr. Uriel Halbreich, for example, has shown these [changes in motor coordination and slowed reaction times] in studies [of midlife-to-older women] at SUNY Buffalo [the State University of New York at Buffalo]. We know that the dopaminergic [nerve transmission] system [that depends on the neurotransmitter dopamine] is involved in motor coordination and reaction times."

McEwen added, "Neurologist Dr. Stanley Birge has started to study motor coordination in older women. He realized that [some older] women fall and break their hips. And, yes, their hips are fragile [because of osteoporosis], but Dr. Birge wondered, why do they fall? He suspects it may be because of less motor coordination—the neurological consequences of [long-term] reduced estrogen levels in the brain and the rest of the central nervous system. If you are withdrawing estrogen from all of these systems that estrogen is supporting, [all these neurotransmitter systems] that are the sort of the utility systems of the brain I spoke of earlier, you are going to have lots of things that depend on them becoming less efficient. That's what we are really talking about."

I had been surprised to discover that apart from what he knew about rats deprived of estrogen McEwen, a male laboratory researcher after all and not a clinician, was aware of the WHMS impact of estrogen loss on cognitive functioning in some postmenopausal women. During the question-and-answer section of the Mount Sinai "Estrogen and the Brain" conference I attended in 1997 he had noted that when he lectured about his work at medical schools women had told him about their cognitive experiences of menopause, and how they had improved after taking estrogen replacement therapy. When I later asked him about those earlier comments, he said, "High-functioning women who make extensive use of their memory and cognitive skills, they know the difference. They know something has happened. It is very common [these changes]. I said at the conference that if you looked at Barbara Sherwin's data [of studies showing memory decline in tests of verbal memory and learning in postmenopausal women and other women with estrogen loss] the differences are not huge [though reliable and statistically significant]. If you looked at them and didn't realize what they meant you might not be that impressed. But when you know women's stories about those changes it really makes a difference. They are irritated by it."

Did he think this was widely recognized? I asked. "No, it hasn't been," McEwen said. "The people who study cognition [psychologists mainly] have been totally ignorant of hormones. And that's largely because sex hormones were only thought to work on the [brain's] hypothalamus and affect reproduction. Now we know they affect all these other functions and the phenomena of the memory changes. So they [the researchers who study cognition] are beginning to realize this is an important aspect they've neglected up to this point."

And ob/gyns? "Over the past [several] years I've been invited to two different meetings of the North American Menopause Society and a meeting of the International Menopause Society and I've given talks there. [I've found that] people who are practitioners [doctors who attend the meetings] tend to be quite amazed by the facts about what estrogen does to brain function because they haven't heard about it. Menopause experts are more likely to be aware of it."

When I voiced my concern that most ob/gyns, however, seem to be not automatically menopause experts McEwen concurred with my appraisal. "I know," he said, "and that's one of the problems that needs to be corrected."

Lastly, I asked him if he agreed with Dr. Frederick Naftolin's sweeping statement about the pervasive effects of estrogen on the brain. Was this his view? McEwen then proceeded to review out loud the many brain areas, the hippocampus, the cortex, and on and on that he knew to be associated with the effects of estrogen and finally stopped. "I agree with Fred," he said. Almost as if surprised himself by this "take" on the topic, he said "That [summary] sort of indicates that there is no part of the brain that escapes the influence of the ovarian hormones."

Specific Categories of What Estrogen Has Been Found to Do

Labeled by some as a "memory molecule," estrogen is now seen by some as "preserv[ing] and even improv[ing] some of the brain's highest functions," as "empower[ing] brain cells involved in thinking in man," as having widespread influence in the brain through both different estrogen *receptor* pathways that directly bind to estrogen and through multiple *nonreceptor* estrogen pathways, many only now being uncovered.

Through its effects on multiple systems in the brain, estrogen is now seen by researchers in this field as having the potential for affecting memory, learning, speech, language, movement, mood, and emotions, to give you the short list.

It is not surprising therefore that so many different kinds of symptoms in WHMS could be accounted for by the changes in estrogen levels produced by changing ovary function, the hallmark feature of perimenopause and menopause.

Although critics not infrequently try to minimize or dismiss human studies of estrogen's effects as being difficult to interpret clearly because so many other things are often going on concurrently in women's lives at the time of perimenopause and menopause, animal studies of estrogen's effects leave less room for this form of confounding and might serve as useful tools for clarifying results in human studies.

Below are the different categories of what estrogen has been found to do by researchers in recent years.

- **Estrogen alters the neurochemistry of the brain in learning and memory-forming/cognitive functions**
  - by affecting the supplies of multiple neurotransmitters: serotonin, dopamine, acetylcholine, glutamate, GABA, noradrenaline
  - by affecting critical enzymes (i.e., choline acetyltransferase)
  - by stimulating the presence of nerve growth factors
  - by affecting substances known as neuropeptides, which act in neural tissues

— by reducing the formation of toxic brain-destroying proteins implicated in Alzheimer's disease
— by promoting uptake of the brain's fuel—glucose

• **Estrogen alters the architecture and structure of the brain in memory- and learning-associated areas—the anatomy of brain neurons**
— by increasing the surface area of potential "docking sites" for connections to incoming messages *on nerve cell "arms"* via monthly sprouting of new spines and potential synapses
— by stimulating the growth of *more dense branches* (as on a shrub) on nerve cells (arborization) that potentially increase connectivity and complexity

• **Estrogen maintains the interconnections of the brain and supports nerve growth**
— by maintaining a denser mesh of nerve fiber outgrowths for potential connections than when it is not there
— by increasing synapse formation *after neuronal damage*
— by inducing nerve growth via induced release of different nerve growth factors in a complex feedback loop

• **Estrogen affects widespread areas of the brain, by affecting their "workout tone," acting to enable nerve-communication pathways that fan out all over the cortex and important memory centers of the brain**
— by stimulating and promoting the function of the brain's cholinergic projecting system
— the brain's serotonergic projecting system
— the brain's dopaminergic projecting system
— the brain's adrenergic projecting system
— the neurotransmitter projecting system that depends on the neurotransmitter GABA (gamma-aminobutyric acid)

• **Estrogen increases the neuronal plasticity of the brain**
— by regulating the formation and breakdown of synapses and branches
— by facilitating response to injury after strokes
— by having the ability to orchestrate the turning on of different genes

- **Estrogen acts as a potent neuroprotector shielding nerves from multiple forms of damage**
  - by acting as a natural antioxidant helping brain cells "skirt death" by oxidation, protecting nerve cells against free-radical damage that can destroy cell function
  - by boosting the body's own natural antioxidant defense system
  - by protecting brain cells from different toxins including proteins that "clog up brain works" in Alzheimer's patients (beta-amyloid plaque deposits)
  - by helping brain cells survive deprivation of vital classes of substances longer
  - by increasing the expression of more nerve growth factor receptors or "catching mitts"
  - by recruiting the aid of nerve growth factors
  - by decreasing the toxicity of substances known as excitotoxins such as glutamate in cultured neurons, known to produce added damage to neurons after stroke and brain injury
  - by acting as an anti-inflammatory agent that appears to moderate the inflammation damage of the plaques known to form on neurons in Alzheimer's disease

- **Estrogen boosts the metabolic functioning of the brain and body in different ways**
  - by increasing availability of the brain's major energy source, glucose (the brain can't store reserve glucose)
  - by increasing cerebral blood flow and preventing cerebral ischemia (blood deficiency) damage
  - by maintaining the elasticity of blood vessels, which can maximize the body's demands for metabolic "deliveries" of blood, oxygen, nutrients, etc.
  - becoming menopausal is associated with a reduced resting rate of metabolism in women

- **Estrogen acts as an "activator" and performance enhancer of many brain and body activities**
  - by increasing speed of rapid limb-coordinated movements in animals

— by increasing other measures of coordinated limb movements in animals, i.e., hurdle negotiation task, treadmill, balance beam walking, running in square wheel
— by increasing finger-tapping skills and manual speed and dexterity in women
— by increasing in women verbal fluency (ability to generate names/words), speech articulation agility, syllable repetition, speeded counting, word reading
— by increasing sensory perception for a variety of modalities: hearing, smell, visual signal detection, fine touch
— by maintaining central processing motor integration in such tasks as driving
— by markedly boosting metabolic activity of most areas in the brain and spinal cord within hours of administration
— by acting as an "upper" to increase feelings of energy and well-being, mood, feelings of elation, and euphoria in human studies and, paradoxically in some, anxiety during the preovulation rise of estrogen
— by reversing in some instances severe depression resistant to other forms of treatment (when given in high doses)
— by boosting attention to tasks in monkeys
— by decreasing distractability
— by increasing reaction time in premenopausal women during estrogen-dominant stage of cycle
— by increasing short-term memory
— by increasing performance and speed of learning in rats on sensorimotor tasks

- **Estrogen acts as a neuromodulator altering the responsiveness (or gain) of brain regions and messages**
  — by turning on many but not all progesterone receptors
  — by boosting neurotransmitter response (tripling the amounts of at least one kind of neurotransmitter)
  — by amplifying the sensitivity of a nerve cell
  — by strengthening the electrical pathways that "etch the groove" for retaining memories—long-term potentiation—for at least six to eight hours

— by making neurons more sensitive to a helpful protein substance believed to play a role in sustaining, and growth of, reaching-out arms (dendrites and axons) of nerve cells

- **Estrogen turns on other genes or alters gene expression**
  - by hooking up with estrogen receptors in the cell's nucleus estrogen can turn on or change the expression of a host of genes inside the nucleus of cells
  - by modulating the expression of the apolipoprotein E gene estrogen may possibly affect in some the risk of developing Alzheimer's disease since one form of the ApoE gene is considered a major risk factor for Alzheimer's disease and for early cognitive changes

- **Estrogen affects the integrity of learning, memory, and old knowledge**
  - by boosting by 30 percent special receptors in the hippocampus, NMDA receptors, now believed to be important in maintaining the strength or durability of synapse connections involved in creating longer-term memories or learning
  - by producing effects on the learning and memory-coding center, the hippocampus (shown to date mainly in animal studies)
  - by building and maintaining synapses, the structures through which one neuron communicates with another for learning and memory
  - by maintaining verbal memory, verbal learning, and spatial memory in women

- **Estrogen can affect mood and emotions via its neurotransmitter effects: "nature's psychoprotectant"**
  - estrogen stimulates a significant increase in receptors—dopamine 2 receptors—whose disregulation is associated with mood disorders and the thought disorder schizophrenia
  - estrogen affects the synthesis, release, reuptake, and breakdown of one of the major neurotransmitters associated with depression—serotonin

— studies have shown that blood levels of serotonin are decreased in postmenopausal women compared with premenopausal women and that estrogen levels vary or correlate with blood levels of serotonin in women.

— administering estrogen to rats with ovaries removed has been shown to significantly increase serotonin-binding sites in many areas of the brain associated with mood, emotion, mental state, cognition

— giving a high dose, up to 25 mg, of estrogen (Premarin) to severely depressed pre- and postmenopausal women who did not respond to antidepressant treatments was shown to lead to significant improvement in depression scores and behavioral improvement compared to placebo treatment

• **Estrogen can moderate the effects of stress**

— by reducing harmful stress hormone elevations (glucocorticoids) evoked by stress

— by likely buffering the hippocampus from the "hammering" effects of stress hormones on the survival of the neurons there (the hippocampus has many receptors for stress hormones)

MECHANISMS BY WHICH ESTROGEN MAY MAINTAIN INTELLECTUAL STATUS QUO OR AFFECT COGNITION

In what ways might variably faltering or plummeting estrogen supplies during perimenopause and menopause possibly affect the brain, cognition, and behavior of women? The possibilities are obviously many given all the functions that estrogen has been found to have. Though which ones are the right ones will have to await more research.

As one author put it, "The [research] implies that when estrogen levels drop sharply upon menopause, the complexity of connections could slowly diminish, perhaps making neurons—brain cells—more likely to degenerate or atrophy, or die." Or work less efficiently.

It may be that irregular estrogen supplies during perimenopause and even less after menopause may "down regulate" or diminish the number of estrogen receptors and thereby the ripple of effects—metabolic, modulating, gene "turn-on," and others—that depend on such receptors.

"Maybe without estrogen," speculates Dr. Janice Juraska, a research biopsychologist studying aging in female rats at the University of Illinois, "a link in the interacting circuits is missing in the old engrams [the presumed "grooves" or circuits of memory]. Maybe after menopause some of those special synapses that estrogen supported and are connected to facts and [neural] circuits aren't as hooked up to each other any longer" she speculates.

Reduced supplies of the neurotransmitter acetylcholine, which are influenced by estrogen's direct regulation of the enzyme ChAT (choline acetyltransferase), may make scarce supplies of the memory "juice" or "ink" for memory processing that the neurotransmitter is known to supply.

Estrogen's decline and fall may lead to diminished supplies to the brain of blood and the "goodies" it brings with it, a condition known in extreme form as cerebral ischemia. Related to this may be estrogen's known ability to increase the vasodilation of blood vessels as a means for boosting cerebral blood flow.

By maintaining a more complex "mesh" among communicating nerve fibers, estrogen may make possible more complex connections among "circuits" involved in storing information and perhaps boost the reserve capacity or potential of the brain, before memory- or skill-agility lapses take hold, i.e., there may be more redundancy in the brain in where and how information is stored with estrogen, leaving the brain less vulnerable to age-associated losses.

Perhaps, suggests Dr. Stanley Birge, "By promoting expression of neurotrophic factors, [nerve-growth promoting factors] estrogen may better equip . . . sensitive regions of the central nervous system [the brain and spinal cord] to resist or repair . . . insults resulting from the aging process or conditions such as Alzheimer's disease."

Echoing this theme in a 1997 article titled "Estrogens and Memory Protection" Dr. James Simpkins of the Center for the Neurobiology of Aging at the College of Pharmacy at the University of Florida in Gainesville, together with his coauthors write: "Estrogens are potent neuroprotective agents. We and others have shown that estrogens protect cultured neurons and neuronal cell lines [grown in test tubes] from a variety of insults. . . . Further, estrogens are potent antioxidants and this action . . . can account in part for their neuroprotective actions. Finally, estrogens have a marked effect on the transport of glucose into the brain and this action of the estrogens may explain the acute memory enhancing effects of the [hormone]. Recent evidence supports a role for ovarian [hormones] in the normal maintenance of brain function and suggests that the loss of these steroids at the time of menopause may play a role in the cognitive decline and neurodegeneration found in aging and Alzheimer's disease."

While estrogen loss may not directly cause the degeneration of neurons, it has been suggested that by pruning the architecture of nerve cells in important memory and learning regions of the brain or by reducing the supplies of major enzymes, the end effect may be to make brain cells more vulnerable to insults.

It has even been proposed that the cardiovascular-protecting effects of estrogen—reducing the "bad" low-density cholesterol (LDL) and increasing the "good" high-density cholesterol (HDL)—might similarly act in the brain to keep the "works" unclogged: to "slow progression of cerebral atherosclerosis and prevent vascular dementia and other cognitive decline."

As knowledge about the specific symptoms of WHMS becomes more widespread, it is likely that brain researchers will have more substantive pieces of the estrogen/cognition puzzle to work with in figuring out which *potential* mechanisms associated with estrogen's roles are *actually* at work.

WHICH FUNCTIONS OF ESTROGEN ARE MOST IMPORTANT?

Which functions of estrogen are most important? Ask different researchers and you will get different responses. McEwen: "It remains to be seen which of the mechanisms found in animal studies may explain the effects of ovarian hormones in humans, but it is likely that the structural changes produced by estradiol [estrogen] and the actions of estradiol on the [neurotransmitter-dependent] dopaminergic, cholinergic,

GABA and various neuropepetide systems will be found to be important in explaining changes in neurological, affective [emotional] state and cognitive function which occur in some women after natural or surgical menopause."

If you ask researcher Dr. James Simpkins, whose research articles in this area comprise a three-inch thick pile, he will probably suggest that the multiple neuroprotective functions of estrogen along with its potent antioxidant effects in mopping up free-radical damage, and its energy or fuel-supplying glucose transports to the brain across the blood-brain barrier are the most important.

Dr. Simpkins and Dr. Birge both suspect that the intermittent aspects of the WHMS symptoms I described to them—why the symptoms don't just stay but come and go—might be accounted for, at least in part, by temporary shortages in the brain of its major fuel source, glucose. Dr. Birge said, "There may be a rational basis for that intermittency. We have become interested in the role of estrogen in glucose transport. The brain is the only tissue in the body in which glucose transport is estrogen-dependent. So the hypothesis was developed by Dr. James Simpkins in Florida that as a result of the abrupt change in estrogen at the time of menopause [a woman] has a decrease in glucose transport into the brain. This results in the brain's sensing glucose deprivation and then through an autonomic [nervous system] discharge attempting to stimulate the liver to release glucose. This would then raise [the body's] systemic glucose and restore glucose levels in the brain. The liver is one source [of such glucose production]. Another source is muscle."

Dr. Birge pointed out that Dr. Simpkins's experimental work had revealed that by blocking glucose from getting to the brain of animals, measurable "hot flashes and palpitations in rodents could be produced" [as measured in their tail temperatures]. He further noted that research by Dr. Robert Greene (Polly Van Benthusen's ob/gyn) and his colleagues "has demonstrated that in the PET scans of [women] patients having hot flashes there is significant evidence of a decrease in glucose uptake during that hot flush. He hasn't published this yet."

Dr. Birge added, "You asked about the episodic nature of these

[WHMS] symptoms. Obviously if the brain is deprived of glucose it's not going to function very well. There is a group of cells in the brain that are uniquely sensitive to glucose deprivation. And those cells reside in the hippocampus—specifically in the dentate gyrus within the hippocampus. Of course," he says, "these are the same cells that subserve the function of memory. This is also the region of the brain that is the primary target for Alzheimer's disease. We don't know why these cells are uniquely sensitive to glucose. But they are. This was learned purely from observation. A neuroanatomist recognized that diabetic patients treated with insulin who had brittle diabetes would end up with memory impairments. And at autopsy he found they would have a loss of [neurons] within this region of the brain. We also know that if you infuse glucose you can improve cognitive function in patients with mild to moderate Alzheimer's disease. Glucose does affect memory!" (For more about glucose and memory see chapter 11.)

Could this provide a potential "candy-bar cure" for WHMS symptoms? I asked Dr. Birge, only half jokingly. "I can't verify this," he said, "but anecdotal information I've heard from both women and gynecologists suggests that if a woman drinks a coke [nondiet sugar-rich Coca-Cola] during a hot flush she can ameliorate the hot flush. I don't know whether this is true or an old wives' tale, but if it is true, it might support the cognitive picture we've just been discussing too."

WHAT UNRELATED RESEARCH SUGGESTS ABOUT THE BASIS FOR SOME WHMS SYMPTOMS

Just as estrogen's relationship to glucose may offer a scientific rationale for what might be occurring during WHMS symptoms in women experiencing estrogen loss or variable hormonal supplies, so too other experimental research suggests clues as to what might be occurring during specific WHMS symptoms, and what might help specific symptoms in women *apart from estrogen replacement therapy.*

For example, it has been shown that "clinically significant" impairments in "reading, spelling, verbal fluency and object naming" not unrelated to those in WHMS could *be produced* in twenty-two healthy young women in a dose-dependent manner, by "cholinergic block-ade"—blocking activity of the neurotransmitter acetylcholine via a specific drug treatment, scopolamine, the drug that prevents motion sickness. That is, the more of an acetylcholine "blocking" drug these young healthy women received the worse their impairments became. The researchers showed that these same impairments could be reversed by restoring normal acetylcholine activity. Since estrogen loss is known to affect supplies of the neurotransmitter acetylcholine and the cholinergic system that depends on it, could drugs that safely stimulate acetylcholine production or prevent the breakdown of available acetylcholine supplies, such as some of those drugs now being used to treat Alzheimer's patients, help restore such skills in perimenopausal and menopausal women, if they were shown to be safe? It's worth a try in my book—namely, this one!

It has also been found that symptoms of attention deficit disorder (ADD), known these days also as attention deficit hyperactivity disorder (ADHD), can be associated with deficiencies in supplies of the neurotransmitter dopamine. Since more than a few symptoms of WHMS involve symptoms not unlike the attention-deficit symptoms of ADD, and since estrogen loss can be associated with alterations in dopamine supplies, might treatments with dopamine-restoring or dopamine non-degrading agents (such as Ritalin) help women reluctant to risk estrogen treatments?

Here, by the way, is a list of the "inattention" half of the symptoms necessary for a diagnosis of ADHD (six symptoms present for at least six months are necessary for the diagnosis; the other "half" of symptoms relate to possible hyperactivity symptoms):

- Fails to give close attention to details or makes careless mistakes in schoolwork, work, or other activities
- Has difficulty sustaining attention in tasks or play activities
- Does not seem to listen when spoken to directly
- Does not follow through on instructions and fails to finish schoolwork chores or duties in the workplace
- Has difficulty organizing tasks and activities

- Avoids, dislikes, or is reluctant to engage in tasks that require sustained mental effort
- Loses things necessary for tasks or activities
- Is easily distracted by extraneous stimuli
- Is forgetful in daily activities

(Source: Russell A. Barkley, Attention-Deficit Hyperactivity Disorder, *Scientific American,* September 1998, pp. 66–71.)

This list overlaps considerably with more than a few of WHMS symptoms and may make plausible a dopamine deficiency or disregulation hypothesis as a basis for some of WHMS symptoms with estrogen loss.

Another of WHMS symptoms involves uncharacteristic scheduling errors such as those that Polly Van Benthusen and NOW's president Patricia Ireland (see Introduction) began to make before estrogen replacement corrected their problem: "Forgetting appointments more or not anticipating events of importance with the same accuracy as before." Interestingly, however, a constellation of research unrelated to estrogen has suggested that inaccurate functioning of a so-called internal time-monitoring anticipatory "interval stopwatch" is associated with deficient amounts of the neurotransmitter dopamine and abnormal temperature regulation in the body (hot flashes would fit this bill), both features plausibly associated with estrogen loss. Could, therefore, some of the WHMS symptoms that involve time-estimation or scheduling deficits be amenable to treatments that boost dopamine supplies and/or help the body to resist temperature irregularities such as hot flashes? It will be worthwhile to find out once WHMS research gets going.

Dopamine is also considered to be a neurotransmitter involved in working memory, the "scratch-pad" kind of memory skill associated with the prefrontal cortex region of the brain, i.e., holding something in mind while you perform some other operation or deed, such as carrying a number from one column while adding up the second, or not "keeping in mind" what you intended to do while walking from one room to another, or in losing your train of thought—losing sight of the bigger idea—after beginning to express a thought. Again, could boosting dopamine supplies without giving replacement estrogen do the trick in reversing these symptoms?

Other scientifically plausible possibilities for treating WHMS symptoms without estrogen suggest themselves. Since we know that estrogen is a potent antioxidant, and since it's been found that treatment with the antioxidant vitamin E helps prevent Alzheimer's disease, could replacing during perimenopause or menopause the declining antioxidant supplies of estrogen with other antioxidants such as vitamin E similarly produce beneficial effects on cognitive symptoms, only this time not in Alzheimer's patients but in younger women?

Since estrogen is known to increase oxygen availability to the brain and to boost cerebral blood flow, could the antioxidant tree-derivative agent, ginkgo biloba, known to increase oxygen supplies to the brain and reported to improve memory in some studies, perhaps help some WHMS symptoms in women experiencing estrogen loss?

The many newly discovered functions of estrogen, as you can see, provide a potential wealth of scientifically rational inroads for exploring treatments for WHMS that may not necessarily require replacement estrogen per se but an understanding of what may be causing the symptoms at multiple levels. What remains to be seen, however, is whether only estrogen-to-the-rescue remedies will rush to be marketed as worthwhile or whether these less obvious, potentially more risk free and conceivably brain-sparing alternative routes to possibly treating WHMS symptoms will also be found to merit investigation and investment research dollars.

However, even more research evidence exists affirming estrogen's major roles with respect to brain function: research on that most feared and debilitating of cognitive impairments, Alzheimer's disease.

4

Estrogen and Alzheimer's Disease Research Evidence

O nly a few years ago the outlook for preventing Alzheimer's disease or helping those already with the disease appeared unrelentingly grim with few signs of promise on the horizon. Today that picture, at least to researchers, appears considerably changed as multiple promising associations and clues have emerged from a variety of studies in recent years showing potential avenues for intervention into this most devastating of diseases.

Estrogen now is part of that hopeful picture. And some researchers, at least in private, wonder if estrogen could ultimately prevent *not only* osteoporosis in the bones of women uniquely susceptible to it (only 25 percent of women are considered to be at elevated risk) but also what some think of as a kind of "osteoporosis of the brain" in women.

In order to understand better the societal picture into which the Alzheimer's/estrogen news fits in, it's useful to know that the same hopeful research I am referring to has also done much in tandem to buoy the hearts and minds of public policy planners. Until recently they could be described not entirely inaccurately as wringing their hands collectively, projecting and grimly anticipating what will happen to our economy when today's fifty-year-old population bubble of baby boomers reach the peak years of Alzheimer's incidence in thirty-something years (most of them likely women). And begin then to produce a hemorrhage in dollars on the economy for supportive public resources, which could persist for some twenty years, as layers upon layers of new baby boomer Alzheimer's cases emerge. A recent study projected that the 2.32 million Americans with Alzheimer's in 1997 could by 2047 quadruple to 8.64 million people so that one in every forty-five Americans—again mainly women—would have the disease. "If we don't get something to treat and prevent Alzheimer's disease, the numbers will get astronomical," says Neil Buckholtz of the National Institute of Aging. "We are now spending $100 billion a year caring for patients with Alzheimer's disease," says Richard Mayeux, M.D., Gertrude Sergievsky Professor of Neurology, Psychiatry, and Public Health at Columbia University's College of Physicians and Surgeons and one of the multiple authors of a recent study, which indicated that estrogen use can significantly reduce and delay the risk of later developing Alzheimer's disease. "Projecting [those dollar amounts] into the future . . . could break a country financially. If we could simply delay the disease by just a few years" we could avert such an economic tidal wave, he and others reason, as death by lifespan aging out would intervene to limit the enormous toll in needed services on the economy and reduce the numbers requiring direct care.

And to an extent such dreams have come true.

Over the last several years in study after study it has been repeatedly found that the use of estrogen during a woman's lifetime can significantly reduce the risk of developing Alzheimer's disease by an astounding 33 to 60 percent across the different studies. Altogether some twelve studies have assessed this relationship with most recent studies confirming this strong association

In one such 1996 study researchers found a 54 percent reduction in the risk of developing Alzheimer's disease in those who had taken estrogen. They had been studying 514 women who were part of the Baltimore Longitudinal Study on aging and who had been tracked for up to sixteen years.

In another 1996 study published in *Lancet,* in which Mayeux was a lead author, it was found that estrogen reduced significantly, by 50 percent, not only the risk of developing Alzheimer's disease but delayed the onset of the disease, even in those at increased hereditary risk of developing the disease—those with the ApoE4 form of the apolipoprotein gene. In studying an ethnically diverse population of 1,124 women in New York City, the researchers found that only 1.7 percent of those who had taken estrogen for more than a year developed Alzheimer's disease while 7.5 percent of those who had taken estrogen for up to one year developed Alzheimer's, and 16.3 percent who had *never* taken it developed Alzheimer's disease. The authors wrote at the end of their report: "These results suggest that a history of oestrogen use during the postmenopausal period significantly delays the onset of Alzheimer's disease and lowers the risk of disease. The duration of oestrogen use seems to be important because women with a history of long-term use had the lowest risk."

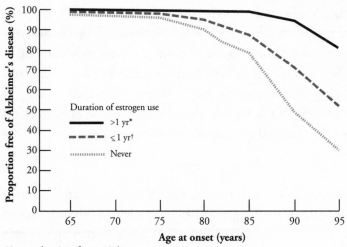

*Average duration of use = 13.6 years
†Average duration of use = 4 months

Figure 3

Estrogen use in women 65 and over reduces later risk of developing Alzheimer's disease.

Source: M. X Tang, D. Jacobs, Y Stern, R. Mayeux, et al. Effect of oestrogen during menopause on risk at onset of Alzheimer's disease. *Lancet* 348 (1996): 429–32.

In another 1996 study of 3,760 women, researchers found that those who took the highest estrogen dose and for the longest amount of time had the lowest risk of developing Alzheimer's disease, data that some contend argues for a causal relationship between estrogen and Alzheimer's disease. In this study those with the greatest exposure to estrogen had half the risk of developing Alzheimer's disease.

The studies examining the relationship between taking estrogen and the risk of developing Alzheimer's disease to date have been typically large *observational* studies, the kind that say "let's see what exists out there observing people without manipulating groups experimentally." Such studies are usually easier to carry out than gold-standard double-blind, randomized, placebo-controlled studies, which offer the advantage of being able to "nail" cause and effect associations between variables in science with fewer ambiguities in the interpretation of results. Despite this limitation, however, in reviewing studies of estrogen and the risk of developing Alzheimer's disease, one of the major researchers in this field Annlia Paganini-Hill, a professor within the Department of Preventive Medicine at the University of Southern California School of Medicine at Los Angeles, nevertheless summed up the collective findings in this way: "Although limited [by being observational], the epidemiological data are becoming increasingly consistent, showing a strong association [between estrogen use and a reduced later risk of developing Alzheimer's disease], a dose-response effect [higher doses are associated with more protective effects], and the greatest effect in current users [as opposed to past users of estrogen]."

———

In addition to these findings involving estrogen use in *healthy* women there have also been promising findings from some twelve studies in which small numbers of patients in various stages of Alzheimer's disease have been given estrogen as an experimental treatment for *already existing* diagnosed Alzheimer's disease.

The earliest of these studies took place in 1985 in the clinical research center at New York City's Rockefeller University when Dr. Howard Fillet, a physician/scientist who had been studying aging, dementia, and the use of estrogen for osteoporosis, hooked up with neuroscientists Dr. Victoria Liune (then working at Rockefeller University with Dr. Bruce McEwen) and with McEwen himself, in an "Aha!" moment of cross-fertilization between disciplines, during rounds of a new Alzheimer's unit at Rockefeller University in 1984. Liune had already shown in *basic research* that estrogen in rats protects and stimulates acetylcholine-based activity in neurons in the very parts of the brain where Alzheimer's patients were known to lose such memory-associated neurons—the basal forebrain. Why not see in *applied research* if estrogen could help "turn on" the activity of these acetylcholine-based neurons and perhaps help boost memory capacity in actual Alzheimer's patients, the group mused. The three collaborated with still others and in 1985 using seven patients, three with *mild* early dementia and four with *advanced* dementia, they did just that, in a trial of estrogen use without any control group. Fillet gave all seven patients an oral form of the body's predominant estrogen—17 beta-estradiol [Estrace] without any progesterone. He says, "All three mild cases showed a good response after three to six weeks. We noticed that from being quiet and apathetic they became more activated, that their memory was definitely better on objective standardized tests," i.e., learning pairs of words. The results were "fairly dramatic" in several instances according to Fillet and the patients' families were eager to keep the patients on the estrogen. But "when we tried to get funding from the National Institutes of Health and other funding sources at that time," Fillet says, "we had no luck." His applications for funding came back with the comments that they had "no scientific merit." Today, ironically, the same kind of research is considered front-burner "hot." Frustrated at the difficulty in trying to be a funded physician/researcher while also trying to raise a family, Fillet eventually left academia for more traditional medical work as a physician.

However, since then some eleven other small studies using estrogen for the treatment of Alzheimer's disease have been done, with ten of the eleven replicating Fillet's and colleagues' earlier findings, namely that some or all the women on estrogen improved on at least some of the measures they were assessed on. Four of these eleven studies used placebo control groups, with sizes of the groups in the studies varying between four and fifteen women per group. For those of you interested, the women with Alzheimer's disease received typically standard estrogen doses, either 0.625 or 1.25 milligrams of either conjugated equine estrogen (Premarin) or the equivalent doses of 17 beta-estradiol, for intervals that ranged from three weeks up to nine months.

In one of the most recent double-blind, randomized, placebo-controlled trials Dr. Sanjay Asthana and his colleagues at the Veterans Affairs Medical Center in Tacoma, Washington, gave twelve mild-to-moderately impaired women with a diagnosis of Alzheimer's disease living at home with caregivers either an estrogen patch (releasing 50 micrograms per day) for two months or a placebo patch. The women were then evaluated at four intervals over the two months on six types of tests. "We found improvement in five of the six women given estrogen on two specific types of tests," says Asthana, "on a test of verbal memory [Bushkie] and on the most difficult parts of an attention test [Stroop]. Performance on the verbal memory test," Asthana notes, "improved at the end of the first week of treatment!" The women could for example remember twice as many words presented to them twenty minutes earlier than they could when the study began. "We found a direct relationship between the level of estrogen in the blood and improvement in memory," he added. Interestingly, however, Asthana found "The caregivers didn't notice any improvement [initially]. They only noticed changes when the subjects were taken off the estrogen." Asthana suspects that the caregivers "may not have had the language to describe what was going on" or the ability to sense what the women internally were experiencing.

These optimistic findings have been fueling an eagerness for outcomes from larger similar studies on the effects of estrogen on Alzheimer's disease risk, its onset, or the progression of symptoms once the disease has been diagnosed. Two studies examining some of these aspects are already underway. One involves the Women's Health Initiative, where results are expected in the year 2006, and the second involves a National Institutes of Health Alzheimer's study of estrogen's effects in outpatient elderly women with the disease, with results expected by 1999.

There have been still other estrogen/Alzheimer's findings. It has been found, for example, that women diagnosed with Alzheimer's disease on hormone replacement therapy "show better cognitive skills than women with Alzheimer's disease who are not taking estrogen," particularly "on a naming (semantic) memory task," a finding which may have relevance to the change in naming efficiency I have associated with estrogen loss in the WHM Syndrome.

It has also been found that though *healthy* women overall tend to perform *better* than men on many verbal tests, women with Alzheimer's disease tend to do *poorer* than men with Alzheimer's disease on certain verbal tests, especially those that involve naming skills. What might account for this turnaround in verbal advantage? The supposition considered by some is that estrogen probably underlies and supports verbal fluency (meaning the ability to generate the names of lists of things), and that women after menopause experience long years of estrogen deprivation, which might affect this fluency, while men's brains, which also depend on estrogen, (their body's testosterone is converted to estrogen by an enzyme known as aromatase) don't experience the same precipitous dropoff in estrogen supplies over a lifetime (but a more gradual decline with time). According to researcher Barbara Sherwin, by age seventy-two, women's blood levels and presumably brains too contain less estrogen than men's blood levels and, likely, brains.

Perhaps related to this picture as well is the finding that women are twice as likely as men to develop Alzheimer's disease (some estimates hold that women are three times as likely), even when women's longer survival is taken into account. Longer years of having estrogen around to protect brain neurons from harm and to carry out its many supportive brain functions are suspected here too of being a factor in men's reduced likelihood to develop Alzheimer's disease.

So should women *with* Alzheimer's be put on estrogen? According to neurologist Victor Henderson, a leading researcher in this field, the results of the existing studies to date are limited by their small size, the short spans of treatment, and some of the weaknesses in design of the studies. "Nevertheless," he writes, "*[Findings to date] lend credence to the role of estrogen replacement in the treatment of the disease . . . particularly for women with relatively mild cognitive deficits* [emphasis added]."

And for women *without* Alzheimer's disease who are postmeno-pausal, should they take estrogen? Henderson, writing for a professional audience, says, "There are compelling reasons why a postmenopausal woman and her physician would consider hormone replacement ther-apy. For most women risk reductions for cardiovascular disease, overall mortality and osteoporosis appear to outweigh the recognized hazards of hormone replacement therapy, including endometrial cancer and the probable risk of breast cancer. Given current uncertainties as to the role of estrogen in Alzheimer's disease," he says, "one cautious approach is to consider hormone replacement therapy in post-menopausal women who are asymptomatic for Alzheimer's disease and in women who al-ready have symptoms of Alzheimer's disease without regard to putative effects on Alzheimer's disease."

What Henderson appears to be saying is that there are many good reasons to consider taking estrogen apart from any factors having to do with Alzheimer's disease, and if you are considering taking estrogen for preventing or moderating Alzheimer's, use the evidence-based rationale that you are really taking it for all its other more clearly substantiated beneficial effects.

Mayeux says, "No one knows whether to advise older women to take estrogen at the moment for preventing Alzheimer's disease. We only have [studies with] observational data to go on at the moment [as opposed to studies designed to prove a direct cause-and-effect relation-ship]. Given *that,* women have to go to their doctors and review all per-sonal risks and make a choice. Estrogen is a potent drug and it does have side effects. It's complicated. We aren't sure that anything happens to the brain immediately [after estrogen loss]. Abrupt loss of estrogen may not have any immediate effects." (Mayeux was not aware of WHMS symp-toms when I interviewed him.)

A student of both osteoporosis and dementia, Howard Fillet sees the situation, theoretically, as follows: "The mean age when osteoporosis becomes a disease [by virtue of] the increased incidence of hip fractures is seventy-nine. We know that [some] women need to start taking es-trogen at fifty-one [the mean age of menopause] to prevent hip fractures at seventy-nine. If they don't during those years they are in an estrogen-deficient state which can be chronic and progressive in leading to bone loss. The mean age of Alzheimer's onset," he says, "*is also seventy-nine*. It may take thirty years of estrogen deficiency to lead to bone fractures or heart attacks. Similarly, it may take thirty years of estrogen deficiency to lead to enough brain loss to produce a state of Alzheimer's disease, a state that, just as with hip fractures, might be preventable with starting estrogen use also at fifty-one [after the onset of menopause]."

What specific aspects of estrogen might conceivably be involved in reducing the risk of Alzheimer's disease? Fillet says, "Keeping neuronal cells in the brain alive; helping them survive injury from free radicals via [estrogen's] role as an antioxidant; reducing the possible effects of inflammation in the brain; increasing blood flow to the brain and improving the vasculature of the brain as [estrogen] does in heart disease; also [estrogen's] influence on many [brain] neurotransmitters; and its role in helping neurons to grow."

Others point to estrogen's known neuroprotective roles, such as the ability to keep clearing away the potentially toxic amyloid protein buildup that is characteristic of the distinctive beta amyloid plaques associated with Alzheimer's disease and the death of neurons; or estrogen's ability to increase glucose uptake, metabolism, and use; or its ability to help the brain adapt to injury, to bounce back from the various assaults of age, illness, or stress, by means of stimulating regeneration of axons and restoring a dense network of synaptic connections by various means, including the recruitment of different brain growth factors, so-called neurotrophic factors.

"Studies in experimental animal models provide a convincing rationale for a role for ERT [estrogen replacement therapy] in the treatment and prevention of dementia," aging expert and researcher Stanley Birge wrote not long ago in an article titled "Is There a Role for ERT in the Prevention and Treatment of Dementia?" "These studies establish the role of estrogen in the regeneration and preservation of [brain neurons] that are analogous to those [very] regions of the brain most sensitive to the neurodegenerative changes associated with AD [Alzheimer's disease] . . . We do not know [now]," he writes, "what factors contribute to the selective neuronal injury which over time eventually leads to the neuronal loss and reduced synaptic density that result in the cognitive impairment of AD. At this time we can only speculate as to estrogen's role in modifying this process. Data from experimental animal models suggest that estrogen deficiency selectively increases the vulnerability of estrogen responsive [nerve cells in the brain]."

Stating it more simply, James Simpkins, of the University of Florida's Center for the Neurobiology of Aging and the Department of Pharmacodynamics, and his colleagues, reporting recently on exciting animal and test-tube research demonstrating estrogen's memory-boosting, and acetylcholine-boosting activity in nerve cells in the hippocampus and frontal cortex, and its nerve-growth-promoting effects, say, "Women are two times more likely to develop AD [Alzheimer's disease] than men, and the mean lifespan for women is seventy-eight years. Considering the normal age of menopause . . . , it is probable that women will spend 25 to 33 percent of their lives in an estrogen-deprived state. This highlights the prospect that estrogens may participate in normal brain maintenance and that estrogen deprivation plays a role in age-related neurodegenerative diseases." After reviewing their research findings they write "These findings indicate that estrogens are behaviorally active, affect the function of basal forebrain cholinergic neurons [the ones devastated in Alzheimer's disease], and reduce neuronal vulnerability to a variety of insults. These multiple actions of estrogens and the wealth of data with ERT in postmenopausal subjects warrant clinical trials of estrogens in AD [Alzheimer's disease]."

These findings on replacement estrogen's role in (1) reducing the risk of developing Alzheimer's disease in often a dose- and duration-related manner (2) in delaying progression of the disease (3) in reversing cognitive decline in some domains in some of those with mild to moderate cases of Alzheimer's, and (4) in bolstering verbal naming skills in those already diagnosed with the disease, are certainly of independent interest in the hope they offer for staving off Alzheimer's disease or its progression, and in the hope they offer that one day Alzheimer's disease may no longer be the death-while-living scourge that so many fear today. However, my main purpose for presenting them is to argue that these findings collectively support the estrogen loss/WHMS connection I point to in this book, to emphasize that there is a plausible connection between estrogen and changes in cognitive functioning (i.e., speech, naming abilities, memory), between estrogen and multiple facets of behavior, to hammer home the message of the Alzheimer's-estrogen research: namely that both estrogen loss and estrogen replacement can, for some, have significant cognitive consequences.

Collectively all the research on estrogen and the brain also points to still other conclusions that are of significant relevance to understanding the possibilities inherent in WHMS. I address these in the next chapter.

5

Evidence the Symptoms
Can Be Reversed

M uch of the collective research on estrogen and the brain suggests either implicitly or explicitly that changes produced by estrogen loss are not necessarily always immutable. Rather, they can often be reversed considerably or partially with replacement estrogen.

Indeed one of the intriguing aspects of the discovery of estrogen-dependent dendritic spines that Catherine Wooley, Bruce McEwen, and their colleagues made in the hippocampal memory and learning neurons of rats (the potential added docking sites for incoming information) was the apparent ever readiness of these spines to return, after disappearing, even in adulthood. The spines would predictably shrink and disappear when the rats' ovaries and therefore estrogen supplies were removed. But as predictably they could be made to sprout and "blossom" again within forty-eight hours by replacing the hormone.

The unexpected plastic potential in the adult brain discovered by neuroscientists in the 1990s accounts in part for this picture of reversibility.

This same potential for reversibility is also evident from years of women's experiences with estrogen, namely that many of the symptoms produced in some women during perimenopause and menopause with estrogen loss—the hot flashes, vaginal dryness, the thinning of vaginal and urinary tissues—can often be readily reversed with replacement estrogen (given most often today together with progesterone).

I present in this chapter more research evidence pointing to the possibilities of reversal of cognitive changes associated with estrogen loss in older, middle-aged, and younger women, and in animal studies.

ESTROGEN-REPLACEMENT RESEARCH WITH OLDER WOMEN SHOWS ESTROGEN CAN REVERSE SYMPTOMS

Here now are some "strobe-light" glimpses of studies with women that demonstrate the reversing potential effects of estrogen replacement on cognition.

To show that reversals in cognitive functioning are possible even after many years of estrogen deprivation let me begin with two estrogen-replacement studies of older women done in the 1950s to 1970s when progesterone was not routinely given with estrogen therapy. In a 1952 placebo-controlled study of twenty-eight normal, nondemented seventy-five-year-old women living in a home for the aged and receiving weekly muscle injections of either 2 milligrams of a form of estrogen (estradiol benzoate) or a placebo, the researchers found that after twelve months, the women receiving estrogen *had increased significantly on the verbal IQ score* of the Wechsler-Bellevue Intelligence Scale. (This is a composite score reflecting performance on various subtests assessing abstract reasoning, vocabulary, attention, comprehension, etc.) The group receiving placebo injections for twelve months over the same time span actually *declined* on the measures that make up the verbal IQ score and *had lower verbal IQ scores.* Furthermore, the women who had been receiving estrogen also scored significantly better on the Wechsler Memory Scale, another test comprised of different subtests, while the placebo-treated women's scores had fallen below where they had been a year before. As noteworthy were the findings that estrogen *improved memory only while it was being given.* It did not have lingering effects: A year after all women had stopped receiving any kind of treatment, when again tested on the Wechsler Memory Scale the scores of the women had fallen below where they had been *two* years earlier, i.e., with age and no treatment there had been gradually declining cognitive functioning.

Some twenty-three years later, another placebo-controlled study of seventy-five-year-old nondemented women living in another home for the elderly was done again using only estrogen. Twenty-five randomly selected women daily received a low dose (0.625 milligrams) of the kind of estrogen that is in Premarin—conjugated equine (horse) estrogen—for three years while twenty-five randomly selected women received a placebo during the same time. All the women were rated every three months on the Hospital Adjustment Scale, which evaluated their skills on self-care, their communication and interpersonal skills, and their work activities. The scores of women treated with estrogen improved steadily with time on these measures *over a period of eighteen months* and then remained at the same stable level throughout the rest of the study while the placebo-treated women were rated *as steadily decreasing on these skills over the same time interval.*

It is interesting that in women this age, it took eighteen months at that dosage level to get to a plateauing stable level. We saw that with Polly Van Benthusen it took some seven months for her to get back not everything she had lost but a good part of it. It's interesting to speculate whether higher doses of estrogen would have led to a quicker return of function in the older women, or a greater return of function, or if the eighteen months it took to get to a plateauing level of functioning was related to the age of the women. Studies to address these issues obviously will need to be done in developing ideal treatment regimens for WHMS that involve replacement estrogen.

ESTROGEN-REPLACEMENT RESEARCH WITH YOUNGER WOMEN SHOWS ESTROGEN CAN REVERSE SYMPTOMS

That similar reversals—improvements in memory—can occur in young women is evident in a 1996 study by leading estrogen/cognition researcher Dr. Barbara Sherwin, a psychologist/behavioral neuroendocrinologist who is both professor of psychology and obstetrics and gynecology at McGill University in Montreal and codirector of McGill's Menopause Clinic. Probably more than anyone, Sherwin has helped make credible to the medical and scientific world, and hence to the world at large, the plausibility of the human connection between estrogen and cognition. Sherwin has done this by being a highly methodical and rigorous experimenter who has designed and implemented many near-flawless experiments that don't easily lend themselves to ambiguous interpretations. The robustness of her experimental designs and her carefully weighed comments about her findings has meant that even rather paternalistic and staid old-line medical pros in the worlds of research and obstetrics and gynecology almost reflexively speak of her work—the work of a woman researcher from the sometimes seen as soft field of psychology—as "the highly respectable work of Barbara Sherwin."

In this particular recent study thirty-four-year-old women were given estrogen-suppressing medication to treat infertility due to fibroids. The women were tested before beginning estrogen-suppressing treatment on measures of verbal memory, and again after twelve weeks of being estrogen deprived. Then while remaining on the same estrogen-suppressing medication, half the women were randomly assigned to receive either a placebo for eight weeks, or replacement estrogen (0.625 milligrams Premarin, conjugated equine estrogen, daily). Both groups were then tested a third time at the end of the eight weeks on the same verbal memory measures. Here is what happened to their verbal memory scores. The twelve weeks of estrogen-suppressing medication alone led to statistically significantly decreased performance on the tests of verbal memory in these young women compared to their baseline memory scores before being deprived of estrogen, i.e., estrogen loss led to poorer verbal memory. Verbal memory scores *remained* depressed in those estrogen-deprived women who were only given a placebo for the next eight weeks. However, in the estrogen-deprived women given replacement estrogen for the next eight weeks, the "memory deficits were reversed," writes Barbara Sherwin. "These results," she said, "provide further compelling evidence that [estrogen] plays a role in maintaining verbal memory in women," or stated differently, that estrogen loss leads to declining verbal memory that can be reversed with "add-back" replacement estrogen.

Sherwin has found similar reversible results in many other studies including studies of *middle-aged postmenopausal women* experiencing estrogen loss. She has found the same essential results in three different studies of younger *premenopausal* women who have had to have complete hysterectomies with ovary removal. Estrogen loss consistently led to reduced scores on verbal learning and memory measures compared with baseline measures—having to remember a paragraph or paired sets of words immediately afterward, or after a delay—and a return to baseline levels when estrogen-replacement therapy was given—*sometimes to better than baseline levels.*

"Overall," Sherwin writes in a 1998 review article summarizing her and others' work, "the findings of studies that have investigated the association between estrogen and memory provide increasing support for the hypothesis that estrogen helps maintain aspects of short- and long-term verbal memory."

Sherwin has also reported a study in which postmenopausal women given 1.25 milligrams of conjugated equine estrogen for a year with or without progesterone "had a higher energy level and a more enhanced sense of well being" than women not receiving replacement estrogen. (A lower dose, 0.625, of this form of estrogen, *did not* produce such results, showing the need for more such studies exploring what levels of estrogen constitute effective doses for what kinds of women.)

The previous year, 1997, I asked Sherwin at a Society for Behavioral Neuroendocrinology meeting in Baltimore, "Your studies seem to have shown constant reversibility, no?" "Yes," she said, "in all our studies estrogen replacement brought on reversibility of the cognitive function that was deficient. These changes are reversible. They are clearly reversible. There is brain plasticity. Catherine Wooley [and those who worked with her have shown] that there is enormous plasticity of the adult brain."

What did Sherwin think might be occurring in perimenopausal and menopausal women losing estrogen? "Can we assume that women's brains are subtly changing to some degree with the loss of estrogen, or could it be that as with puberty, a period of chaotic destabilization might be followed by a return to normal equanimity again?" I asked. "I don't know why they [women] would stabilize," Sherwin responded. "They would stabilize at a lower level of functioning. . . . If we are right that estrogen maintains aspects of memory then it [cognitive function- ing] shouldn't get better on its own. Reproductive tissues for the pur- poses of conception don't get better with time if you don't treat them. Bone density doesn't. Look at any other organ system in which estrogen is doing something. Does it get better on its own? Why should it get better here?" she reasoned.

Based on her studies to date of women experiencing estrogen loss for different reasons, Sherwin has found statistically significant evidence of decline in short-term and delayed *verbal* memory and verbal learning as reflected in diminished recall of paragraph content and paired-word new learning tests. Other studies as well have reported statistically sig- nificant findings with respect to enhanced verbal skills with estrogen: improved proper name recall in older women on ERT, statistically sig- nificant improvements in concept formation (Similarities Subtest), de- layed and immediate verbal memory, and performance on a naming task in older women (mean age of seventy-four) who had been on ERT for at least one year in the past compared to women who had not.

Sherwin has not, however, found detectable differences in measures of visual and spatial memory in women deprived of estrogen. (Her tests in this area may not have been sensitive enough or her subjects too vari- able on these measures.) Unaware of the range of possible WHMS symptoms, to date Sherwin has believed that estrogen-based loss is spe- cific to the *verbal* arena and is not more global, that estrogen loss doesn't affect broader areas of function.

However, very recently other researchers have begun to report *other than verbal* differences in cognition in women after menopause and with replacement estrogen. In 1995 another long-term hormones-and-cognition researcher, Canadian psychologist Doreen Kimura, in a research paper titled "Estrogen Replacement Therapy May Protect Against Intellectual Decline in Postmenopausal Women," reported that twenty-one postmenopausal women over the age of fifty and on estrogen therapy for at least several years, and matched on several variables with thirty-three women who were not, "had better scores than those not on therapy" to a statistically significant degree: on two tests of perceptual speed, two tests of spatial perception, one verbal articulation tongue-twister test, a test of hand-movement speed and accuracy, two tests of facility in thinking rapidly (verbal fluency)—naming colors, generating sentences), and a logical inference test. "Estrogen may guard against some of the intellectual decline which is to be expected [sic] postmenopausal," Kimura wrote in that paper. "Perhaps some minimum or optimum level of estrogen is needed to maintain neural circuits for a number of behaviors," she speculated. Kimura, however, also noted that many of her tests were time-limited "so conceivably estrogen therapy may simply have improved a general speed-of-processing factor" that may have affected the outcome of the other tests.

In 1997 Dr. Susan Resnick, a senior staff fellow in the Laboratory of Personality and Cognition at the National Institute of Aging, in Bethesda, Maryland, and her colleagues also reported statistically significant differences in spatial memory skills with estrogen-replacement therapy, using subjects from the Baltimore Longitudinal Study of Aging. They found that 116 women with a mean age of sixty-two (age range forty-two to eighty plus) on estrogen-replacement therapy made fewer errors on a spatial memory test involving recalling geometric designs, the Benton Visual Retention Test, than 172 women not on such treatment though of comparable age and matched on different variables.

In a second part of the study Resnick looked at the successive performance on this same test of spatial memory of eighteen women of perimenopausal/menopausal years who had *never* had ERT with eighteen age-matched women who over a six-year span had gone from taking no estrogen to taking estrogen. Resnick says, "Women who were treated with estrogen showed no change over the two time periods" of being tested on the spatial memory tests. However, "in women who were never treated there was an increase in the number of errors on the Benton Visual Retention Test [when they were tested six years later]. They had poorer memory by a couple of points on the test."

Still other researchers have reported differences in reaction-time tasks and complex motor-coordination tasks favoring women of menopausal years taking estrogen-replacement treatment.

Laboratory studies, however, are formal, often artificial, settings. The real question of significance is how do these test differences play out in women's actual daily lives? Sherwin used to question whether the differences in short-term and long-term verbal memory and new learning she found in her studies had any practical relevance to women's daily lives and invariably would add such a written disclaimer to her published reports. In May of 1997 I asked Sherwin for her current "take" on this matter. "Are the differences you've found in your studies clinically *insignificant* in menopausal women as you've often suggested in print?" I asked. She said, "Well I have said that until people started to point out to me recently that I am in error and that I am underestimating my own data. I'm starting to look at that because there are hints, and I think that they [those pointing this out to me] are right. Because when you actually look at the effect size in my data [how statistically robust the data are], particularly in the women over fifty using estrogen or even in some of these studies where the women were forty-four but premenopausal and had their ovaries removed, the effect size is on the order of two standard deviations. [Those findings] are not small or modest. That's a fairly robust effect. . . . Perhaps I have been underestimating the effect size of my own studies." During the same interview when I asked Sherwin what proportion of women report problems with cognition around menopause she said, "Some significant proportion are subjectively aware of the change in memory around the time of menopause. These changes seem to be even more profound in perimenopausal women. Hormone levels are changing rather abruptly at that time. When they stabilize at low levels after the menopause you find that women have less symptomatology."

Nearly a year later I again asked Sherwin in a telephone interview how her findings translate into the actual lives of women. She said,

"From women I hear 'Not being able to remember things that I need to do that day,' 'Not being able to remember a new phone number in the way I could before.' I could use one hundred examples," she said. "I think my test scores [the changes in performance with and without estrogen in women] have a lot of correlation with everyday life. Paragraph recall [the verbal memory test I use] is correlated with not being able to recall material you just heard. . . . It could be less verbal fluency [a test she uses that measures the ability to think quickly of words], the sense of 'it will come to me.' I do see women come into our clinic with memory complaints. The fifty-one-year-olds are saying 'I notice changes in my memory that are disturbing to me and worrisome.' I see perimenopausal women say this too between the ages of forty-eight and fifty-two. [But] [t]hey [women of this age] also come in without memory symptoms."

STUDIES OF COGNITIVE/BEHAVIORAL SKILLS DURING A NORMAL MENSTRUAL CYCLE INDICATE COME-AND-GO EFFECTS OF HIGH AND LOW ESTROGEN LEVELS

In a series of studies Doreen Kimura alone or with her colleague Elizabeth Hampson has studied proficiency of different skills during different hormonal phases of the normal menstrual cycle in young women that come and go. "We found that over the course of the menstrual cycle there were mild but consistent differences in certain skills," Kimura told me. "Higher levels of estrogen," she said, "are associated with more accurate performance on articulatory [pronunciation] speed and accuracy, verbal fluency—the ability to think quickly and accurately of the intended word, and perceptual speed and accuracy—the visual skill of scanning an array and picking out fine details. The changes are small but consistent. We found that in the case of *spatial abilities,* women [perform] best at the lowest estrogen levels." (Sherwin and an associate also found this in 1992.)* What these findings suggest is that higher estrogen levels may actually interfere with spatial skills.

*S. Philips and B. Sherwin, Variations in Memory Function and Sex Steroid Hormones Across the Menstrual Cycle, *Psychoneuroendocrinology,* October 1992, 17 (5), 496–506.

The average gynecologist, Kimura notes, "is unaware of studies in this field."

ANIMAL STUDIES OF EFFECTS OF ESTROGEN LOSS AND REPLACEMENT SHOW REVERSAL POTENTIAL OF COGNITIVE SKILLS

Animal studies too have shown the potential for reversal of memory or learning deficits in female animals deprived of estrogen with add-back estrogen. The effects, however, sometimes depend on the type of memory task involved and on the length or schedule (chronic versus acute) of the estrogen replacement given.

"Ovarian Steroid Deprivation [estrogen loss] Results in a Reversible Learning Impairment and Compromised Cholinergic Function in Female Sprague-Dawley Rats" was the title of a published 1994 report in the journal *Brain Research,* in which researchers found that normal levels of estrogen replacement resulted not only in *"superior performance"* compared to estrogen-deprived rats but also an *"accelerated rate of learning"* compared to normal intact animals with estrogen. (Replacement estrogen made them "smarter than normal.")

In a later 1997 study of memory-related behaviors in female adult rats some of the same authors found that on a learning task involving avoidance of punishment "OVX [estrogen deprivation] caused a decline in avoidance behavior [worse learning] and estrogen replacement normalized the response." The researchers found that on a task of spatial memory—the Morris water task—that "OVX animals showed normal spatial learning [they mastered the task involved] but were deficient in spatial memory [in remembering what they learned], an effect that was prevented by estrogen treatment. Together these data indicate that OVX in rats results in an estrogen-reversible impairment of learning/memory behavior."

P. Dohanich and colleagues reported research in which estrogen administration to rats improved working memory. ("Working memory" is the "keep in mind while doing something" memory that is lacking when you can't remember what you came into a room to get—a WHMS symptom.) They gave estrogen for thirty days to female rats with removed ovaries and tested them before and after estrogen, on a test of working memory (the radial arm maze—"guess which radiating arm has the food"). They found in the estrogen-treated rats "significantly improved working memory performance compared to females treated with [a placebo type of treatment]." Discussing their many studies collectively the authors say, "Estrogen improves performance on tasks that depend on working memory . . . but impairs performance on tasks that are highly spatial. Our results have some parallels to the selective effects of estrogen on learning and memory reported in humans."

Others too have reported related "reversible" findings. Particularly intriguing is the work of Gillian Einstein and Christina Williams, professors of psychology at Duke University Medical Center, for what it suggests about the subtleties that may have to be attended to in giving women estrogen replacement for cognitive improvement or status quo stability. These researchers have been studying the effects of estrogen exposure on learning and memory in both young and old female rats. What they have found is that "estrogen replacement to *adult* ovariectomized rats improves working memory of [where] food [is] on a radial-arm maze. This memory-enhancing effect of estradiol [an estrogen] is most dramatic if estradiol is administered short-term (i.e., several weeks) and can be seen in both young (three months) and old (fifteen months) rats. In contrast *chronic replacement of estradiol for nine months at either a low or high dose does not appear to cause savings in memory* [emphasis added]. . . . These data suggest that the aging female rat brain is still responsive to estradiol but requires estradiol exposure acutely [in limited bursts] rather than chronically. We believe that the temporal pattern [timing] of estradiol exposure may be the key to estrogen's effectiveness. [The] remarkable plasticity of spines in the hippocampus is a possible mechanism underlying estradiol's . . . enhancement of working memory."

Others too have recently reported that *specific regimens* of replacement estrogen were necessary to produce in rats the maximal brain neurochemical benefits associated with memory improvement. "These findings demonstrate that (1) estrogen replacement produces regionally selective effects on basal forebrain cholinergic neurons which vary as a function of both the dose and duration of estrogen treatment, and (2) estrogen has both short-term and longer-term effects on basal forebrain cholinergic neurons, each of which may contribute to the effects of estrogen on learning and memory process [sic] and the development of age and disease-related cognitive decline."

Given this animal and human research, it is now up to researchers to get busy and figure out how these clues translate into treatments that can maximally benefit women with WHMS symptoms. In view of the human studies reported above with estrogen-replacement therapy, it does seem that reversibility as a concept is possible at all ages. Among the many questions that remain, however, are: Is *total* reversibility of self-detectable changes in function possible at all ages in all women? Is total reversibility for most menopausal women *necessary*—are the changes in *most* women with WHMS symptoms not important enough to make a big difference, practically and functionally, in life? Are there time-limited windows of opportunity that need to be taken advantage of to get maximal return? Are there "critical periods" when the rate of estrogen-associated brain changes are most rapid and when temporary treatment might be most beneficial? Is it possible to get back *some* of the many things that estrogen normally does in the brain, but not *all* of the things it does? Can replacement estrogen only prevent decline or produce "arrest" of further decline, as one leading researcher in this field suspects, but *not* necessarily produce reversibility? These are all open questions at the moment, in need of answers.

PRESENT HUMAN RESEARCH IN THIS FIELD IS PROBLEMATIC IN DETECTING WHMS SYMPTOMS

Before turning from this topic, I believe it is highly important to emphasize that some accommodations in interpretation may be necessary in thinking about some of the *human* studies I have just reported in view of what I know about the WHMS syndrome: I suspect that the *design of many of the human studies above may not have been sufficiently sensitive to detect all the WHMS-like changes* that may have been present in some women and evaluated in some studies. Because of this, some of the findings may have underestimated—not reflected fully—changes with estrogen loss that women were actually experiencing. It is my belief that to ably identify existing WHMS symptoms in women who have them *different* kinds of studies than the ones I have just described may be necessary in the future. Special studies may need to be designed to accommodate WHMS special features. What do I mean?

Almost all of the human studies I have described above have not taken into account features that are specific to WHMS. WHMS symptoms tend to be *intermittent* and not continuously present as you've seen in the cases presented so far. Second, many of the symptoms seem to occur most often when women are *"just being"* rather than focusing directed effort on tasks.

However, in most of the studies that have been done till now women have been given "formal" tests in formal test-taking experimental situations.

What do most people do when they are given formal tests? They *try*. They bring effort and directed attention to a task. Particularly if they are women with a long history, typically, of being "good girls," of trying to do their best, of pleasing. What does this mean? It means that the standard situation in which women with estrogen loss have been tested in research to date may actually have impeded detection of the pattern of their symptoms as they occur in the naturalistic environment, in life. Thus, the formal research designs used to date in their implicit demand for effort and attention may have actually served to override and obscure detection of existing WHMS symptoms. Research studies done to date with tests that have *not* detected changes in women with estrogen loss may be inconclusive. They may be open to mixed interpretations. There truly may have been no changes in women with estrogen loss in these studies, or they may have been present in life, but not present during the testing situation. The test situation may have been invalid for the purposes for which it was being applied.

Even if we were to overlook this particular flaw in existing research other problems exist: The nature of WHMS symptoms is such that they are sometimes there and often not. So the research problem of detecting an *intermittent* symptom itself poses a problem to the typical formal experimental situation and to the studies done to date on estrogen and cognition. In most research, the researcher typically does not move in and live with subjects (though I actually did this once while doing formal sleep research) but rather tests subjects on one, two, or at most several occasions. So in view of what we know about how WHMS shows up in most women's lives—intermittently—the kind of research done to date may not have detected the symptoms at the time they were present because it did not sample "behavior" frequently enough or continually and missed the symptoms at the time when the research was going on. Thus, research studies in the field of estrogen and cognition done to date that have not detected changes in women with estrogen loss may be inconclusive for a second reason. They may be open to mixed interpretations. There truly may have been no changes in women with estrogen loss in the tests posed, or changes may have been there in the lives of those tested, but not present during the testing situation. Again the test situation may not have been valid for the purposes to which it was being applied by virtue of the *intermittent* nature of WHMS symptoms.

A third problem with the research on estrogen and cognition is that the neuropsychological batteries of tests now commonly used in cognitive and brain research to assess brain damage or brain changes may not be *sufficiently sensitive* to the subtle but internally evident changes that women with WHMS experience as a result of estrogen changes. As noted before more than a few of the tests commonly used in neuropsychological batteries are used because they proved their worth in assessing people with heavy-duty brain injuries—victims of war injuries or car accidents, etc. That they are sensitive to the subtle changes implied by WHMS remains to be proven.

The fourth problem area that needs to be better addressed in future studies of estrogen and cognition is the need for developing a test battery (or test situations) that reflects the *full span or scope of the possible kinds of changes in cognitive functioning* represented by Warga's Hormonal Misconnection Syndrome, i.e., spelling tests, reading comprehension tests, pronunciation tests, face recall tests, etc.—the whole spectrum of symptoms in Table 1, since some women only have a few or one kind of symptom(s) while others have a full panoply of them. Without tests for such *an array* of symptoms, studies may conclude that women tested have no cognitive changes when they may not have sampled the kinds of changes that were present in the women.

The fifth and last problem I see as critical that future research take into account, in terms of research design, is the enormous known *variability* that typically exists among women when it comes to "reproduction associated changes": how some women long suffer PMS while others don't at all; how some women have almost no symptoms in the years surrounding menopause while others have many. The high degree of variability among women together with the frequent use of small numbers of subjects in many of the studies done to date means that true "signals" of cognitive change with estrogen loss, present in some of the women evaluated, could too easily be drowned out statistically by all the "noise" of the variability among women. This would lead to studies with results that do not reach statistical significance and that misrepresent the true state of nature with respect to WHMS symptoms. Studies that do not recognize this great amount of variability, as I see it, lead science astray with wrong conclusions or lead to studies with inconsistent sometimes-yes, sometimes-no outcomes and waste research funds. Because of these methodological problems, I believe the positive findings that have been found to date in the estrogen/cognition research above likely are valid while the absence of positive findings in these studies may need to be held in abeyance as possibly inconclusive at present.

What is there to say about studies that *did* detect improvement in performance in women with estrogen loss given replacement estrogen, compared with comparable women not given replacement estrogen? Why were differences found in those instances? My guess is that those symptoms that were detected on the tests are probably more prevalent or intense WHMS symptoms, or less easily overridden with directed effort.

What is needed to get around some of these problems with current research studies? The answer is research designs that reflect and accommodate the realities of WHMS symptoms as they occur in life. This might mean research designs that ethically "catch" those with WHMS symptoms unawares, that ostensibly ask subjects to come into a room and introduce themselves to the experimenter, but later ask questions related to the real goal of the experiment: "How many objects were you aware of in that room? What was the time on the clock opposite you? How many historical faces in pictures on the wall in that room can you identify on the sheet here?" and even better variants of tests of this kind.

It might mean having those with self-professed WHMS tested via brain scans of one kind or another while subjects are asked to wait ("just being") and noting changes over time in regional activity of glucose, or oxygen, or evoked potentials compared with those not professing WHMS symptoms. It might mean doing brain "scanning" while subjects are asked to engage in tasks that also lend themselves to "just being" or to "blinking" wavering attention, such as being asked to count to a thousand or to estimate when five minutes is up. It could mean trying to develop a symptom-sensitive test battery: giving women who profess to have many WHMS symptoms a sufficient number of different kinds of tests on repeated testings, until researchers could identify a set of *valid tests* sensitive enough to detect changes in women who said they experienced WHMS symptoms during the tests. That would make the tests at least valid to a degree, if not necessarily consistently reliable (the symptoms might be present during testing on some occasions but not on many others, thus producing inconsistent results). Studies could be done with larger numbers of women, prescreening or selecting women for estrogen/cognition research on some known relevant biological variables so they start out less variable as a group. For example, some studies would use only women who have a history of PMS (premenstrual syndrome).

Without such accommodations, research in this field will continue to be inconclusive and open to ambiguous interpretations.

However, as important as assuring that *researchers* will be able to validate WHMS in future research is the goal of assuring that *women themselves* are familiar with the different forms the WHM Syndrome can take.

III

DO YOU HAVE
THE SYNDROME?

6

Who Suffers from Warga's Hormonal Misconnection Syndrome (WHMS)?

What can you expect? What do different women experience when the cognitive/speech/behavioral symptoms of WHMS begin to blink on and off in the midst of an otherwise busy normal life? It can feel as if the "da-da da-da" refrains of a *Twilight Zone* hallucination have privately taken hold, as unexplainable symptoms "possess" one's body, mind, and/or mouth, or as if the "engine trouble" light on the dashboard of a car had suddenly begun to glow an ominous red on an unfamiliar unlit mountain road. "What in the world is going on?" women think. "What will happen next if these weird things are already happening now?"

My goal is to present as best I can the range of experiences that constitute the WHM Syndrome for different women, walking the tightrope between not overstating the impact of the symptoms in some women and not minimizing the dislocation and fear they can arouse in others.

After first presenting an overview of WHMS, I will describe in this chapter the different subgroups of women that exist in relation to WHMS symptoms.

KEEPING THE BIGGER PICTURE IN MIND

I must first warn readers that the list of WHMS symptoms and their apparent strangeness can convey the wrong impression: The symptoms and the syndrome as a whole can appear much more menacing and incapacitating than is inevitably the case in the lives of many of the women who experience them. It is important to remember the bigger picture with respect to this syndrome: *The WHM Syndrome has escaped detection by others for all these years because it does not for the most part produce enormous decrements in performance. In most women it represents a disorder of fine-tuning, not a breakdown.* Most women keep on leading quite normal lives around the symptoms. Women's reactions that they are "losing it" can come as much from not knowing what is happening and dire fears of what their momentary glitches will ultimately lead to as from the direct impact of the symptoms themselves. "I'm falling apart at the seams" declarations are often a form of appropriate "catastrophizing" projections of what may plausibly happen in the future in light of what is unexpectedly happening at the moment—fears of Alzheimer's disease or brain tumors, or losing a critical balance of self-control over one's life, or a reaction to a particularly distressing WHMS symptom episode.

Once women know what the symptoms represent they are mainly manageable and tolerable for many but not all women, except for certain left-over common residues: the anticipatory anxiety their unpredictability can evoke over a span of time in important situations—the fear of saying something wrong when standing up to speak; the occasional momentary embarrassment they can produce; the temporary sense of frustration they can evoke in people who want to get things done the right way "this exact moment"; the lack of self-command they imply to oneself and, women fear, to others; the sense of annoyance and self-diminishment they can evoke when they are more than minimally persistent.

One forty-nine-year-old woman I interviewed told me, after she read my *New York* magazine article, that she hated her verbal and memory "slips" and was full of self-loathing because of them. A lecturer on music at a community college who valued precision and loved her work, she said, "After I read the article I was much kinder to myself since I now felt the symptoms were understandable, excusable, and forgivable."

Another woman, a highly successful take-charge fifty-two-year-old businesswoman who prides herself on a whirlwind involvement in multiple projects on several fronts at once, told me after reading my article that whenever she misplaced something at home "in an instant" after putting it down, rather than customarily ranting and raving at herself in frustration at her seeming stupidity, she now instead shouted out loudly to her husband in self-vindication, "Hormones!" As if to say, "You see, it isn't me but this thing I'm going through that's making me act in this strange way." Thus, understanding the basis for the symptoms can lead to tolerance and self-forgiveness, replacing a reflexive sense of revulsion over encounters with an unfamiliar and ego-alien self.

OVERVIEW ON WHMS

As I've explained in chapter 1, Warga's Hormonal Misconnection Syndrome (WHMS) is a previously undescribed, as yet unrecognized, set of *subtle,* unusual, but *normal* symptoms that frequently occur in varying combinations in association with each other in the *inner* experiences of a significant proportion of normal women. The symptoms can *intermittently* affect the fine-tuning of multiple aspects of speech, and/or specific aspects of attention, concentration, thinking, memory-storage/encoding and retrieval, perception, face recognition, time awareness, and a wide range of other subtle behaviors, in *normal* women. The symptoms of the syndrome occur in association with estrogen loss *due to any cause* and may be the first and possibly only indicators of changes in ovarian functioning and estrogen loss. The symptoms are outward markers heralding the progression to perimenopause and menopause, though the progression to menopause can take upward of a decade in some women.

These symptoms occur in many *but not all women.* They can most easily be understood in their *variability, pattern,* and *intermittency* of occurrence, by comparing them to another estrogen-loss–based symptom associated with the years surrounding menopause—hot flashes.

Hot flashes occur in some women not at all. In some they occur once, or only fleetingly and never again. In some women they occur frequently over an interval of months or years in an unpredictable intermittent manner that is an inner annoyance but not a major impediment to otherwise normal functioning. In some women they occur (when untreated) in great frequency for many, many years in a pattern that significantly disturbs, interferes with, and sometimes appreciably erodes a woman's quality of life. In some women they last for a few years while some continue to experience them intermittently into their seventies in an unpredictable manner or in association with stress.

WHMS IS OFTEN SELF-WITNESSED BUT OBSCURE TO MOST OTHERS

In contrast to hot flashes, most WHMS symptoms are not directly evident to outsiders, but are experienced by women only internally. This may lead some to doubt their existence. "Women who have none of the symptoms are often intolerant and doubt those that do," notes Long Island menopause expert Dr. Maurice Cohen. In the elaborated list of symptoms in the next chapter I indicate which symptoms can remain outside the awareness of others.

When the symptoms first occur it is not uncommon for women with WHMS to have the experience of stark amazement in watching themselves suddenly "putting on a bad show," behaving unintentionally, having unintended words pop out, or exhibiting off-the-mark momentary behaviors. Most outsiders, however, discount the symptoms they detect as momentary "glitches" due to fatigue or some other innocuous cause. Spouses, close coworkers, friends, or other family members seen daily often do become aware of the outward signs of some of the symptoms. They too can experience a sense of annoyance, frustration—and in the case of a spouse, life partner, or child—embarrassment through association from observing what is going on, without understanding what the "glitchy" behaviors mean, beyond personal fallibility or insufficient attention or motivation.

SYMPTOMS OCCUR MOST WHEN WOMEN ARE "JUST BEING"

The symptoms tend to occur most commonly but not exclusively when women are engaged in casual, "just coasting," or "automatic pilot" behaviors that don't involve much direct effort or active attention, such as walking from one room to another, walking on the street, doing laundry, or entering the house after an outing. The symptoms can frequently, but not invariably, be overridden by applying focused attention to what one is doing, through directed effort and active striving. For this reason the symptoms tend to occur with greater frequency in women's personal lives than in the workplace. It is quite possible therefore for women to manifest these symptoms at home or in other aspects of their personal lives while still performing more than capably in their professional lives or in jobs.

BASIS FOR THE SYMPTOMS IS ESTROGEN LOSS

The symptoms appear to result from the direct and indirect effects of estrogen loss on the thinking, perceiving, attention-bringing, speech-producing, retrieving, information-storing-and-processing parts of the brain. The many far-reaching direct and indirect new roles discovered for estrogen in the brain in recent years are consistent with potentially producing the broad spectrum of "ripples" in normal functioning, represented by the symptoms of the WHM Syndrome. (Because estrogen often "turns on" or "induces" the presence of many but not all progesterone receptors in the brain, some of the effects of estrogen may also be related to progesterone's joint action. Progesterone, however, for the most part, but not exclusively, is known to act biologically to "tone down" or down-regulate what estrogen "revs up." Both are ovarian hormones whose function declines with perimenopause and menopause. So when I am speaking about estrogen's actions it is plausible that progesterone to varying degrees may also be involved. Much still remains to be known about the subtleties of action of both of these hormones separately and together.)

CHANGES IN PRE-EXISTING INTEGRITY OF BRAIN SYSTEMS APPEAR TO UNDERLIE SYMPTOMS

The intermittent symptoms of WHMS appear to reflect "off the mark" or desynchronized "connections" in parts of the mind and/or brain: alterations in the agility of the mind or brain to "access" necessary memory "files" and "commands" for carrying out specific behaviors and cognitive or perceptual processes with the same consistent "online" facility as previously experienced. This suggests changes in the integrity or "wholeness" of the subsystems involved in these functions. These alterations in "wholeness" may reflect changes in the "wiring" patterns or circuitry of brain neurons; changes in the chemistry underlying these functions, such as changes in neurotransmitter availability; changes in the supportive architectural structures of the brain underlying these specific behaviors and the processing of information and thinking subroutines; or combinations of such changes. These different types of proposed change are not inconsistent with what scientists now know to be associated with estrogen loss.

TYPES OF WHMS SYMPTOMS

The resulting "misconnections" can lead to different types of episodic or intermittent symptoms:

(1) *timing errors in retrieval:* halting, delayed, or absent retrieval ("forgetting") from memory, of information such as well-known names, old well-drilled knowledge such as spelling, one's Social Security and ATM numbers, faces, facts, words, ideas, long-established behaviors, location "maps" from one's experience

(2) *disordered execution of the mind's intent by the brain:* poor follow-through of what one's mind intends to say and do, a seeming change in the efficiency of the support "staff" serving a mind that has intentions; errors in the content of speech and behavior that appear to represent

"retrieval from a neighboring, related, but ultimately wrong 'bin' in the brain"; what I term as verbal and behavioral and navigational "malapropisms" (see below)

(3) *episodes of defective storage of new information:* due either to inconsistent "blinking" attention, or insufficient memory "ink" to imprint new learning or storage of information in the brain ("What did you just say?")

(4) *episodes of uncertainty in the realms of long-entrenched knowledge:* uncertainty about spelling, simple arithmetic, the names of one's children, etc.; tremors in the firmament of one's old fund of knowledge

(5) *less-consistently active monitoring than before of one's self, one's "I,"* within one's environment and of one's context; amnesia-like blackouts of short duration ("Where did 'I' just put my . . .?")

(6) *temporary "tremors" in the "automaticness" of behaviors* long considered almost "reflex" (within an overall pattern of ongoing competence); brief tremors in the usual coordination of driving skill routines, how to turn on one's computer, how to work one's microscope, etc.

(7) *changes in internal "clock-watching" agility* for anticipating or monitoring or recalling events of personal relevance

(8) *changes in one's baseline pattern of subtle motivations or predilections*

WHAT THE SYNDROME IS NOT AND WHAT IT MIGHT BE

WHMS typically does not affect or dominate a woman's overall judgment, reasoning, or logic. The symptoms represent a disorder of fine-tuning, in the sense of a functioning complex machine being in need of a "tune-up." The synchronization and timing involved in some *restricted* aspects of thinking, speaking, and behaving may be affected *intermittently,* though *the overall ability to think, act, and function in the necessary realms of daily life persist* in most women.

The syndrome also does not typically affect a woman's core personality except when emotional reactions to the symptoms, fears about their cause or meaning, or their effects on daily life profoundly color a woman's prevailing mood. Depression and anxiety can arise as a result of experiencing the symptoms, in addition to potential mood changes brought about by the neurotransmitter changes induced by estrogen loss alone.

Unlike early Alzheimer's disease patients, women with WHMS typically are not "confused" per se in the face of their mistakes. They are most often aware of their symptoms and are usually embarrassed front-seat spectators to their unusual performance rather than unmindful or uncaring about it.

It is possible that the symptoms of WHMS may somehow reflect a positive rearrangement, a shift to an altered balance of cognitive, perceptual skills in women that offer their own adaptive compensations: perhaps seeing better the "bigger picture" more than the specific details, or becoming better at spatial learning if not necessarily spatial memory, or other such shifts. I do not know if this is inevitably the case, but in view of available research related to this area I urge both women and researchers to be on the lookout for such possibilities in trying to understand what may be occurring in association with WHMS symptoms. One fifty-two-year-old woman I interviewed for this book, a music professor with a "three-ring circus" of life-disrupting perimenopausal symptoms, reported being amazed to have suddenly hit upon multiple effective new ways of teaching material she has taught for twenty-five years. She actively speculated about the possibility of some such shift in her own case. She could think of no ready explanations for her new problem-solving facility in this well-rehearsed area.

ONSET/DURATION OF THE SYMPTOMS

Based on the present extent of my interviews, it appears that WHMS symptoms can occur up to twelve years before the onset of menopause (defined here and commonly as twelve months without a period) and can either fade over time or persist in varying combinations and patterns of frequency for variable lengths of time, and in some women for decades after the onset of menopause.

At present no one knows how long the symptoms of the syndrome typically last. Given the normal degree of variability among women in the area of reproduction-associated biological changes, large numbers of women need to be evaluated before estimates on "average length of symptom duration" can be made. It is now not known whether the symptoms represent temporary "adjustment" reactions to a period of changing and unstable hormonal activity, as with adolescent hormonal changes around the time of puberty, or if they represent an enduring hormone deficiency state. No one really knows yet if the symptoms in some women progress over time, fade, and reappear years later, as do hot flashes in some women, or are associated in a predictive manner with any other disease state, just as no one yet knows what frequent hot flashes predict. At present insufficient information exists about whether the symptoms as they occur in women naturalistically are permanent, temporary, cyclic, or progressive.

In terms of my own observations I have witnessed verbal mala-propisms as a symptom persisting relatively unchanged in frequency over the span of thirty-five years without noticeable progression in one woman now in her eighties. I have also observed a relatively stable form of absentminded forgetfulness in misplacing objects, dating to at least forty years that has remained relatively stable in another woman now aged eighty-three.

At present no one knows whether any of the changes associated with the WHM Syndrome as they occur in midlife are at all predictive of developing Alzheimer's disease later in life. This is an important added reason for drawing attention to this syndrome. It is conceivable that knowledge about the consequences associated with the WHM Syndrome might *theoretically*—only theoretically—play a role in preventing later Alzheimer's disease and in averting the expected public health disaster epidemiologists now anticipate thirty or so years from now.

TYPES OF WOMEN WITH RESPECT TO WHMS SYMPTOMS

As with hot flashes, there are different types of perimenopausal and menopausal women with respect to WHMS symptoms:

The "Nevers"

There are women who never experience WHMS symptoms just as some perimenopausal and menopausal women never experience hot flashes or nighttime awakenings, etc.

The "Almost-Nevers"

These are the women who get flashes of WHMS symptoms only once, or so intermittently that the symptoms have little or no impact on their lives. Even this category of very mildly affected women can nonetheless worry about incipient Alzheimer's disease. The even fleeting tremors in their cognitive firmament set off worries of looming Alzheimer's disease. One women who fits this category, an educational consultant, now fifty-seven, with fleeting WHMS symptoms over a ten-year span, explained her reaction to me in this way. She said, "You know, you read about Alzheimer's in the news all the time. People talk about their parents. It's a real scare. I still get a jolt thinking it might be Alzheimer's disease, even after all these years [of getting only occasional symptoms that haven't gotten worse over time, e.g., spelling uncertainty episodes in a formerly great speller, forgetting a child's name, etc.]"

The "Worried Well" (Without Major Quality-of-Life Changes)

These women experience an on/off flutter of symptoms regularly that aren't evident to most outsiders and that don't disrupt the overall quality of life in any *major* way, but who are distressed by the symptoms nevertheless and may experience added stress coping and managing well around them. Such women often begin to circumscribe their lives, by protectively guarding themselves against situations that may reveal to themselves and others what limitations they might have. They worry where all this will lead.

The "Worried Not-Well" (Suffering Major Quality-of-Life Changes)

These are women whose combination of, or frequency of, symptoms are interfering with their personal and/or professional lives and who can't successfully "cover for" or work around their symptoms. Their sense of effectiveness of self is significantly compromised by the symptoms (possibly interacting with the high demands of their lives). This group can include those who are forced to significantly change their jobs or personal lives as a result of the symptoms and who live with realistic fears that this may happen, or with the chronic fear that they may not be able to hold it all together in some foreseeable frightening future and become insentient. High demands for precision performance in the lives of some of these women may make their otherwise not-terrible symptoms have more serious costs and consequences.

In regard to this latter category of women I think of the rather shocking statistic brought to my attention by Dr. Johanna S. Archer of the Department of Obstetrics and Gynecology of the Medical University of South Carolina, in Charleston. In a forthcoming article elucidating in part some of the neurotransmitter changes biologically associated with estrogen loss she writes: "Investigators [discussing perimenopause] have shown a greater incidence of psychological symptoms in women forty-five to forty-nine years of age with *a peak suicide rate during this period*. There is no corresponding suicide peak in men at the same age [emphasis added]."

While speculative interpretations of this statistic are possible, it is not entirely implausible to wonder whether these "psychological symptoms" and the peak suicide rate during these years of high WHMS likelihood may not reflect the experiences of "Worried Not-Well" (Suffering Major Quality-of-Life Changes) women with WHMS symptoms whose lives are going under, who don't understand what is happening to them and feel helpless and hopeless about their prospects in the present and future. My suspicion is that women who are self-supporting, or in precision-demanding jobs, or who are highly vested in continued high-level cognitive functioning would be most at risk for such suicidal ideation. Since WHMS has never been identified before, it may be an overlooked causative or disposing factor in women of this age group who have committed or unsuccessfully attempted suicide and warrants both active retrospective and prospective investigation. It is also possible that during this time of life biologically induced depression resulting from the effects of estrogen loss on the neurotransmitters specifically associated with depression may also be a direct or interacting factor in this sad statistic, disposing women to more suicidal ideation at this time of life or more hopelessness in reaction to experiencing WHMS symptoms.

Based on my interviews with women to date, I estimate that the least common groups of women with respect to WHMS symptoms are the two extreme groups, the "Nevers" and the "Worried Not-Well." Dr. Maurice Cohen, who specializes in treating perimenopausal and menopausal women on the North Shore of Long Island in New York and is in my view "tuned in" to the subtle experiences of women at this time, estimates on the basis of his experience of women who complain of cognitive/behavioral symptoms at this time of life that "One third experience no symptoms—they just breeze right through perimenopause and menopause, one third experience mild, not very distressing, symptoms, while one third experience more than mild symptoms that are more than mildly disruptive in their lives."

IS IT A ONE-RING, TWO-RING, OR THREE-RING CIRCUS OF SYMPTOMS?

In order to understand the experiences of women with respect to WHMS during the perimenopausal and menopausal years, it's critical to know whether women are experiencing predominantly only WHMS symptoms as Katherine Kennedy did, or a combination of other potential classes of symptoms associated with estrogen loss that can produce vastly different kinds of subjective and disruptive experiences: namely *physical symptoms,* such as hot flashes, sleep disruptions unrelated to hot flashes, heart palpitations, panic disorder, fatigue of unknown cause, vaginal dryness and itchiness, urinary incontinence, new aches in hips and joints, and/or a variety of potential *mood-altering symptoms,* such as short-temperedness or irritability, grouchiness or anger, emotional flatness or depression, unpredictable bouts of tearfulness or crying, suicidal thoughts, disaffiliation (wanting to be alone), etc.

I consider having any one set of symptoms "a one-ring circus," two sets of symptoms "a two-ring circus," and all three types of symptoms "a three-ring circus." Some women experience *only* WHMS, or *only* emotional, or *only* physical symptoms during these years. Some experience two of these categories sequentially, but not at the same time (i.e., peri-menopausal and menopausal changes can shift over a span of years somewhat like weather fronts). Some experience all three categories—WHMS, *and* physical, *and* emotional symptoms, at different but not overlapping times.

For some women experiencing even *all three* categories of symptoms at overlapping times may produce nonetheless only a mild "bigger" picture overall—again because the symptoms aren't present most of the time or because they may be inconsequential in terms of their impact on daily living.

For some women, however, having all three sets of symptoms at once can be highly destructive to a sense of control over one's life and can sometimes be associated with thoughts of suicide: either as a result of suffering from experiencing the interference of all the symptoms, or as a potential estrogen-loss–based mood-altering symptom itself. (Author Marcia Lawrence in her book *Menopause and Madness* describes what this can feel like.)

The case of Patricia Estrich vividly demonstrates what a "three-ring circus" of perimenopausal or menopausal symptoms can feel like from within, in association with WHMS symptoms. The "three-ring circus" includes accompanying thyroid dysfunction and suicidal thoughts.

A Case of a Three-Ring Circus of Symptoms

Case 5: Patricia Estrich: "Worried Not-Well" (Suffering Major Quality-of-Life Changes)

The following case is intriguing because it illustrates what a three-ring circus of symptoms can feel like but also because thyroid complications, themselves not uncommon during the age-span of menopause, were intermixed in the total picture.

Patricia Estrich (an alias) is now forty-nine. Her symptoms began at age forty-three. She now works full-time providing direct care to infants for a state agency. She is married and the mother of four children, two adult children from a first marriage and two children from a second marriage, now aged seven and eight. She was referred to me by a menopause expert, a physician familiar with the cognitive symptoms that can accompany perimenopause and menopause.

Reproductive State: perimenopausal when WHMS began.

For me it all began with irritability at age forty-three. Everything made me critical—the dog barking, a car horn going off. I wanted to scream when I heard these. My older kids were then young adults and the sound of the motor running when they got in the car felt unusually loud and irritated me to no end. They said I was very short-tempered with them and yelled at them for practically anything. This was not how I had been before.

I also started to get depressed for no reason at this time. My husband would try to get me out of it—he's a bit of a comedian but I didn't *want* to get out of it. Just a dark mood would come over me so that I felt sorry for myself. I wanted to cry and didn't know why. I wanted to be left alone to brood till I was ready to come out of it. I had no idea what to make of it. I thought it would all pass and be gone.

When this began I was still menstruating regularly. Then at age forty-four, one month I just stopped for three months and then it came back. First I thought I was pregnant—bad news—my older kids were sixteen and seventeen. Then I thought it was an illness, a tumor, a cancer or something. I wanted the doctor to just fix what was wrong with me.

Then new symptoms started. Sleeplessness. I'd go for three days and three nights and not sleep. I didn't have hot flashes at this point. I could have these sleepless bouts every other week regularly. I was tired and wanted to sleep but couldn't. Later on I started having hot flashes too. I'd sleep for five minutes, get hot, and feel as if there was a pile of hot ashes on the bed—like someone had set a fire under the bed. Once it was five degrees outside and I had the air conditioner on.

When I started to experience palpitations and chest pain my husband said maybe I needed a vacation and we went to Nassau for one week where all I did was sleep the whole week. I felt relaxed. But when we returned at the airport the minute we landed suddenly the palpitations and chest pain returned.

I thought maybe this was all about stress though that didn't make sense in my life overall. Nothing much had changed. What was real stressful were these *things* happening to me. So when we came back I went to a heart specialist. He came up with a diagnosis of hyperthyroidism, and I got treated for two years for that and lost sixty pounds. The palpitations went away when I had radiation treatments for the hyperthyroidism.

Between the ages of forty-four and forty-eight I would have tests for menopause every six months. I'd have my period, then it would go away again. Last year the tests said I was menopausal.

Even after I got treated for hyperthyroidism I was still restless. I just couldn't relax and watch TV. I would just jump up all the time to do something. It was unreal and I knew it. I felt guilty; I had to be doing something. Doing laundry I'd done before. In the middle of the night I would mop the kitchen floor and clean out cabinets and fold laundry. My mind would be racing, planning what I would do next. I felt like my mind wouldn't shut down. The hot flashes were going on at this time and I would open the freezer and stick my head in. My husband thought I was nuts. He'd be buried under a blanket and I'd be drenched on top of it. I was working as a cosmetician then and I could barely concentrate on any one thing because my mind was racing. It didn't affect my work, however. At work with the hot flashes I had an assistant who would mop my face. It was like in an operating room.

Around this time I got disinterested in sex. It was something to see the change in me. I also started forgetting my kids' names. I would call all their names before I'd get to the right one and I had never done that before. I'd go to call someone [on the telephone] and then forget who I went to call by the time I picked up the phone. Often I'd be calling my best friend. For eight years we talked daily. By the time I'd realize who I went to call I'd forget my best friend's telephone number. So I had to go to the book and look it up. I started figuring maybe it's just old age. It started getting scary.

Around this time I also started having problems with being in crowds and going to the mall and I stopped doing it. Just to be in a crowd got me paranoid. I felt people were watching me, or if I heard laughing in a crowd I thought it was directed at me. I got so anxious in crowds I couldn't breathe and would have to go outside. It happened if I was alone.

Another time I got lost in the mall and cried like a child. *I used to work in that mall.* I knew it like the back of my hand. I saw kids watching me and got embarrassed. It lasted five minutes. I stopped going to the mall after that. I had been at that mall for ten years and worked there for one year.

A doctor I was going to then gave me a videotape about estrogen because he thought I might want to go on it. But I heard all the controversy about taking it and was afraid to. I would talk to the women I worked with as a cosmetician. A friend there told me she felt better than ever in her life after she started taking it. She said she had so much energy. She said she was able to sleep finally. She had no more hot flashes. She said, "I'd rather feel good now and take my chances with cancer later." But I still was afraid of taking it.

Then I started getting more symptoms. Since I was thirteen I've read one novel a week. All of a sudden I couldn't concentrate enough to read. I would have five books waiting to be read and just started reading less. I'm not a TV watcher and don't go to movies so it was a problem.

Then I started having more of what I call the "What am I doing here? phenomenon." I'd go upstairs to get what I want, forget what it was when I got there, backtrack, remember, and go up again and maybe do that again. I'd done this before every now and then but it just got more noticeable and common. The strange thing is that I'd do that at home but not at work. At work everything has to be just right even more than at home. I'm a perfectionist and if a vase or coffee table is not in the right place I get irritated and have to have it be in the right spot. My family likes things lived in but I don't.

I forgot to tell you that when all these symptoms started it got so that my words got jumbled. I thought at first it was a stroke—they run in my family. But it wasn't. With my adult daughter if I tried to tell her a story the words didn't seem to come out right. I'd be jumping around. I couldn't put a sentence together. I thought I was crazy.

Another thing that happened was I wanted to leave my husband.

For no reason. Just because of the way I was feeling. I didn't want to be around anyone. I wanted to be by myself where no one knew me. It didn't make sense logically. My husband is a wonderful guy but I just didn't want to be around him. I wanted to leave him. I was telling this to a friend at the time and she confessed she felt the same way. She wanted to leave her kids who meant everything to her. She was as crazy as I was.

I confessed these feelings to my old doctor and he sent me to a doctor for psychotherapy and told me not to act on what I felt till I spoke to the doctor. I told my husband what I was feeling and he said, "Fight it, fight it, fight it." I didn't act on my feelings.

The symptoms went on for five years till last year, when I went on estrogen therapy. To me those years were hell. I thought that I would be like that the rest of my life. I thought about suicide a lot. I didn't want to feel like that. I knew I hadn't felt that way before so why now? I disliked my kids—my kids are my life—but I disliked them so much. They were noisy, they had fun. I wasn't having any. I didn't like my husband. He's very relaxed and a comedian. I felt he should be feeling what I was feeling. With wanting to kill myself I thought maybe if I killed myself they would feel sorry for me. I wanted to make them feel what I was feeling. I had no plan but I did go so far as to write a note to my husband and children one time. I wanted to die but was afraid to die.

A lot of this was the depression. The hot flashes and the depression were the worst part of it. One year it lasted like that at its worst with wanting to kill myself.

An endocrinologist eventually turned me on to Dr. D. who saved my life. The endocrinologist first put me on thyroid medication for some of my symptoms. But they found I was losing so much estrogen, even though I wasn't really menopausal yet, that they put me on low-dose replacement estrogen and that slowed down my thyroid into the normal range. Somehow they work together. That's how I got to Dr. D. He gave me a low-dose weekly patch of estrogen and had me take Provera [a progesterone] the first twelve days of the month. I hadn't had a period for a long time and suddenly had one again on the fifteenth of the month. Within a month I felt better, like my old self—100 percent better. The hot flashes stopped. I wasn't tired. I wasn't irritable. I was smiling. I could go to the mall. The depression lifted as well. I had been taking everything too seriously. It was my body. I said to Dr. D. I feel I could kiss you. I feel great now. So far I haven't had any side effects from the estrogen.

During those years I felt like I wasn't myself. I also didn't like myself the way I was. I felt like I was on the outside looking on at what was happening to me.

Another gynecologist I went to before I got to Dr. D. wasn't at all sympathetic. He felt it was me, not my body, that was causing all the trouble.

It was distressing to see my mind wasn't working well. Sometimes I felt hazy a little. My older son said to me one time, "I'm talking to you but you don't hear me." I wasn't concentrating. I did that a lot. He always let me know what he was feeling. He'd point that out to me. He'd say "Talk to me. Talk to me" when I was like that. The memory problems were interesting but not very bothersome. I could work around them in my everyday life. I thought they were a sign of aging. I didn't think along the lines of menopause. I have an aunt who raised me who had Alzheimer's and I thought maybe it was that. During that time, I would have sold my soul to the devil for a good night's sleep when it was at its worst. I would sleep for five minutes and feel like I'd slept all night and then I'd wake up. But the next day I'd feel exhausted. My mind felt as if it were telling me I'd had enough sleep but my mind and body were sending different signals and drawing different conclusions. My friend had this too.

TREATMENT OF WHMS IS AN ART

As you've seen in the case of Polly Van Benthusen and the accounts of different women cited so far, WHMS symptoms are frequently responsive to either estrogen-replacement therapy (usually taken in association with progesterone) or, in the case of some perimenopausal women, to low-dose birth-control estrogen/progesterone pills (they have considerably higher doses of estrogen in them). However, not infrequently women require adjustments to different doses over the course of perimenopause or menopause, or to different brands, or to different balances between estrogen and progesterone. Among those few physicians who are familiar with WHMS symptoms, it appears to be the rule that treatment in this area is an art rather than a science in which women's *symptoms* are the target of treatment and not their "numbers"—their blood test or hormone test numbers.

At present much remains to be known about which intensities and forms of estrogen work best for which kinds of women, or for which specific WHMS symptoms.

Although plant-based estrogens, phytoestrogens, such as those in soy-based products, have not specifically been used to address WHMS-like symptoms to my knowledge, there is reason to suspect that such forms of treatment may prove helpful in relieving WHMS symptoms. Time and further research will tell. (See chapter 11 for more discussions of these treatment options.)

In view of the growing list of roles and functions of estrogen in the brain, it is quite possible that nonhormonal and even over-the-counter substances that replace the functions typically served by estrogen in the brain in women experiencing estrogen loss may also help reverse WHMS symptoms. I hope future research will examine these options. I describe some of these possibilities in chapter 11.

There is also reason to suspect that thyroid disregulation, both too high as in the case of Patricia Estrich, or too little as in hypothyroidism may in some women affect some WHMS symptoms. Women with WHMS should thus be routinely tested for these possibilities. I also believe that double-blind placebo-controlled studies should be undertaken to establish whether empirical short-term trial treatments with thyroid medications improve WHMS symptoms appreciably.

WHO ELSE CAN GET WHMS SYNDROME?

While WHMS most commonly occurs in perimenopausal and menopausal women, I believe it can occur among *any women experiencing estrogen loss*. These can include: (1) women experiencing a total hysterectomy in which the estrogen-producing ovaries also are removed—a procedure known as oophorectomy; (2) women with premature ovarian failure—their ovaries simply stop working; (3) women being treated for fibroids with anti-estrogenic medications; (4) women with cancer being treated with chemotherapy or radiation treatments that compromise the functioning of their ovaries and therefore estrogen production (not all women treated with chemotherapy or radiation, however, inevitably develop ovarian/hormonal changes); (5) women being treated for endometriosis with estrogen-suppressing medications; (6) women who have had surgery, such as tubal ligation, that may have compromised the blood supply to, and nerve supply of, their ovaries; and (7) as I have discovered, women who consistently breast-feed after giving birth for the first six to twelve months. (See below for an explanation.)

It is my present untested hypothesis—a suspicion based on a number of interviews and a reading of the research literature—that women with PMS may also routinely experience some or even many features of WHMS symptoms during their premenstrual phase. Research now suggests that despite apparently normal hormonal levels these women may be uniquely sensitive biologically to intervals of their normal menstrual cycle when estrogen levels are routinely low (the luteal phase). I believe this group of women needs to be evaluated to see if they experience WHMS symptoms during this monthly time interval.

The same unique biological sensitivity to low estrogen levels is also suspected as a causative factor in women who develop postpartum depression. These women too are suspected of being biologically distinct in being atypically sensitive to low estrogen levels. They too, I suggest, may need to be screened for possibly experiencing WHMS symptoms. These women, and indeed all women, after delivery experience a sudden sharp drop in estrogen availability after birth when they expel their estrogen-supplying placenta. Women with postpartum depression may be particularly sensitive to such abrupt changes. Pregnant women typically from the end of the third month of pregnancy onward receive their supplies of estrogen from the placenta, not primarily the ovaries as is the case during the first trimester, and before pregnancy. In women with postpartum depression it is suspected that when estrogen supplies (and, I propose, associated neurotransmitter supplies) fall below some "set point" these estrogen-sensitive women may experience mood and physical estrogen-loss symptoms and, I propose, the cognitive/behavioral symptoms of WHMS that are associated with estrogen loss.

BREAST-FEEDING IS ASSOCIATED WITH WHMS SYMPTOMS

It may come as a surprise to read about breast-feeding in a book on peri-menopause and menopause but I believe I have made the discovery that other women who commonly experience many—I don't know yet if all—WHMS symptoms are breast-feeding women who don't use supplemental bottle feedings. In women who feed their infants only with breast milk, unsupplemented by other sources of nourishment, the ovaries typically do not turn "on" to supply women with estrogen after the placenta is expelled, for some eight to ten or twelve months after they begin breast-feeding (this interval apparently varies among women).

I was first alerted to the estrogen-deprived nature of breast-feeding women in an inadvertent comment by ob/gyn and reproductive endocrinologist Dr. John Arpels, associate clinical professor of obstetrics, gynecology and reproductive medicine at the University of California, during an interview in early 1997 and didn't know initially what to make of the fact. An incident with a suddenly forgetful breast-feeding neighbor, however, reminded me of this little-known fact of biology and led to my informal and formal interviews with breast-feeding women. (Others need to confirm these findings but I have a good measure of confidence in their ultimately being proven true.)

My interviews with breast-feeding women who have had multiple children have revealed that women experience WHMS symptoms during the first eight to ten months after they breast-feed and then experience a return to what appears to be, and may actually be, cognitive normality, after each child. (At eight to ten months, infants may be eating solid foods more and/or sleeping longer. The decline in the frequency of suckling is suspected of being a trigger signaling the ovaries to again "kick in.")

I use the existence of WHMS symptoms in breast-feeding women and the successive returns to normality after WHMS in women with multiple children to argue that WHMS symptoms in perimenopausal and menopausal women are "normal" since I think it unlikely that "nature" would harm or impair women in a seriously detrimental manner while engaged in the critical task of nurturing and assuring the survival of the species. Whether breast-feeding women overlap entirely, or predominantly, or only selectively in the symptoms of WHMS they share with perimenopausal and menopausal women remains to be researched.

WHMS and Breast-Feeding "Mommie Mind"

Sharp-witted political pundit Mary Matalin, a major strategist on George Bush's 1988 and 1992 campaigns, the wife of political strategist James Carville and the mother of two young children, not long ago was quoted in the Sunday *New York Times Magazine* about the cognitive surprises after the birth of a child. She was quoted as saying, "There's a new study . . . [that describes brain changes during pregnancy.] So there's a definitive explanation for the stupidity that sets in when you have a baby. . . . But I'd say the brain death is one of the biggest surprises. I remember sitting on the front porch with my new infant in my arms, crying hideously while singing to her. . . . What was that about?"

The illustrative case below—I have more—may offer a clue to what Mary Matalin may have been experiencing. It presents an instance of a breast-feeding woman reporting cognitive WHMS-like changes in association with consistent nonsupplemented breast-feeding.

Some may choose to dismiss this case and others like it as either subjective impressionistic blather, characterizing it as anecdotal instead of clinical evidence, or as the likely consequence of life events such as being sleep-deprived and fatigued from raising small children—and not as biologically based. I say life is complicated and difficult to disentangle; it's hard to detect the biological in the welter of environmental and psychosocial factors *always* operant in a life. If biological factors also exist and are not looked for they won't be found. I suggest it is time to really listen well to women. Women haven't been listened to well enough in the past and are the best candidates for reporting what they experience. They are the most "plugged in" to the nuances of their functioning. For hard-nosed researchers, I suggest that they first gather extensive "firsthand" data (described by some as subjective) on the breadth of the terrain they need to cover and later devise more rigorous validation methods for measuring the variables women tell them are changing with different hormonal stages. If they don't find what women tell them is there I urge them first to doubt the sensitivity of their measures rather than dismiss what women say. It is my suspicion that just as WHMS symptoms in perimenopausal and menopausal women have been too often "written off" as due to life events, diet, or other nonbiological factors, the tendency to not look further than the obvious disruptions of raising young children has obscured the discovery by others of WHMS-like symptoms in breast-feeding women too. I strongly suspect that researchers (I hope to be among them) who compare breast-feeding women with those who only bottle-feed their infants will discover important differences between these groups on WHMS symptoms, if they use appropriately sensitive tests to look for differences or conduct in-depth standardized interviews.

I also think it is worth wondering actively whether the lack of interest in sex after childbirth that some women experience, certainly understandable in terms of the physical trauma of birth and preoccupation with child rearing, may not also possibly be related to estrogen loss and the similar lack of interest in sex some women experience during perimenopause and menopause also in relation to estrogen deprivation. Consistently breast-feeding women too are estrogen-deprived, for at least a good part of the first year after delivery. Comparing breast-feeding women with nonbreast-feeding women with young children, on their comparative interest in sex, would be yet another important study for researchers to do.

The Solution to WHMS During Continual Breast-feeding

The solution to WHMS symptoms during continual breast-feeding, it would seem (for those women who find it too compromising an experience), is to get their ovaries to "turn on" and start supplying estrogen again to the brain. How? Very simply. By starting out supplementing their breast-feeding with bottles early on—formula milk or quite possibly even self-expressed milk. They can return to full-time breast-feeding again, I suspect, after their ovaries have turned on. Breast-feeding, to judge by my interviews and the account below, apparently still "works" well even after women's periods return, i.e., their ovaries turn on and produce estrogen again.

Women who work and don't breast-feed exclusively, judging by my interviews, appear to have their ovaries "kick in" early and don't experience WHMS symptoms to the same degree or for lengthy intervals. This of course needs to be evaluated too with research.

Pregnant women need to be informed about what they are likely to experience after childbirth if they plan to breast-feed consistently. They need to be informed of their options, so they can exert control in their lives and not plan, as one consistently breast-feeding new mother with WHMS did, to set the date to defend her doctoral dissertation shortly after the birth of her child when she discovered she had a mind in a state of drifting fog.

The Case of a Breast-feeding Woman

Olivia Johan is a thirty-five-year-old, former talk-show radio producer who has breast-fed two children, her daughter now four and a half, for twenty-eight months, and a fourteen-month-old son she has been breast-feeding since birth and was still doing at the time of our interview.

We call it "mommie mind," my friends and I [the cognitive/behavioral/speech symptoms]. I don't know any woman who is breast-feeding who hasn't had it and I know about fifteen women who have or are now breast-feeding. I don't have a complete thought now. I lose my train of thought in an instant, and it's the same whether I get a good night's sleep or not. I don't think it has much at all to do with sleep. When I was breast-feeding my daughter the veil on how my mind was working lifted slightly after the first twelve months. I had some of the same symptoms during pregnancy—probably during the third to fourth month it started. But breast-feeding forgetfulness is different from pregnancy forgetfulness. It's much more severe and drastic than in pregnancy. My husband will ask me to pick something up during the day and I just forget over and over. You feel stupid. I find that husbands don't understand [what's happening]. They think you're not as smart as you used to be.

My husband is quite wonderful but I don't feel now I'm capable of being as organized as he expects me to be. Organization has never been one of my strong suits but with a regular brain I could do things. Now I often feel I can't think of where to begin a project. I used to be able to do this. Other women, we say to each other, we're not clear thinkers anymore. And it's not sleep deprivation. I can try to stay focused—that helps—the effort. But I try to get into a conversation with my husband and not drift, but I drift. He gets irritated and aggravated.

I feel when I'm forced to do something that I need to do I'm able to do it. In fact it's a good experience for my brain to do this interview. I find that women who go back to work part-time, their "mommie mind" is not as intense as mine. Something, the work or the effort, forces them to tune in more and they do. I lose my train of thought in a minute. I walk into a room and end up saying, "I came to get something, what was it?" When my train of thought is on its way out I can usually complete it; but if I have a thought and others are talking, if I don't jump on it I lose it. With friends I'm likely to say "let me just say this before I forget."

I got my period back after ten months of breast-feeding my daughter, and with my son now it came back at eight months. I'm very sensitive to my body. When I ovulate I find that I have a great fashion sense and a great vocabulary, and after ovulation, when whatever changes, I won't remember words and don't ask me to go shopping. I come back with the frumpiest outfits. Biologically what I think is happening is that my body is geared up to attract a mate during the first two weeks and then afterward when my fertile period is over I can look like Dowdy Dora. My spelling is fine the first two weeks of my cycle [estrogen high] and the last two weeks [estrogen low] it's awful. I recently couldn't remember how to spell "fourteen." I had to write our mortgage check and I couldn't remember how to spell it. This happens right before I get my period. I have PMS and I'm getting it again now that my period is back [even though she is breast-feeding].

With my daughter things got better cognitively; I became more like myself after twelve months of breast-feeding. I felt I wanted to stop then but my daughter developed allergies and she needed me to continue to avoid the allergies. Most everything came back after that year. I feared then that I'd be this way the rest of my life; I feared that I wouldn't have all of my faculties. I really worried about it. It was shocking to me [the first time breast-feeding] to go from being an independent productive person to being a mom who can't even have a grown-up conversation. It was very scary and depressing, this mind business. Not all my faculties came back. The first few years there were still the jokes "Well, I'd love to tell you that but I can't remember." But by the time my daughter was two I was a lot better.

In my [social] group I have two friends who aren't affected like the other three are this way, and they don't believe in this hormone thing or the PMS symptoms. They think it's all a matter of mind over matter. But they have both given birth in recent months and both become weepy when their milk comes in. They now believe that hormones can affect you. The experience can be like feeling wonderful and then in a turnaround second the lowest low. After my daughter was born I recall not being able to make my mom's airline reservations on the phone for her to come out to me because I couldn't—get this—say the words "departing flight." I would just burst out crying at the idea of the word "departing." I know it sounds crazy. I should tell you also that when I was breast-feeding my daughter during her first year I had the strangest experience. I had difficulty understanding speech in the movies and on the radio—anything that was broadcast. It sounded garbled. I just couldn't make sense of it. I saw lips moving but didn't understand the words. I didn't have this trouble with people speaking in real life. At first I thought there was something wrong with my hearing. But that didn't seem to be it. It went away when I got my period back. I thought maybe I was going to need a hearing aid at one point. It hasn't happened with my son.

My friend who's breast-feeding—we laughed the other day. She said about her son, "I like to give him carrots for the 'ketaberateen.'" She meant beta-carotene. I don't do that but I find myself saying "whatchamacallit" a lot more than I used to and having either words or ideas I want to get out be stuck on the "tip of my tongue." I lose my train of thought now at the drop of a hat. I also keep putting crazy things into the refrigerator and say to myself "Stop that—that doesn't go in the refrigerator." When I fill up the baby bottle with apple juice I'm constantly putting the wrong caps on the bottle and the juice."

There's more: I was always great at recognizing faces but this year I can't remember them. I also can't seem to decode "space spelling." My husband will ask me "Did you pick up the c-a-n-d-y?" and I can't decode what he's spelling. All this chips away at your self-esteem and makes you feel bad about yourself.

I'm reading more with this baby than the last but I will read an article and want to talk about it and can't remember anything about it. I have to really focus and review it to remember anything. Other times it's like the top of my head is cotton-headed. Like I'm in a fog. It's scary not to be able to make it go away when I want to. My father is irritated with my mother's difficulty in thinking clearly. She had six children and did not nurse any of us. She's sixty-eight. She's been that way for a long time. Our spouses are reflections of ourselves and if they look stupid we think *we* look stupid. My father says to my mother, "I'm mortified at your being this way." She's really very smart. She pronounces things incorrectly sometimes and my sister gets irritated at her. She thinks my mother's being sloppy in her speech and expects more from her. My mother had a hysterectomy at forty-one. I don't know if she ever took estrogen or not. What having this has done to my mom is that it inhibits her trying to learn new things. She's afraid of looking foolish and stupid. She seems to be afraid of challenging herself now. She won't try to figure out how to use the new washing machine, or how to pump gas. I was trying to teach her at a gas station so she wouldn't have to depend on my father, but she wouldn't do it. I know from being with her that she could but she won't.

Breast-feeding and WHMS Conclusions

The above facts and case provide added credibility to my contention that WHMS-like symptoms can occur in any state associated with estrogen deprivation (or in the instances of PMS and postpartum depression, in response to unusual sensitivity to estrogen-low states). However, I would greatly caution readers—and the public—or anyone in a position to discriminate against breast-feeding women against blatantly assuming that *all* breast-feeding women routinely experience WHMS symptoms. My contention is that this is likely to happen only in consistently breast-feeding women and not to all breast-feeding women. And it is likely to be easily remediable. Moreover, since women tend to vary enormously in so many different facets of reproduction-associated stages, there is likely to be considerable variability even among consistently breast-feeding women, in the extent to which WHMS symptoms are likely to become manifest.

My statements here are meant to be preliminary to further research in this area. It is my hope that knowledge about this important topic will empower women with knowledge and effective self-management choices, that it will leave them and their partners less in the dark about what may be occurring within the context of family life, with less potential loss of regard and self-regard, and with greater tolerance for the biology of the human condition.

7

The Symptoms: Warga's Hormonal Misconnection Syndrome (WHMS)

Now that you know who is at risk for WHMS, from a breast-feeding mother to a perimenopausal forty-two-year-old, to a woman in the flush of menopause at fifty-two, what are the symptoms and how do you recognize them? Here I will detail the *possible* symptoms that may occur during perimenopause and menopause. *Having one symptom need not imply that you will have any of the others.* Having several symptoms need not imply that you will have many of the others. The experiences of perimenopause and menopause, as noted earlier, are highly variable among women. The experience of your mother during perimenopause or menopause may or may not be relevant to what your experience of these stages will be. (However, checking out your mother's, sister's, or aunt's experiences with perimenopause and menopause may not be a bad idea, to give you a framework for possibilities and a sense of the range of variations possible among women.)

I believe that no one as yet knows how long WHMS symptoms persist and in what pattern and to what degree, in a *large* population of women. Anyone who tells you differently is basing an opinion on their own limited sample of experience. I also suspect that there are more symptoms yet to be discovered by others and myself. This is an emerging field. Before you assume you are crazy for suspecting that a symptom you have, which is not listed here, is associated with hormonal changes, assume instead that it has not yet been identified. There is much to be discovered and doctors, at least for now, do not in my experience have the last word in knowledge about this topic.

Awareness of WHMS-like symptoms as a *new* intermittent *pattern* in your life without plausible explanation should prompt you to go to an ob/gyn to start monitoring your hormone levels (1) as an external diagnostic "check" for what might be causing these symptoms and (2) to guide you in different possible treatment options, including the option of doing nothing but watching nature unfold. I discuss what diagnostic blood tests some experts believe are relevant to detecting hormonal changes in chapter 10 in a section on how doctors treat WHMS symptoms, and I discuss different treatment options for women who experience significant quality-of-life changes in association with WHMS symptoms in chapters 10, 11, and 12.

The reality seems to be that for some women, WHMS symptoms can occur before doctors can reliably detect the hormone changes *now* used to declare a woman is in perimenopause. So external confirmation of the hormone changes that may be causing a WHMS symptom may not always be possible, at least for now. More sensitive indicators of a woman's evolution from full fertility, to waning fertility, to absent fertility may need to be developed for such confirmation. If you do go for such tests it is important for you to be aware that perimenopause in general is known for highly fluctuating hormonal levels from month to month, so that the blood test readings of one month may hold little relationship to the hormonal readings the next month. Not all doctors, however, consistently give repeated tests. (This is why women who are told their hormones indicate they are perimenopausal sometimes find themselves unexpectedly pregnant. Several weeks after the last tests, their hormones may have reverted from the perimenopausal range to levels consistent with fertility for a time. Repeated testing over a span of months or years is a surer way of knowing if you are perimenopausal or menopausal.)

In the future, however, once WHMS-like symptoms are widely accepted, it is likely that other diagnostic tests for WHMS will be newly developed to supplant hormonal tests. These will, I suspect, be tests of brain function that will incorporate noninvasive brain-imaging scanning tests such as PET (positron emission tomography), functional MRI (magnetic resonance imaging), SPECT (single photon emission computed tomography), and yet other noninvasive brain scans. Together with standardized protocols these will be used to routinely watch the brain in action as it thinks, learns, "speaks," and "retrieves" information and memories. Such tests will be used for assessing over time the effectiveness of the mind and brain functionally and at the biological level, for establishing baseline "norms" for later comparisons, and for follow-up diagnostic and evaluation purposes, much in the way women are now evaluated on bone scans for their baseline and ongoing risks for osteoporosis at different body sites.

When I asked experts while researching this book if it would be desirable for younger women now to establish some "baseline hormonal profile readings" during their years of maximum ovarian/hormonal functioning, in the way we now ask women to get baseline mammograms, to use as a reference point for comparisons with later possible changes or to know what a woman's unique personal hormonal "best" was, they told me this would be difficult at present. It would be a cumbersome task requiring repeated testing over the course of a month, since women's estrogen and progesterone levels normally vary enormously during a typical monthly menstrual cycle in the peak years of fertility. Such tests would have to be taken numerous times over the course of a month to develop a reliable representative profile.

What all this means is that determining if your WHMS-like symptoms are due to hormonal changes may not now be an exact science. Medicine will have to catch up in finding objective measures to confirm the experiences of women when they say they are experiencing WHMS-like symptoms.

Here then are the symptoms of Warga's Hormonal Misconnection Syndrome. The symptoms fall into seven main categories: changes in thinking, speech, attention, short- and long-term memory, behavior, spatial/perceptual skills, and time sense. Individual symptoms could conceivably be shuffled into different patterns of organization.

THE SYMPTOMS OF WHMS

I. THINKING CHANGES

Flash episodes of:

1. Losing One's Train of Thought Midstream

Drawing "blanks" on what one was intending to say after having already begun to speak. This may represent greater distractability in attention or greater difficulty keeping something stored "in mind" (on the "scratch pad" of working memory) while following the train of one's thoughts. This symptom may be related in its underlying mechanism to the symptom of walking into a room and forgetting what one went to get. (See below.)

Example: Professor Katherine Kennedy, as described earlier, finds it frustrating to argue with her husband because she now finds she will lose her train of thought in the middle and be unable to make her point.

Example: Education professor Sally W., now sixty-four, says she has been losing her train of thought while teaching since before she became menopausal at fifty-four. When this happens in class now, she jokes about it and says she is having a "senior moment." In a cooperative venture, her students help set her back on course by "feeding her" her previous statements. "They know I'm a good teacher and we all laugh about it. It's humanizing," she says. "I take it in stride. I wish it didn't happen but it does." She says this doesn't deter her from continuing teaching, which she loves.

(Can be observed by others, but can be passed off as due to fatigue or sleep deprivation, etc.)

2. The "What Did I Come In Here For?" Sensation

A pattern of more frequent episodes of not being able to keep things in mind momentarily as efficiently while you do something else, i.e., walking into a room and forgetting what you came in to get or holding a series of numbers in your mind when asked to repeat them backward. The "scratch pad" of what is called "working memory" doesn't seem to hang on to what is briefly "put" on it. It sometimes erases what is on it quicker than in the past. This symptom may be related to losing one's train of thought in the act of speaking or thinking.

Example: Polly Van Benthusen says, "I'd be standing in the kitchen and yell to my husband 'Why am I here at the cupboard?' And he'd yell back, 'You needed oil for the skillet.' Or I'd go into the bedroom and say 'Why am I coming through here?' and eventually realize it was to put some things in the closet. It's like your mind goes out of gear."

Example: Dr. Elizabeth G., a forty-nine-year-old research scientist/physician with a twelve-year-old son says, "I found that as I walked from my lab to my office I would forget as many as eight times a day what I went in to get. It was becoming increasingly frustrating. I couldn't think of the words I needed when I needed them."

(Frequently not observable to others as a symptom.)

3. Less Consistent Agility in Concentrating with Focused Effort

Episodes of not being able to concentrate when one wants to "in an instant" as consistently as before. This symptom has been described as being not as intense a disruption as the next two symptoms: feeling foggy and thought blockade.

Example: Mona S., forty-eight, now finds that occasionally she can't get herself "in gear" when she specifically wants to concentrate on something she wants to dwell on. "It's almost as if my mind is in a 'daydreaming state,'" she says, "but I'm not daydreaming. It's sort of like spring fever. If I wait awhile it passes."

Example: Grace D., forty-seven, says, "I'm sort of struggling to figure out how to get my mind sharp [during moments when I can't concentrate]. It's really a nice feeling when the mind is sharp. It's a little unsettling to have it not be."

(Often not observable to others.)

4. Feeling "Foggy," "Hazy," "Cotton-Headed"

Episodes of feeling as though one is "thinking through cobwebs," experiencing "cloudiness." Not being able to think clearly when one wants to.

Example: Polly Van Benthusen: "It was like being drowsy. Almost like you want to shake your head to think. It was hard when I really needed to focus. Like being in a funk. I had to read things three times and I would get lost. It improved a great deal with the estrogen. Now I get a lot of stuff into my office and get on it and I don't even have to take a break; I can focus so well."

Example: Grace D., menopausal at forty-four, now forty-seven, says, "There are different tones to the fogginess. I have it now and feel tired and spacey. [She doesn't sound or look it.] Sometimes I'll feel like 'there's nothing up there.' I just have nothing to add to a group discussion. I just can't think [at that moment]. I probably should be asking people to repeat something . . . because I'm really not following. But I know it's not imperative to follow. So I just let it slide. People don't notice. After all, nobody talks all the time. So it's more internal. It's not readily apparent to others. It's another example of feeling like you're on the edge of craziness like I used to get with PMS. It's like more in your head, the craziness, than stuff people would know about."

(Often not observable to others.)

5. Thought Blockade: Inability to Think of Ideas on Demand

Experiencing flash moments when you feel that you can't access the part of your mind that lets you generate ideas at the moment you need to. Experiencing a thought blockade.

Example: Dr. Fredericka Xerov, now fifty-four, says, "There were times when I was first interning [as a genetics counselor], when I couldn't write notes on the sessions I had just had with patients. It was scary not being able to summon my ideas when I needed to. When I was being supervised I couldn't contribute to the group. I couldn't pull what was in me out. It was a great relief to see things change with estrogen."

Example: Polly Van Benthusen: "I've always been a great brainstormer, the ideas person, and I'd be in a meeting and for the moment felt as though I couldn't come up with a different idea. People would be stunned that I didn't have an idea. Now [after being on estrogen] I can come up with ideas all over the place and meet deadlines. It feels great to be able to do these things in the same way again."

(May be, but need not be, always observable to others. One can pass it off as due to fatigue, other isolated events that belie the presence of an intermittent pattern.)

6. Changes in Prioritizing Agility

Discrete episodes of experiencing oneself as requiring more conscious thought or time to sequence the necessary steps in a task requiring prioritizing skills. Less of an intuited sense of "This is the way I'm going to go about organizing *X*." Less of a "fully conceived answer" popping out or presenting itself. Those who experience this report that the ability to succeed in one's efforts is not necessarily diminished. The *approach* to going about this seems intermittently altered, however, compared to the past.

Example: Sherry Strumph says, "I feel I have more difficulty prioritizing things than before. I'm still very good at it but I feel there's a change in the directness with which I organized a task before."

Example: Phyllis R., forty-five, lives in a small studio apartment and reports never being a very organized person, but now she feels more overwhelmed by how to make order in her realm. "I don't seem to know where to begin and how to proceed at first."

(Often not detected by others when it occurs.)

II. CHANGES IN SPEECH

"Flash" episodes of:

1. Naming Difficulties

A pattern of brief episodes of not being able to think of the long-known names of things or people from one's *old fund of knowledge:* the name for geraniums, your children's names, your best friends' names (dysnomia). In these instances women say they don't have a clue as to what the right name might be but find instead a void with seemingly no associative links.

Example: Writer Anna Quindlen at age forty-five wrote: "[W]hen I began to wake bolt upright in the middle of the night and started forgetting the names of my children, I initially thought I was losing my mind not simply my fertility. . . ."

Example: Elizabeth Q., fifty, told me she walked into her long-ongoing reading group one evening and discovered she couldn't think of anyone's name. She had to wait till someone mentioned a member's name to "get" names that evening. She was shaken by this one event and worried it would happen again. Afterward she became anxious that this blanket loss of naming ability would be repeated and publicly revealed when it came to making social introductions.

Example: Mary W., at thirty-eight, found she suddenly had to run through each of her children's names before hitting upon the correct one more than in the past.

(This symptom can be detected by others but can often be attributed to social anxiety.)

2. Episodes of Finding Oneself at a Loss for Words

Finding oneself temporarily speechless—at a loss for words. Aberrant bouts of absent or halting speech when one intends to speak. Not being able to think of how to say what one wants to say. Not being able to find the words to express an intended idea. The words don't come the way they always have in the past. Sometimes other words can be found that approximate one's intent. Sometimes one remains stumped at how to convey the intended idea. Sometimes in one's struggle to convey the idea, off-the-mark approximations come out. There is less of a sense of precision in "knowing" what one wants to say than in the "tip of the tongue" sensation below.

Example: Katherine Kennedy, thirty-eight, says, "[A]t times I'm grasping for words in the middle of a conversation and I just can't find the words I need—it's like I'm running up against a brick wall. I know what I want to say but I can't. My mind feels like I'm shuffling around not finding what I want."

Example: Banker Cheryl Calhoun, fifty-two, says, "Before [taking estrogen] nothing would come to me in the split second that I needed it. You start looking for words and shuffling for other words. I would become afraid that I'd end up without a job staying at home in a bathrobe and chewing bonbons all day.

Example: Mary G., a graphic designer, age forty-three, was at an awards dinner at an elegant restaurant in connection with her husband's position as an editor. The organizer of the party, dressed in an evoca-tively romantic gown, had done an excellent job presenting awards and had been particularly charming to everyone. Upon leaving, Mary wanted to compliment the organizer on her fine performance and in-tended to say something like, "You seemed like the gracious hostess of an intimate salon." As she stood in front of her she suddenly found her-self at a loss for words, and in the awkwardness of the face-to-face situ-ation, grasping desperately for *any* words to express this idea, she heard herself say, "You looked like a . . . a . . . a . . . courtesan" to the some-what startled organizer.

(This symptom is sometimes observable to others, but often it is not. Those who experience it describe the experience from within as very strange and dislocating.)

3. "Tip of the Tongue" Phenomenon Difficulties

An increased frequency of brief episodes of the experience "I've got it right there on the tip of my tongue but I can't get it out." In this in-stance a nearly palpable sense of the word is present but the person can't get to it. The experience here is that the intended word is very close to being retrieved, more so than in other forms of word-finding difficulty.

Example: Harriet F., fifty-four, a homemaker, says, "Sometimes I've got what I want to say on the tip of my tongue only I can't get it out. It feels like it's sitting *right there* but I can't reach in and get it out. It can be incredibly frustrating to feel so helpless in doing such a simple thing."

Example: Elizabeth L., fifty-six, college administrator: "One week I thought I was going crazy. I had what I wanted to say on the tip of my tongue but over and over I couldn't get it out. I was certain I had Alzheimer's disease."

(Not often observable to others.)

4. Malapropisms: Wrong Words Popping Out

These are slips of the tongue that are related to the intended word in concept but are "off the mark." I think of these errors as misconnected retrieval, i.e., "retrieval from the wrong bin in the brain," retrieval from a neighboring but ultimately wrong *specific* bin in the brain.

The wrong word that pops out sometimes sounds similar (phonologically) to the intended word but need not always do so. Sometimes the two words sound different but still have related meanings (semantically). The malapropisms usually don't result from an effortful struggle to find the right word but are more reflexive and spontaneous than with word-loss symptoms. Malapropisms appear to differ from Freudian slips in that they don't usually have a truth-leaking, witty edge to them. Playwright Richard Sheridan who created the nearly fifty-year-old character Mrs. Malaprop, was apparently an astute observer!

Example: Sherry Strumph: "I said to myself [internally] 'You used to have a photogenic memory and then said 'You fool, you mean photographic. . . ." (The common concept is "photo.")

Example: Writer Letty Cottin Pogrebin, in her early fifties, stood up and said on one occasion before a different group, "Low-birth-weight babies tend to be born to women who have had no prenuptial care." She meant to say "prenatal." On another occasion she heard herself say, "In our synagogue we do a lot of congressional singing." She meant to say "congregational." The common concept is "large assemblies of people."

Example: Marilyn Evans, forty-seven, saw on TV the church in which her father had his funeral and announced to a friend: "That's where my father was euthanized." She meant to say "eulogized." The common concept is "death."

Example: Psychiatrist Janice S., fifty-one, was leaving her apartment and internally said to herself "I've got to take the elevator" instead of the intended "I've got to take an umbrella." The common concept is "leaving-home self-instructions," only it is the wrong specific "leaving-home instruction."

Other Examples:
- Saying "Stop jumping on that chair" instead of saying "couch"
- Saying "She turned onto the wrong river" instead of saying "highway"
- Saying "Ingmar Bergman" when intending to say "Ingrid Bergman"
- Saying "Queen Easter" when intending to say Queen Esther (of the Jewish Purim holiday at the same time of year as Easter)
- Saying "Queen Elizabeth" instead of "Queen Victoria" in a discussion of a film

(This symptom is potentially observable to others but usually is interpreted as signifying a momentary slip or a sign of being tired and thus appears relatively innocuous. Those who hear it don't realize that making malapropisms has become a more frequent occurrence for the person involved.)

5. Reversing Words While Speaking

An increased frequency of reversing the sequence of words one intends to say.

Example: Polly Van Benthusen, experiencing WHMS symptoms while taping a radio show for work, heard herself say instead of a "fast buck" a "bast f——k" and had to do another take.

Example: Psychologist, Susan E., forty-seven, would call out to her eight-year-old daughter in the morning, "Go brush your face and wash your teeth."

Example: Sheryl L., fifty-six, said, "You'll see it will lead to a "flashback" when she meant to say "backlash."
(Observable but usually not interpreted by others as signifying anything but a momentary slip and thus relatively innocuous in its impact.)

6. Reversing the First Letters of Words While Speaking

An increased frequency of reversing the first letters of words one intends to say.

Example: Mary S., fifty-five, said to her son "Go tot your knie" for "Go knot your tie."

Example: Leslie V., forty-two, driving past a farm, said, "What great hales of bay" instead of "bales of hay."
(Observable but usually not interpreted by others as signifying anything but a momentary slip and thus relatively innocuous.)

7. "Echo" Intrusions of Unintended Words into Speech (as Distinct from Word Reversals)

Unintended words popping out that are lingering echoes of a word that was recently thought, or a behavior very recently engaged in. The "echoes" produce intrusive "slips of the tongue." This has been described as "Whatever was in my hand came out of my mouth." Or "Whatever was in my mind came out of my mouth." Sometimes it is a word or a sentence popping out that is inappropriate but related to an immediately preceding conversation. This appears to represent the "loosening" of a normal mechanism of "holding on to" or "grasping on to" a thought that more typically acts to screen out intrusive competing thoughts; it represents greater distractability in staying focused on an intended statement. It appears to represent as well diminished powers of appropriate inhibition.

Example: Polly Van Benthusen went to make room reservations and meant to ask for "One room with two beds" but instead said "Two rooms with one bed." This may be a word reversal or it may be the result of preparing in thought to ask for "One room with two beds," with the "two" in her thought rehearsal intruding into her speech.

Example: Miriam D., age fifty-one, went up to a subway toll booth agent in New York City to ask for *two* tokens. She handed over the requisite *three* dollars. Instead of saying "Two tokens please," however, she said, "*Three* tokens please." Handing over three dollars intruded itself as an echo and replaced the intended word she meant to say, "two."

Example: Ellie V., age forty-six, went to her hairdresser and was chatting with him at length about her upcoming trip to Hawaii. When she had paid her bill she meant to say "Bye, have a great month" with the unvoiced thought "While I'm away on vacation." Instead she heard herself inappropriately say, "Have a great vacation." The earlier discussion about her upcoming vacation or the unvoiced part of her farewell intruded inappropriately as an echo.

8. Resorting to Filler "Whatchamacallit" Phrases with Greater Frequency Than in the Past

Having to use nonspecific filler words such as "whatchamacallit," "you know what I mean," "whatsisname," "that thing," etc., to replace the word you want to say in the course of speaking due to retrieval problems more often than in the past. A specific kind of word-finding difficulty. Lack of access to one's verbal repertoire: a specific word or name one needs in the course of speaking.

Example: English professor Katherine Kennedy, thirty-eight, said, ". . . and what drives me mad these days is that in the middle of talking I'll forget the name of a certain noun I want to use and wind up saying 'that thing' when I mean to say 'diploma' . . . I wind up using the generic 'doing' instead of the more subtle action word I want to use."

Example: Valerie S., forty-four, says, "I have conversations with my sister now where we both can't think of the names of the people we're talking about or how to identify the situations we are referring to but we know exactly what we are talking about. It's very funny but also bizarre." (Observable but usually not interpreted by others as signifying anything but a momentary slip and thus relatively innocuous, unless they are with you most of the time.)

9. Speech That Is Not As Well Organized As Usual

Momentary "flashes" of experiencing oneself as having less coherence than usual in the organization of content of a sentence or in "telling a tale." What this symptom suggests is that we apparently have a word-order/thought-order "sequencer" that prioritizes the order or unfolding of content of a thought or sentence or "tale" we intend to spout. This mechanism can apparently undergo occasional "tremors" during this time interval. (This was not a frequent symptom in the course of my interviews.)

Example: Patricia Estrich said, "[W]hen all these symptoms started [age forty-three] it got so that my words got jumbled. I thought at first it was a stroke—they run in my family. But it wasn't. With my adult daughter if I tried to tell her a story the words didn't seem to come out right. I'd be jumping around. I couldn't put a sentence together. I thought I was crazy."

Example: Esther D., forty-five, a highly verbal woman, suddenly noticed that occasionally an incident or a story she was describing to her family was more than usually disjointed in the telling. In the sense that some people are just naturally great storytellers and others are not, Esther felt she now was not as consistently a wonderful storyteller as she typically had been. Most of the time, however, this symptom did not affect her. She didn't know what to make of it when it was present.
(Depending on the severity of the specific example, this symptom may be detected by others or it may not, since people vary on this dimension naturally anyhow.)

III. CHANGES IN THE "BEAM" OF ATTENTION OR ENCODING OF SHORT-TERM MEMORIES

1. Listening but Not Always Attending: Blinking Social Attention (Milder Than Following Symptom)

Intermittent episodes of wavering baseline attention, i.e., realizing in the midst of a conversation with someone that you have no idea what the person was just talking about even though you didn't mean to "tune out" on the conversation. Transient loss of awareness with respect to social interactions. These episodes are more frequent than in the past. A detectable pattern of having to ask to have things repeated more often than in the past. Not taking "in" what's been said with the same consistency as before. Not being able to count on your baseline passive attention—the attention you have when you are not "trying"—to "take in" or absorb the same chunks of input as consistently as before.

Example: Sherry Strumph says, "I half focus on things. People will be speaking and I'll have no idea what we just spoke of. My friend Michele was speaking the other day and I realized I had no idea what the conversation was about."

Example: Patricia Estrich: "My older son said to me one time 'I'm talking to you but you don't hear me.' I wasn't concentrating. I did that a lot. He always let me know what he was feeling. He'd point that out to me. He'd say, 'Talk to me. Talk to me' when I was like that."

Example: Polly Van Benthusen: "Sometimes in one-on-one conversations my mind would wander. It would be really embarrassing and I'd say 'Could you repeat that?'. . . . Sometimes . . . I would say, 'I'm sorry, I was gone a minute but I'm back now.' My husband at times like these would say to me, 'Were we in ozone?'"
(Often not detected by others.)

2. Absentmindedness Concerning What Just Happened; Blanking Out; The Missing "I"; The Missing Context; "Not Being There"; Not Being Present; "Where was I?"
(Can be more intense than above symptom and relates more to non-social aspects).

Episodes of amnesia: behaving with less active self-awareness, particularly in the *physical* sense of self-monitoring what one's "I" has been up to within one's environment or context; "I was here," "I just did that," "I just put that down there." More of "just being" without a monitoring vigilance to one's physical self, internal self, and features of the context. Being less aware of one's awareness; transient loss of self-awareness. The absentmindedness tends to occur more often but not exclusively while engaging in "automatic pilot" behavior or while performing automatic chores of not great inherent interest, i.e., doing laundry, running errands, or "idling," when one is "just being" rather than striving with active engaged effort for a specific goal. The symptom tends to occur less often at work, where one is typically more actively striving, than in one's private life when one has more occasion to "just be."

Example: Grace K., now forty-seven and menopausal: "Over the last few years I've become a basket case mentally. I forget things in a most amazing way. . . . For example, I came home from work, parked the car, walked in the house, and suddenly I couldn't find the backpack I carry that contains my whole life, you could say. I always put it under the table in the hall but it wasn't there. I went back and searched the car. . . . I went to the sidewalk and looked again. I had put it in the closet in a new place and totally forgot I'd just done it. I completely blacked out on what happened to it. That's what happens all the time [now]."

Example: Virginia D., fifty-five, lives in the suburbs and drives nearly everywhere. At a four-way intersection, she looked for oncoming cars in one direction, then the other, and was nearly rammed by an oncoming car from the first direction she looked at. She had blanked out on what she had seen coming. She fears she may have to stop driving for her own safety.

Example: Kelly V., a forty-eight-year-old physical therapist has gone back to school for an advanced degree and writes reams of pages of notes during class. When she checks them at the end of class she finds she sometimes thinks to herself "He [the professor] said that? I can't remember that at all." (Taking notes here is the directed effort; one can "just be" in terms of the processing of what's being said while one is taking notes.)

More Examples:
- Misplacing (anything one has touched) in an instant
- Having *no* recall where one just parked one's car
- Stepping out of the shower having only shaved one leg
- Not remembering in the shower if you used conditioner or not or which body parts you've washed
- Putting things in strange places: shampoo in the refrigerator
- Loading the washing machine twice with soap and bleach and forgetting to put the wash in

- Not remembering the amount of money you gave the cashier or if you got cash or your credit card back
- Absentmindedly making a wrong turn on a familiar road while driving
- Episodes of things not being where they typically have been for years and you are the only one who could have moved them somewhere else; no recall of where they might be

(Often can occur without others realizing it has become an intermittent pattern.)

3. Increased Distractability

Intermittent behaviors (see above symptoms) that reflect a less tight intrinsic "hold" or "fix" on the "beam" or "focus" of one's attention or on one's intended words or actions. Some women explicitly experience themselves as more distractable but not all symptomatic women do. Rather their symptom behaviors appear sometimes to reflect this possibility. For example: the verbal intrusion symptom, blanking out on the self's behavior, losing one's train of thought midstream, walking into a room and forgetting what one went to get, reading less than before for no apparent reason.

Example: Cheryl Calhoun: "I can't tune things out the way I once used to."

Example: Polly Van Benthusen: "Whatever was in my mind came out of my mouth." "Whatever was in my hand came out of my mouth." (Often can occur outside of awareness of others.)

IV. CHANGES IN MEMORY: SHORT- AND/OR LONG-TERM

1. No Threads of Association Forgetting: Missing Connections

The experience of forgetting with a sense that there are no threads of association by which to get back to the memory one seeks to recall. A sense of missing associative links, ties, or connections to events or memories one wishes to recall or reconstruct.

Example: Katherine Kennedy says, "In our marriage I'm the treasurer who handles all the practical things. . . . Recently I thought we had cash in the bank and it turns out we had less than I remembered. I just couldn't recall where I had spent it. It's scary. . . . Last month I lost my wallet, which I never do. But what had me really worried was I couldn't even think where I might have lost it—my mind just blanked out on any possibilities—I drew a total blank. That was weird."

Example: Polly Van Benthusen, forty-eight: "I didn't remember whole conversations I had with people. People would say 'Don't you remember that?' and I didn't . . . It would feel as though someone had kidnapped me from my life . . ."

Example: Debbie R., thirty-seven, cannot recall by memory alone on which breast she had surgery a number of years ago without resorting to looking at her breast for the scar.

Example: Sherry Strumph: "My concentration also changed. I would start to read a book and pick it up two weeks later and have absolutely no memory of any of it. As though not a trace had stayed with me."

(Often not observable to others.)

2. Episodic Changes in Spelling Certainty

Looking at a word and not being as certain how it should be spelled in formerly excellent spellers. Recognizing that a word is wrong but not knowing how it should be corrected.

Example: Polly Van Benthusen: "My spelling . . . during my forties had gotten worse and [now after taking estrogen] it's not back 100 percent. I'd look at a word and it would not look right; I'd have to get a dictionary out or use spell-check [on the computer]. Even when I looked the words up they didn't look right. I couldn't explain the loss. It was just so absurd. I'd think "I have spelled this word nine hundred times!"

Example: Sherry Strumph says, "I used to be a great speller. I didn't have to think about it. Now I have to think about it. I was looking at something someone wrote with the word "comrade" in it and I couldn't remember if it had an *e* at the end or not. Working with language has been my business and this is not like me."

Example: Marylou G., forty-two, sat down to write her husband a quick note about arranging for a baby-sitter for their six-year-old while she would be away and couldn't remember if "baby-sitter" was spelled "baybe" or what exactly. A minute later she realized the correct spelling and the knowledge felt "locked in" once again. She has always been a great speller and these "glitches" don't make any sense to her.

Example: Georgina H., forty-seven and menopausal for three years, says, "[I] used to be a very good speller and now I find I'm having this spelling problem. I laughed when Dan Quayle, the vice president, didn't know how to spell potato. I thought he was stupid. Now *I'm* not sure how to spell it."
(Can occur outside of awareness of others.)

3. Difficulty Calculating Numbers and Visually Registering Quantities

Taking longer than usual to "figure" easy numerical things, or having short-term "blackouts" in how to do once-simple arithmetic skills. These symptoms appear to represent defective connections for accessing or retrieving "math computation and/or memory files" and to parts of the brain that visually tally, scan, or process images for numerical purposes. The "math" knowledge is still apparently there because the symptoms in most people are intermittent.

Example: Businesswoman Sherry Strumph says, "I used to be able to compute things mentally and now I have to write them down and have someone check them for me."

Example: Denise X., fifty-two, menopausal for two years, was at her mother's house trying to set the table for dinner for her mother, her aunt, and the three members of her family and couldn't figure out how many placemats to set down. She says, "I looked at everybody present but I couldn't come up with '5.' I just couldn't figure it out. The next minute I could. I don't understand what happened. I've been fine since."

Example: Evelyn Schein: Now forty-seven, menopausal at forty-three: "I was always OK at math. Now sometimes I have to add simple things and I have to count on my fingers for simple addition. I had to tally up like 5 and 4 and 3 and 3 and I had to add it up three times to make sure I was getting it right. No, I don't ever find myself feeling hazy, or cloudy, or foggy."

Example: Marilyn P., forty-eight and menopausal, says, "I always was great at dividing up dinner bills when I went out with my friends. I was proud of my skill in doing this. Now I don't leave home without one of those thin credit-card pocket calculators. I'm not certain I can do it anymore and I've become afraid to find out I can't; so I rely on the calculator."

Example: Betty L., an accountant in perimenopause, was shocked to find that she had suddenly forgotten which number comes after 16. (Can occur outside the awareness of others.)

4. Changes in Memory-Retrieval Accessing Speed and Agility

An intermittent pattern of more frequent delays in accessing and/or retrieving information or names or words from the warehouses of one's memory. This can reflect retrieval of one's *old* fund of knowledge or more *recently acquired* information.

Example: Writer Letty Cottin Pogrebin developed many WHMS-like symptoms around age fifty but attributed her symptoms to aging. She writes in *Getting Over Getting Older:* "The mind is the Bermuda Triangle of aging. You never know when a shipshape fragment of knowledge—someone's name, a movie title, a simple word—will sail into treacherous waters and disappear without a trace, or when a raft of information given up for lost will suddenly wash up on the shores of memory."

(Often can be just an interior experience, not observable to others.)

5. Forgetting the Content of an Immediately Recent Experience While Retaining One's Emotional Reaction to It

Forgetting the content but not one's emotional reaction to an immediately prior event. This reminds us that there are two "recording" tracks laying down or registering information in our brains: the "factual," or content, track and the emotional track. This symptom suggests that our emotional reactions, our "take" on a situation ("Is it safe to be here or not?" "Should I avoid this situation next time?") (1) have primacy in being preserved over the specific details of a situation and (2) are probably under the control of different brain mechanisms. The work of neurosurgeon Wilder Penfield also revealed these "two tracks" of recording in memory. When Penfield operated on people with intractable epilepsy and stimulated parts of their brains during surgery, the patients reported memories together with the *emotions* associated with them ("I am playing the piano in our parlor and *feel . . .*").

Example: Georgette H., menopausal at forty-four, now forty-seven, says, "[I]f I go to a movie now I can come out and not know what I just saw. I only remember if I liked it or not."

Example: Evelyn Schein: Menopausal at age forty-three. Symptoms began at thirty-seven. "If I'll go to a movie I can walk out and not remember what it was about. I'll just remember if I liked it or not. It's like a blackout." [Yes, these nearly identical quotes do come from two different people!]

(Often not observable to others.)

V. BEHAVIORAL CHANGES

Intermittent episodes of:

1. Behavioral Malapropisms: Unintended Behavioral Slips Related Conceptually to the Intended Behavior

Off-the-mark "slips" in behavior occurring. "Unmindful" behavioral errors that depart from what the mind really intended to do. The misguided behavior is related in concept to the intended behavior but is "off the mark" from the *specific* intended behavior. The errors appear to represent misconnected or misguided follow-through of the mind's intent by the brain: going into a neighboring but ultimately "wrong bin in the brain" for an act intended by the mind. These tend to occur more typically when the person is on "automatic pilot" behavior—in a state of "just being" without actively monitoring or directing her behavior.

Example: Letty Cottin Pogrebin in her book *Getting Over Getting Older* describes a woman throwing soiled underwear into the wrong type of receptacle or container—the garbage instead of the hamper (both are "receptacles" at the concept level; the specific receptacle is wrong). She also describes a woman unpacking groceries and placing shampoo in the refrigerator rather than in the bathroom. The concept of "storage area" is the same but it is the wrong kind of specific storage area.

Example: Sherry Strumph, as cited earlier, got into her car and sat in the passenger seat waiting to be driven instead of getting into the driver's seat to pick up her business associate on the day it was her turn to do so. The similar concept involves "getting into a car to sit so as to go somewhere." It was the wrong *specific* seat to go somewhere.

Example: Susan V., fifty-one, gave the thruway toll booth agent an envelope instead of the toll ticket. Both have similar concepts of "rectangular-shaped pieces of paper you divest yourself of," only it's the wrong specific type of rectangular paper. Another time Susan reported attempting to change channels on TV with her cordless phone instead of the remote. Both are small remote-control rectangular devices one presses to selectively obtain new input, only it is the wrong device for changing the specific input.

(The behaviors are often undetected by others, because they are so brief and usually self-corrected. They can, however, be detected as a pattern of slips by those who live or work closely with the person.)

2. "Praxis" Blank-outs: Briefly Forgetting How to Do Things

Forgetting in flash episodes how to do things, procedures one has been doing "forever," with the information coming back as mysteriously as it left. This appears to occur most frequently in isolated brief episodes, few and very far between, and not in a recurrent on/off pattern. It does not appear to occur in multiple areas of one's life. The experience is more of "What in the world is going on?" when it happens. The destabilization of knowledge that the experience represents and its unusualness make women fearful for their stability, and for their future. Sometimes it happens just once but it compels attention and fears.

Example: Polly Van Benthusen, in her forties, forgot how to shut off the computers in her office that she had long been turning off at the end of the day and considered getting a label-maker machine to mark in red where the switches were.

Example: Sally B., at age forty-eight, forgot one evening how to turn on the headlights of her old car. She thought she was "losing it" and was afraid to drive that night and the next day. She didn't know what she might "lose" next and wanted to be safe.

Example: Esther K., a travel agent, at age forty-nine forgot how to turn on the computer she has worked on every day for years.

Example: Helen, age thirty-eight, a microbiologist, forgot how to work her microscope one day and became very frightened. She spent the next two years trying to find out why, till she discovered her hormones were abnormally low.

(This symptom usually is not detected by others, though it can sometimes be. The temporary "glitch" can usually be "covered up" through some elision.)

3. Subtle Self-Perceived "Glitches" in One's Familiar Sense of Coordination While Driving. (Deficits in performance are not necessarily implied)

Self-observed "flash" changes in the "automaticness" of aspects of driving that one hasn't had to "think" about for a long time. Observing changes in one's typical coordination of driving, learned long ago, that have become "automatic" and are more like "just being." The outward effectiveness of driving may remain competent but the inner experience of "automaticness" is shaken in flash moments. "Tremors" in the reflex nature of coordinated behaviors present in driving. This does not involve changes in navigational memory.

Example: Polly Van Benthusen: A few times when I was driving, things . . . seemed to be different somehow . . . I would pull out into traffic and concentrate on one thing but not another. I didn't turn on my blinker the way I always do religiously. I misjudged the length of a car . . . This hasn't happened since but it was strange when it happened. It had never happened before.

Example: Cheryl Calhoun says, "One time I simply forgot to put the car in "park" when I got out. I had never done that before and I haven't again."

Example: As forty-four-year-old Harriet P. was driving up a winding coastal mountain road she suddenly noted that she was producing an uncharacteristically unsmooth ride. The pattern of steering the car around the mountain and braking at curves was less smooth than usual. Something about the rhythm of coordinating these skills was not as much a "given" in her repertoire of behavior as it had been in the past. She had to consciously rethink how to go about driving around the mountain more smoothly in terms of braking skills and effectively did so. She reports that no other aspect of her driving seemed aberrant then and or has subsequently. She has never experienced a return of that symptom.

(Often cannot be witnessed by others.)

4. The "Dropsies": Erratic Fine-finger/Hand Coordination

Being less consistently able than in the past to deftly engage in tasks requiring complex "fine" finger-hand coordination. Intermittently dropping "fine-fingered" things more than in the past.

Example: Phyllis B., at forty-three, found that some of the time she felt she was not as agile as she reliably had been in the past in trying to dig out the keys in her purse and open the door to her apartment while holding a coat on one arm and a package of groceries in the other arm. It was no big deal but she didn't know what to make of it.

Example: Susan V. went back to school at fifty-four and found herself embarrassed by all the times pieces of paper would slip from her hands at school. When she went to pick them up something else would drop—her pen or pencil. She didn't know if others noticed, but *she* did. She did not, however, drop big objects at home or things like a kettle or pot requiring larger arm muscles.

(Can be detected by others, but they may attribute behavior to anxiety or fatigue.)

5. Changes in Agility in the Flow of Writing: Leaving Out or Reversing Letters

Intermittently leaving out letters or reversing letters in the midst of writing a word. Doing this without awareness, as an oversight. Observing uncharacteristic "glitches" in one's typical handwriting pattern on and off with a greater frequency of occurrence than in the past. Usually one letter in a word is involved and the ability to decode the word from its landscape features remains present though it is not as easy to read back what one has written. Not a "big deal" as a symptom but evokes "What in the world is going on here?" reaction.

Example: Katherine Kennedy, now thirty-eight, whose WHMS symptoms began very early, says, "In my late twenties if I was writing fast I noticed that I started to reverse letters in words.

Example: Estelle H. is a forty-eight-year-old social worker who takes notes as she works with clients. She found she suddenly had a harder time reading back her notes because she had left out letters in words. Later she became aware that she was leaving out letters *as she wrote* and doesn't understand why she does this. It just happens more than in the past. She can usually decode what she writes and it doesn't represent a major impediment. It is more interesting than an actual inconvenience.

Example: Cynthia K., fifty-six, finds that when she has to address envelopes or sign cards she makes the silliest mistakes in writing. Embarrassed to send out seasonal cards with such silly errors, she tears up many more than she ever would have in the past.
(Might be detected by others in written communications but not detected as a pattern often.)

6. Forgetting How to Spell a Word in the Midst of Writing

Change in writing agility due to a different cause than oversight: the active forgetting of how to spell a word while in the middle of writing it and having to leave blanks to be filled in later. Similar to losing one's train of thought while speaking (see below).

Example: Elizabeth V., a fifty-two-year-old nursing home administrator, finds now that as she writes in longhand she will forget how to spell "speak," for example, in the midst of having begun to do so and will write *sp* and then leave blanks to be filled in later when the "knowledge" returns to her. It hasn't produced any problems but she's noticed it and has wondered what it means.

Example: Polly Van Benthusen: "I'll go spell a word and drop a letter as I write. Because of this I now use an erasable pen. It becomes permanent after awhile."

(Potentially observable to others but easily missed as a new pattern in behavior.)

7. Changes in Agility in Translating or Decoding From Speech to Writing or Across Different Modalities

Episodic difficulty translating spoken words that are numbers into written numerical symbols. Change in the agility of translating or processing different symbol systems (words and numbers) from one channel of communication to another (hearing to writing), i.e., translating heard words into written numbers. This may apply to other cross-modalities of communication, i.e., understanding broadcasted speech—as in the movies or from radio—as contrasted with understanding directly heard speech.

Example: Cynthia H., forty-two, quietly observed that on some occasions recently she has been "stalled" in her usual ability to automatically write down a telephone number someone was conveying to her over the phone. She experienced an uncharacteristic delay somewhere in the pathway between hearing the numbers and being able to automatically convert them into written numerals on a page.

(Usually not a big enough symptom to be observed by others.)

8. Handling Same Amount of Stress Differently

Despite an absence of apparent changes in the external demands being made upon a person, the sense of an altered ability to handle the same amount of or kinds of stress as in the past. The self-perception of not being able to "keep as many balls up in the air" at once as before: handling stress differently. Even with reduced demands compared to the past, a sense of not being able to handle things as well as one would have in the recent past.

Example: Dr. Fredericka Xerov, fifty-four: "I would think to myself this is not the way I used to be. I used to juggle all those responsibilities. I had been director of my own private radiology operation. I had hospital responsibilities, social responsibilities, my husband, the children. Now I had a much simpler life and fewer responsibilities and I was functioning only marginally.

Example: Molly Evans, a sales executive, at forty-seven, is perimenopausal and has just begun to be treated for WHMS and physical symptoms with low-dose birth-control pills. She says, "Before I really wasn't sure whether to attribute [all these WHMS symptoms] to a particular time in my life. Before I would say, 'Well, it's just me being distracted or stressed out or something.' Now I don't know [I suspect it may be related to hormonal changes] because it's been happening now for so many months; and it's intensifying and there's nothing else going on in my life that's particularly stressful. I've had the same job, I've had the same house, I've had the same husband, the same child. I've had the same everything. All of a sudden my mind is going and I'm saying to myself, 'Really, this is not good.' I'm saying that I have to drop out. Like I want to go into my womb, into the cave. Because I keep thinking if I can simplify, simplify, simplify, then I'll be able to get it all in order. But is that the answer? I've thought of quitting my job. I think about it all the time. . . . It's sort of like I can't keep the balls up in the air anymore. That's what I'm feeling. A year or two ago I could have the job, have the kid, have the house, have the husband and all the balls would stay up. Right now I don't seem to have the mental organizational skills to keep all the balls up anymore. That's how I feel . . . I just said to my daughter recently, 'Liz, you don't understand. Mother is losing her mind. I cannot have the demands put on me that you are putting on me. You can't expect me to be good-natured about my responses. I'm just losing it.' I've been eating more healthfully, this Foundation of Youth diet, but I'm not succeeding in improving myself. I exercise religiously one hour a day, every day. Nothing has made a difference."

Example: Menopause expert Dr. Maurice Cohen says, "One of the

earliest signs of hormonal change that I see is women who come to me complaining that they are handling stress differently from before. They say, 'I can't seem to handle stress in the same way as before.' They don't understand why. I've heard it often enough to believe it's an early symptom of hormonal change."
(May or may not be detectable to others.)

VI. CHANGES IN SPATIAL SKILLS: PERCEPTION AND NAVIGATIONAL MEMORY

1. Difficulty Registering/Remembering New Faces of People

A newly present pattern of episodically not recalling or recognizing the faces of people you have met in the past, who know you, and with whom you reportedly interacted (i.e., attended to and "registered"). The feeling is as though you had never met them before. This does not appear to happen with those one knows best. Less frequently this may involve someone one knew on an ongoing basis, i.e., a neighbor across the street who moved away. This may reflect a change in recognizing a spatial configuration, a perceptual skill, or in attention or memory.

Example: Katherine Kennedy, now thirty-eight: "When I entered my thirties I started having these strange symptoms. I would meet people and the next day felt as though I had never seen them before. They'd know me but I had no clue to who they were. Their faces were just not registering . . . I had begun to menstruate copiously around that time . . . Not recognizing faces still happens and I find that slightly scary . . . I met a woman at the radio station a few weeks ago. Then I met her again two nights later and didn't recall her at all."

Example: Polly Van Benthusen: "I saw someone who turned out to be another one of our neighbors from across the street from several years ago but I couldn't remember who she was and where she was from. It was most unusual. I had no recall of having ever met her. My husband had to tell me who she was. There have also been several instances of my meeting people at meetings and I wouldn't have a clue as to who they were. This had never happened to me before."

Example: Marilyn D., sixty-four, college teacher: "My visual memory is very poor now for faces. This has been the case since I hit menopause, in my early fifties. Before menopause I was the memory bank for my four kids, and the memory bank for faces and names who were the members of my husband's club. I remembered everyone. For years now people come up to me on the street and with great fervor say 'Hello Marilyn!' and to myself I say 'Oh my God. I don't know who that is.' 'You don't remember me?' they say.' I comfort myself by saying 'You have a lot on your plate.' I look at people on the street now and think 'That's a familiar face' but I'm not sure. After awhile I'd say hello to anyone who looked vaguely familiar. The same thing happened to me about remembering telephone numbers. But that skill came back after three to four years. This hasn't. . . . I'm still very professionally active on many levels and this is an inconvenience but not a major impediment."

Example: Francine P., forty-seven, menopausal two years: "My daughter had had a play date with a new girl from school. When the girl's mother came to pick her up she was very friendly and we chatted for several minutes. After she left I thought to myself 'Gee, what a nice woman. It might be fun getting to know her better.' A couple of months later she brought her daughter to my daughter's birthday party and I didn't have any idea who she was. She realized it too and said, 'I'm Priscilla's mom.' She was offended. I could tell. I was mortified but didn't know what to tell her. In the past I would never forget faces. This has only happened three to four times in total. It was very embarrassing."

Example: Evelyn Schein, now forty-seven, menopausal since forty-three: "My memory for faces is gone. I don't remember new people I meet. My memory for names has always been bad but this is a new twist on it."

(This symptom is often noticeable but can be covered over at times.)

2. Looking But Not Seeing: More Than in the Past

Not seeing what later turns out to have been right there. Lack of awareness of visual material despite apparently normal visual/perceptual skills. The filter of one's attention appears not to be screening well, and focusing in on, the mind's intent while looking at the "full picture" of reality being viewed. Lack of follow-through on the mind's intent by the supporting scanning "machinery."

Example: Melinda E., forty-nine, perimenopausal: "I recently started taking these low-dose birth-control pills for my memory problems, and last week I had to go to Philadelphia on business. I searched for the pills all over the bathroom. I keep them on the shelf in the medicine cabinet in my bathroom. My husband uses our other bathroom. I searched high and low for them and couldn't find them and turned the house upside down looking for them. I left for Philadelphia, came back, and there they were! I thought I was losing my mind. They were sitting right there. There was no one who could have put them there. My husband was away. The cleaning woman hadn't been there. I couldn't believe it."

Example: Polly Van Benthusen: "I'd gone to the refrigerator and put the juice on the counter and simply didn't remember in an instant that I put it there. And it was apparently sitting there on the counter but I couldn't find it. I looked all over—the fridge, the counter, the kitchen—and just couldn't find it. So . . . I felt I had to jump in the car . . . and get some apple juice for my son. When I came back . . . [t]here was the apple juice right on the counter. [My husband said] 'You set it out on the counter.' I said, 'No, I didn't,' and I was ready to do battle over this apple juice. . . . I said, 'I didn't put that apple juice there.' I said to him, 'I honestly don't recall doing that.'"

Example: Susan D., fifty-five, typically keeps her bank books buried in the back of a closet. She didn't want to forget to go to the bank the next day for an important errand and so left them under her pillow for ready availability. When she awoke the next morning she attended to her usual rituals. When she remembered she had to go to the bank she went to look under her pillow and couldn't find the bank books. She looked everywhere—under the bed, behind the headboard, to no avail. In a state of alarm she immediately went to the bank to sign for replacements. Upon returning home she looked again and *there* the bank books were where she had left them.

(Usually not observable to others.)

3. Changes in Reading Agility: Visual Perception and/or Comprehension

Episodic changes in reading agility. Changes in the visual pattern of digesting and/or comprehending words and sentences while reading. Not reading with the usual automatic intake of words and registration of their meaning. The "train" of words are experienced as not entering one's mind in the usual step-by-step flow, either because the words don't look "right" or the visual pattern doesn't translate into meaning. Disjointedness in this process. A lack of coherence in grasping the meaning of the words as a result of this disjointedness. Much more than usual effort is required to "get" what is being read. Reported as feeling like "suddenly having dyslexia."

Example: Polly Van Benthusen: "Also my reading became so ponderous. I'd reverse words reading and lose the meaning by doing this. I was a big reader and halfway through the paragraph I'd think 'That didn't make any sense.' I'd make things into a question that weren't questions. My reading got so bad I had to read one word at a time. I had taken a speed-reading course and I couldn't skim anymore. I never had ADD [attention deficit disorder] and I had never had problems with this before. I'd think to myself 'Here I am. This is like *The Exorcist*.' I would read things wrong twice. It felt like I was dyslexic. And I'd say 'I really am losing it. It's pre-senile dementia.'"

Example: Evelyn Schein: "With reading, by the time I'm at the bottom of the page I can't recall the first paragraph. *I must read things three times to get them.*"

Example: Marylou F., social worker, now forty-seven and menopausal: "I read something now and realize I don't get it and read it again." (Not usually observable to others.)

4. Less Time Spent Reading by Formerly Heavy-Duty Readers Without Any Apparent Reason

The observation that one is reading less for reasons that seem not at all clear or that can be accounted for by changes in the external aspects of one's life. Often no apparent difficulty in reading per se is experienced by the reader to account for this shift. Some women have a sense that their ability to concentrate is involved.

Example: Denise W., then fifty and recently menopausal, says, ". . . I found last year that I started reading a lot less than I used to. I've always read about three books at a time, and last summer [when I was on vacation with my family] when I should have been able to read a lot, I surprisingly found that I just read one book in little dribs and drabs. I don't know what is causing it, but there's been a change and I can't figure out what's going on." [She says she doesn't experience any difficulty per se in reading.]

Example: Patricia Estrich: "Since I was thirteen I've read one novel a week. All of a sudden I couldn't concentrate enough to read. I would have five books waiting to be read and just started reading less. I'm not a TV watcher and don't go to movies so it was a problem." (Unobservable to others usually.)

5. Close-by Blundering: Malapropisms in Recalling Where Places Are

"Off-the-mark" recall for locations or places long known or recently learned—for "maps" in memory. The errors in navigation that are made are "close" to the actual place one wants to recall, but are specifically "off the mark," not exactly the right place. These "slips" are similar in manner to both verbal and behavioral "malapropisms," apparently involving retrieval of memory from "the wrong bin in the brain." In some instances the errors also represent an unexpected uncertainty over one's old fund of acquired knowledge—about internal "maps" associated with certain places, their internal spatial representations. These changes represent changes in spatial recall.

Example: Cindy G., a fifty-year-old life-long New York City resident, highly familiar with New York City's landmarks, intended to drop off a friend who lived in the suburbs at New York City's Grand Central Station—a train station. Instead she mistakenly drove her friend to another transportation hub, Penn Station, also a train station, and afterward in a second error, to another wrong transportation hub, for buses in New

York City—Port Authority. Her memory for where Grand Central Station was had become uncertain when she was called upon to actively use it. Instead instructions for how to get to two conceptually similar transportation hubs were retrieved. The errors in this example again were instances of retrieval from a conceptually close but specifically "wrong bin in the brain." This particular example also represents a loosening in the *certainty* over old well-entrenched knowledge.

Example: Sally B., a forty-six-year-old social worker who treats patients in her home office, needed to use the car that day for a task of personal importance. Before she left home she asked her husband, who had parked the car the night before, on which block the car was. He called out the information as he left the house but Sally did not write it down. When she went to get the car at noon it was not to be found. She searched up and down the street she thought it was on to no avail and had a sense it was close by but she just couldn't find it. Her husband was unreachable. Very annoyed, Sally missed going where she needed to. The car turned out to be one block over, laterally, from where she had believed it was.

Sally *had* apparently been paying attention and did encode or register the information her husband had given her. However, when it came time to retrieve it, the information had either been stored in the wrong "map" bin in her brain, or she retrieved it in some "off-the-mark" fashion. This example of "close-by blundering" represents a navigational malapropism or "slip-of-the-mind's maps" of newly acquired information or memory.
(Often not observable to others, or if noticed can be "tossed off" as due to fatigue or a momentary "slip.")

6. Brief Bursts of Unfamiliarity in Past Familiar Places

Arriving at a point in a long-familiar setting and for a brief interval realizing that the setting, the gestalt, does not look familiar, or that one surprisingly does not know which way to get to a more familiar setting. A flash episode of a sense of dislocation on a familiar trip.

Example: Patricia Estrich, then perimenopausal, between the ages of forty-four and forty-eight, experienced the following: "Another time I got lost in the mall and cried like a child. *I used to work in that mall.* I knew it like the back of my hand. I saw kids watching me and got embarrassed. It [the feeling of being lost] lasted five minutes. I stopped going to the mall after that. I had been at that mall for ten years and worked there for one year."

Example: Sheryl T., then age fifty, and recently menopausal, was driving back one night from a friend's house in the suburbs. She had been making this trip every few months for many years. When she got to a *T* in the road about a mile from her home, she suddenly didn't know which way to turn. The intersection looked unfamiliar. Her mental map of this setting was not there when she needed it. The landmarks did not seem familiar. She decided to make an arbitrary turn hoping things would suddenly fall into place since she knew she was somewhere near her home. After about a minute or so she again detected familiar landmarks and breathed a sigh of relief. In the three years since, this has not happened again.

(Often not observable to others.)

VII. ALTERED TIME SENSE

1. Time Monitoring/Anticipation Errors

Changes in one's typical pattern of anticipating upcoming events, of tracking elapsed intervals of time. Changes in one's interval clock—the stopwatch, alarm clock, or internal planning calendar that monitors elapsed time for personally relevant events and reminds you "*X* is coming up tonight, or next week." A sense of "time out of mind." Until it stops working consistently, most people don't realize they have such a built-in interval-monitoring/planning mechanism. Possibly related to less self-monitoring.

Example: Polly Van Benthusen: "I'd begun to forget to show up at meetings, which is entirely not like me. I've always been very compunctious about meetings. I sat on a few boards in the community and I was absolutely aghast one evening when the blood center I was on the board of called and said, "You missed that meeting—a meeting that was on my calendar. I just hadn't checked it or recalled it. I was flabbergasted."

Example: Polly Van Benthusen: ". . . Another time stands out. One of my staff members came in and said, 'It's 2:00. Time for a meeting.' I apparently had scheduled one and I didn't have a clue in the world what the meeting was about. So I said, 'OK! Let's have a meeting!' I went with the flow." [In the past her weekly calendar was virtually emblazoned in her memory without effort, or need for cuing.]

Example: Evelyn Schein: "My daughter keeps on reminding me that I have to take her to the airport over and over. My sister keeps reminding me that we have a birthday party for her daughter in two weeks. She knows I won't remember."

Example: Cheryl Calhoun: "I stopped making appointments for Monday mornings because I would miss them. I would forget to look at my appointment book over the weekend."

(Observable to others.)

2. Losing the Continuous Time Line "Thread" of One's Personal History

A less continuous internal historical calendar for past events in one's life, and/or for recent events. The sense that there isn't a continuous ribbon of time connecting the sequential events of one's life. Disconnected events not tethered to an evenly spaced continuum of time.

Example: Letty Cottin Pogrebin writes in *Getting Over Getting Older:* "Forgetting and remembering are critical issues . . . partly because memory is the pathway to personal history wherein lies proof that we have lived and loved and made a difference in the world. Without access to that history . . . we can almost feel ourselves disappear."

Example: Evelyn Schein, now forty-seven, and menopausal at forty-three: "I can't remember the dates of anything. I had a lumpectomy in 1987 and usually I can't remember when or even which breast it was in. I went to the doctor the other day and they were asking for a health history; I couldn't remember which breast I had it in until I looked at the scar. Doctors take a history and I'll say to them 'I know I'm making this difficult but I just don't recall.'"

Example: Melissa C., forty-four and perimenopausal, found she suddenly couldn't remember with certainty any longer the order of the summer vacations of her family over the last eight years without looking at the photographs she had taken. Until recently she loved mentally reviewing the pleasures she had had with her two children and husband in the different places they had traveled to. Now she doesn't have the certainty over which summer they did what. She says she misses having the time line "reel" ready for review.

(Not observable by others.)

3. More "Living in the Moment": a "Spliced-Film-Frames" Sense of Time

Most likely because of blinking attention and concentration, less active self-monitoring, and more forgetting, some of those experiencing WHMS symptoms learn to coast and cope with disconnections in the continuous sense of time that were more implicit in their previous experience. The disconnections from moment to moment are quite tolerable for some people, most of the time, but frustrating for others with less room for slack moments in their lives. An analogy to this experience might be living at times in a film from which segments of frames have been spliced. There is some "jumpiness" in the experience of the film, i.e., the life, but for most women the intermittent "splices" or "glitches" don't disrupt the "story." The overall "picture" of ongoing consistency in one's behavior and functioning makes it possible, surprisingly, for many to coast with this symptom.

Example: Sherry Strumph says, "[K]eys? I no longer carry keys. I never know anymore where they are. I have given new meaning to the phrase 'living in the moment.'"

Example: Charlene F., forty-nine: "You know how you often can't remember what you had for lunch yesterday, or what you did last Thursday exactly and it's no big deal? Well that's what this is like, only more so. I can't remember what I read last night or where I buried the tennis rackets last time—not a clue about both. You could say I'm living from moment to moment but it's not as inconvenient as it could be. I write everything down that's important in my life and keep everything

important in the same place. Maybe this is a way of simplifying life. I don't know."
(Often not observable to others.)

SUMMARY: WHAT WHMS APPEARS TO BE

WHMS appears to be a hormone-related normal *condition*—in the same way that pregnancy is a normal *condition*—associated with declining estrogen supplies. Although estrogen appears to be the primary hormone associated with these changes, it is typically part of a tag-team cascade of "relay" hormone players. Conceivably other hormones or neuroactive substances that estrogen interacts with biologically may also account for some of the symptoms.

The symptoms in summary can variously be characterized as representing *intermittent episodes* of (1) disordered follow-through or implementation of the mind's intent by the brain; (2) altered agility in maintaining "a fix" on one's intended speech, thought, and behavior; (3) altered agility in consistently inhibiting or delaying competing intrusive responses, i.e., a condition of heightened potential distractability; (4) less consistent monitoring of one's self within one's context or environment; (5) altered speed and agility in the retrieval of memories and information long known and/or recently learned; (6) likely alterations in the connectivity of "circuits" of stored knowledge within the brain; (7) a condition of altered verbal agility; (8) alterations in the consistency of one's beam of "online" attention; (9) subtle often innocuous alterations in self-control in various domains of thought, speech, and behavior; (10) potential changes in the sense of certainty over different forms of one's old fund of knowledge; (11) "tremors" in the integrated "automaticness" of highly practiced over-learned, nearly reflex behaviors long ago learned; (12) alterations in the awareness of, internal tracking of, and anticipation of time; (13) alterations in the continous nature of one's internal "time line" of personal history; (14) alterations in the agility of holding information in mind while one is doing something else (a "working memory" problem); (15) alterations in spatial recognition and recall; (16) possibly a new "adult-onset" variant of attention deficit disorder (ADD) with features of dyslexia; (17) a condition of episodic self-amnesia; (18) possibly a condition of diminished hyper-vigilance for "tracking" for safety within one's context from moment-to-moment; (19) a condition of altered "fine-tuning" in aspects of the human organism reflecting an altered hormonal milieu and possibly an altered biological agenda with less focus on a variety of subtle motivations relevant to perpetuating the next generation of the species—species survival.

I would like to emphasize again that though the symptoms can be many, paradoxically, the presence of even *many* intermittent WHMS symptoms does not have to appreciably compromise the overall function and ongoing continuity of a woman's life.

When experienced, however, in sufficient intensity, number, or in combination with emotional and physical symptoms associated with perimenopause and menopause, WHMS symptoms *can,* however, disrupt the quality of life in some it affects. Little is at present known about the typical duration of the symptoms in those it affects or the degree to which all symptoms are always reversible.

Because in the lives of actual women WHMS symptoms often do not occur alone but in flux with physical and/or emotional symptoms, I list in Appendix I: (1) *emotional/mood* symptoms that can accompany WHMS symptoms and (2) *physical* symptoms that can accompany WHMS symptoms. Some of these are new emotional/ mood or physical symptoms that are not as yet formally recognized by the menopause research community. I have identified these based upon my interviews with women. In particular, fatigue and low-grade depression or flattened mood I believe are much more common symptoms during perimenopause and menopause than menopause researchers currently credit.

8

WHMS Screening Instrument and Measuring Tools
Take These to Your Doctor

I suspect that after reading this far about WHMS symptoms you probably have a good sense of whether or not you are experiencing the WHM Syndrome. If you have recognized yourself with a "yes, that's me" response to two or three or four of the symptoms; if you have those symptoms more frequently than in the past; and if, by virtue of your age or situation, you suspect your estrogen supplies and ovary function may be changing, you probably have the WHM Syndrome. Bear in mind that some women's ovaries can stop functioning as early as their twenties—a condition known as premature ovarian failure—and affect their estrogen supply; that perimenopause can start more than a decade before the onset of menopause in some women; and that WHMS symptoms sometimes are the first indication of a beginning shift in estrogen supplies and may not be reflected yet in hormonal blood tests.

MEASURING TOOLS IN THIS CHAPTER

In this chapter I describe several tools for measuring or describing WHMS symptoms and their impact on you, and for offering you and your doctor a quick, memorable "snapshot" of how WHMS together with other possible physical or emotional symptoms associated with perimenopause and menopause are affecting your life over time and/or are responding to treatments. These tools include:

1. WHMS Screening Instrument
2. Perimenopausal or Menopausal Symptom "Circus" Chart
3. The WHMS Golf-Counter Symptom-Change Technique
4. Symptom Diary (optional)

Depending on your needs you could use all of the tools I present or only one or two of them. If you decide to use only one I suggest you use the WHMS Screening Instrument on a repetitive basis as a communication tool, and as a record of your symptoms for yourself over time. You can make photocopies of the pages in this book or order blank copies of it from a supply house in the appendix. If you want to order a complete kit for using the measuring tools in this chapter to evaluate yourself over several years or in response to different treatments, you can order it from the same supplier listed in the index under *WHMS Tools*.

Tracking Symptoms Over Time, with or without Treatment: Are You the Same, Better, or Worse?

Using the same measurement tools over time will help give you an idea whether you are staying the same or getting better or worse with time, no matter what you decide to do. You can use these tools:

(1) if you do *nothing* in the form of treatment but just want to compare yourself from season to season or over a span of years during the years of perimenopause, menopause, or even lifelong, to see if you are changing in your *type* of symptoms or *frequency* of symptoms;

(2) if you start some form of treatment and want to make before-and-after treatment comparisons. This might be with hormone replace-

ment therapy, or one of the non-hormonal forms of treatments and be-haviors I discuss in later chapters;

(3) if you want to change a type of treatment and want to make com-parisons between the two forms of treatment, i.e., compare your symp-tom scores before and after taking each one for three months with perhaps a two-week or longer "washout" interval in between when you don't take anything. Remember, if you are taking a prescribed medication speak to your doctor first about the best way to go off your form of treat-ment and how long the medications are likely to persist in your body. Use that as the length of the "washout" interval between treatments.

Use Tools to Remember Better

Also, since memory problems are a frequent feature of WHMS, the mea-surement tools in this chapter will help you remember better. It is often difficult enough for those with WHMS symptoms to remember what *specific* symptoms occurred yesterday, much less which symptoms were occurring three or six or twelve months ago. So these subjective semi-objective measurement tools will aid your memory and help guide you in deciding what to do.

Use Tools to Prevent Becoming a "Treatment Junkie"

Another reason for using the tools I offer in this chapter is to prevent yourself from unnecessarily becoming what I think of as a "treatment junkie." As I've interviewed women over the last two years I've repeat-edly asked those reporting WHMS symptoms "What has helped?" "What hasn't?" Repeatedly women have told me "I've been taking 'over-the-counter treatment *X*.'" (Though some over-the-counter treatments have not been well researched with regard to their effectiveness in scien-tifically convincing research trials many have not been.) When I've asked if the treatment helped or not, too many times I've heard "I don't know but I'm afraid to stop taking it in case it is helping." It is easy to see how this kind of thinking could lead to ritually taking a daily bowl of over-the-counter treatments with conceivably little benefit that one is simply afraid to stop taking. Measuring your symptoms over time in the ways I suggest may at a minimum encourage "taking stock" and keep you abreast of whether you are benefiting from what you are taking, so you don't become a prisoner of treatments of dubious benefit to you. (I know you may be taking some for preventive purposes and it is harder to assess the benefits of treatments taken for this end goal.)

Lastly, I think it is useful to measure or count certain symptoms because I suspect that people can over time just get used to their symptoms little by little so that gradually they aren't aware of them as "symptoms" anymore but just think "This is the way I am and have been for as long as I can remember." In this regard I am reminded of an interview in which Dr. Susan Love told me about "chemo brain." I had asked if she was aware of the estrogen/brain research and the cognitive symptoms that can occur in association with estrogen loss. She said, "Oh, you mean chemo brain." That was the informal term, she said, used by some cancer specialists to refer to the cognitive changes produced in some women whose ovaries had become damaged by some forms of chemotherapy. (Not all forms of chemotherapy produce this.) Such women could be estrogen deficient as a result, she said. Noting that the topic had been little studied formally, Dr. Love said, "We don't know if it ["chemo brain"] gets better on its own or if women just get used to it."

Dedicate a Loose-leaf Binder for Tracking Symptoms and Treatments

If you are inclined to and have the time I recommend that you get a three-ring loose-leaf binder with paper and dividers with plastic "stuff-in" colored tabs. Alternatively, you can get what is called a "trapper-keeper" containing the above. It's a loose-leaf binder with pockets inside and a zipper around it so papers can't fall out. Set up separate labeled sections to keep track of all the information that relates to your WHMS symptoms, perimenopausal or menopausal symptoms, doctors you have seen, your reactions to them and their recommendations and instructions, and your possible choice of treatments (doctor-recommended or self-recommended) along with prescriptions or photocopies of prescriptions. Keep this book in one spot and return it always to the same spot. You may choose sometimes to take it to your doctor to discuss changes or your treatment history.

In most of the other plastic divider tabs you will write in dates. These sections will contain the results of your symptom measurements from a specific date from the **WHMS Screening Instrument (WHMSSI)**, the **Perimenopausal or Menopausal Symptom "Circus" Chart, and the Symptom Diary.** (You should staple the results of these three onto the loose-leaf pages in this section.) I suggest you keep the results of the **WHMS Golf-counter Symptom-change Technique** in a separate section marked **"Golf Scores"** so you can quickly size up changes in the frequency of your symptoms between measurement intervals.

If you do what I propose, in later months or years as you flip through these dividers containing your measurement tool results you will have a sequential description over time of what has been occurring to your symptoms so that you can assess the "bigger picture" and decide if things are relatively stable or have improved, or if it may be time to take some kind of action.

As you use the measurement tools make sure to fill in the date you used each and list on it what treatments if any you were taking at that time and how long you had been taking them.

Label one of the dividers **"Doctors."** In this folder keep track of what doctors you went to, when, and why. Describe your reaction to the doctor and the visit, how satisfied you were, if you were listened to. Write down or staple in any notes you took—I suggest you routinely plan on bringing written questions to your visits and tape record or take notes while your doctor talks—about what was said and recommended as soon after the visit as possible. In doing this you may realize that you didn't understand something after all, and you can make plans to follow up with questions by phoning the doctor at a time she or he is available. (During your visit ask when is the best time to call for follow-up questions.) If you plan on taking hormone replacement therapy be extra sure to write down what medications you should be taking on what days. It can sometimes get confusing initially to try to remember the names of the different medications—some sound alike—and how often, and when in the day to take them. So having this written down in black and white as a handy reference guide in a dedicated book in a dedicated place can eliminate a certain amount of worry. Don't rely on your memory for this, since it is well known that even for those without memory problems, doctor/patient interactions are often fraught with instant forgetting by the patient. Don't be shy about asking the doctor several times how to take the medication. It is fairly routine and expected. Don't assume it reflects on your mental competence. You could say "I'd like you to reconfirm (or say again) what you said before about how to take these new medications. I want to be certain I'm taking them right." Or bring a small tape recorder and say "I'd like to tape-record your instructions." This way you can always reconfirm the instructions.

Label another divider **"Treatments"** and in this section keep sheets in which you track when you started taking medications, at what dosage levels, how often, at what time of day, and for what reasons. Draw a time line over a span of several years and mark what treatments you took and when you stopped. Also note for each treatment what tips you have been given about possible side effects and how to manage them—from a doctor or from reading. Use a colored pen or highlighter pen to emphasize each treatment so you can scan your treatment notes over time for a quick review. This can help you, over a series of years, stay on top of what regimens you have been through, if you switch doctors or move, or just don't remember. Also, at weekly intervals you might write in if you have noticed any effects of the treatment.

Label another divider **"Golf Scores"** and keep the results of this measuring technique I describe below in this section. Label other possible sections: **"Prescriptions," "Coping Plans."** (The latter might be backup options you could be considering for coping with your symptoms. Having options and alternative plans of action will help you avoid feeling helpless and hopeless and offer you more control.)

When to Use the Different Tools

I suggest you start using the tools in this chapter any time. But if you are going to see a doctor about WHMS symptoms I suggest you start using them at least two to three weeks before so you can record and track what is happening to you and communicate the results in specific detail. I suggest you also start using these tools before you start any treatment so you have a before-treatment baseline frequency of your symptoms that you can use for later comparisons to assess whether the treatment has made a difference in your symptoms.

HOW TO USE THE WHMS SCREENING INSTRUMENT (WHMSSI)

Use the WHMS Screening Instrument below:

- as soon as you read this book to develop a baseline score of what you are experiencing, even if you have very few symptoms
- when you go to your doctor, to show her or him if you think you have WHMS
- before and after starting a form of treatment for WHMS to note any differences
- once a year before your birthday to note any differences over time even if you haven't been taking any kind of treatment

The WHMS Screening Instrument (WHMSSI) below has not yet been formally researched. Its usefulness is as an inventory for taking stock of symptoms that are present, observing changes over time in WHMS symptoms, making relative comparisons between different occasions, and for the purposes of communicating your symptoms to a doctor via a kind of "snapshot."

WHMS Screening Instrument (WHMSSI)

Date: _____   Name: _____

I have been taking: (List how long you have been taking each form of doctor-recommended or self-treatment)_____

Instructions:

- Each statement below should be preceded with the statement **"More than in my early thirties (or the past) I experience episodes of _____."**
- Under the column below marked "Part 1: Frequency" circle the numbered response that fits your experience of **how often this symptom affects you.** Here is what the numbers mean:

Frequency Ratings

0 = Not at all
1 = Occasionally
2 = More than occasionally

- Circle "Yes" in the second column (Part 2) if this symptom **affects your personal life** or **your sense of yourself.** (Do you feel the symptoms are undermining the familiar sense you have of yourself as a person?) Circle "No" if it does not.
- Circle "Yup" under the third column (Part 3) if this symptom **affects you in the work you do.** Circle "No" if it does not affect your work.

Symptom	Part 1 Frequency	Part 2 Affects Personal Life or Sense of Self	Part 3 Affects Work
1. __Having wrong words pop out	0 1 2	No Yes	No Yup
2. __Not finding the words I need	0 1 2	No Yes	No Yup
3. __Using words like "whatchamacallit"	0 1 2	No Yes	No Yup
4. __Forgetting names of people, places, things	0 1 2	No Yes	No Yup
5. __Being more absentminded	0 1 2	No Yes	No Yup

WHMS SCREENING INSTRUMENT AND MEASURING TOOLS

Symptom	Frequency	Affects Personal Life or Sense of Self	Affects Work
6. __Losing my train of thought	0 1 2	No Yes	No Yup
7. __Forgetting what I came into a room for	0 1 2	No Yes	No Yup
8. __Feeling foggy-headed	0 1 2	No Yes	No Yup
9. __Briefly tuning out on what's being said or done	0 1 2	No Yes	No Yup
10. __Forgetting in an instant what I did a second earlier	0 1 2	No Yes	No Yup
11. __Putting things in strange places or picking up wrong things for use	0 1 2	No Yes	No Yup
12. __Briefly forgetting how to do something long known	0 1 2	No Yes	No Yup
13. __Forgetting how to spell words	0 1 2	No Yes	No Yup
14. __Missing appointments or forgetting important dates	0 1 2	No Yes	No Yup
15. __Making errors when I write	0 1 2	No Yes	No Yup
16. __Changes in my concentration skills	0 1 2	No Yes	No Yup
17. __Being more easily distractible	0 1 2	No Yes	No Yup
18. __Handling stress less well	0 1 2	No Yes	No Yup
19. __Not remembering faces as well	0 1 2	No Yes	No Yup
20. __Unexpected changes in my time spent reading or my ease in reading	0 1 2	No Yes	No Yup

197

Symptom	Frequency	Affects Personal Life or Sense of Self	Affects Work
21. __Not remembering how to get someplace	0 1 2	No Yes	No Yup
22. __Not being able to pull out ideas at will	0 1 2	No Yes	No Yup
23. __Dropping things more often	0 1 2	No Yes	No Yup
24. __Forgetting when I did what in the past	0 1 2	No Yes	No Yup
25. __Needing more time or effort to organize a task well	0 1 2	No Yes	No Yup
26. __Changes in my math skills	0 1 2	No Yes	No Yup
27. __Taking longer to retrieve "info" from my memory	0 1 2	No Yes	No Yup
28. __Not seeing a thing that's right there	0 1 2	No Yes	No Yup
29. __Subtle changes in coordination while driving	0 1 2	No Yes	No Yup
30. __Preferring less-challenging tasks	0 1 2	No Yes	No Yup
31. __Feeling like I'm "losing it"	0 1 2	No Yes	No Yup
32. __Worrying that I may have early Alzheimer's disease or a brain tumor	0 1 2	No Yes	No Yup

WHMS Score (0–64): **Personal life/self-sense:** **Work:**
1( ) + 2( ) = ____   **Number of "Yes" answers** ____   **Number of "Yup" answers** ____

To Score:

(1) Add up the number of symptoms you gave a score of 1 to and write that number in the parentheses next to the number 1 (WHMS Score) above. This describes the number of "occasional" WHMS symptoms you experience now.

(2) Then add up the number of symptoms you gave a score of 2 to and put that number in the parentheses next to the number 2 above. This describes the number of "more than occasionally" WHMS symptoms you experience now.

(3) Now multiply that number you just filled in by 2 and add it to the first number. This will give you a total WHMS Score. This score reflects all the WHMS symptoms that affect you now.

(4) Next add up the number of "Yes" answers you circled. This gives you the number of symptoms that affect you in your personal life and/or affect your sense of self.

(5) Next add up the number of "Yup" answers you circled. This gives you the number of symptoms that affect you at work.

(6) Last, on the left side of the sheets put a star (*) next to the symptom or symptoms that concern you the most.

(7) Now transfer the above numbers below.

(8) Over time compare the columns of your successive WHMSSI scores below.

Number of WHMS symptoms that bother me occasionally _____

Number of WHMS symptoms that bother me more than occasionally _____

Total WHMS Score (reflects all the WHMS symptoms affecting me _____

Number of WHMS symptoms that affect my personal life or sense of self _____

Number of WHMS symptoms that affect my work life _____

What the Scores Mean

The scores you have just compiled reflect how often and with what impact WHMS symptoms are affecting your life. The scores are useful as a "snapshot" to make objective to you or your doctor what you are experiencing now. The scores do not yet have a standardized meaning since the WHMSSI has not yet been formally researched in large populations of people. However, the scores will let you determine what category of woman with WHMS you are with respect to the descriptions I presented in chapter 6.

"Never": You are likely to be a "Never" if you scored less than five on the "Number of WHMS symptoms that bother me occasionally."

"Almost Never": You are likely to be an "Almost Never" if you had a score of between 5 and 32 for "Number of WHMS Symptoms that bother me occasionally." (You only checked off symptoms in the 1 column of frequency and didn't check off any "Yes" or "Yup" answers.)

"Worried Well" (Without Major Quality-of-Life Changes): You are likely to be "Worried Well with No Major Quality-of-Life Changes" if you have a score of less than 10 "Yes" or "Yup" answers.

"Worried Not Well" (Suffering Major Quality-of-Life Changes): You are likely to be a "Worried Not Well" (Suffering Major Quality-of-Life Changes) if you have a score of more than 25 on "Number of WHMS symptoms that affect my personal life or sense of self," or a score of more than 25 on "Number of WHMS symptoms that affect my work life."

The scores also prove meaningful when used over different time intervals. You can compare how you filled out the last four lines of the screening instrument at different times. You can ask yourself:

- With passing time do I have many more symptoms (five or more) that are bothering me more than occasionally?
- Is my total WHMS score going up by more than 10 points with passing time?
- Do I have many more symptoms (five or more) that are affecting my personal life or sense of self?
- Are many more symptoms (five or more) affecting my work life?

If the answer to any of these is "yes" WHMS is progressing. You should show these changes on the WHMSSI to a doctor and discuss options. It may mean that it is time to consider some form of treatment—hormonal or non-hormonal—if the symptoms are distressing you. It may mean the amount or type of treatment you are using may not be effective any longer and may need to be reevaluated. If the scores are going down by the same number of points, your WHMS is getting better, perhaps on its own or in response to something you are doing to treat it.

Maria M., an art instructor at fifty-nine, could have saved herself considerable daily worry had she had a WHMSSI to use when her symptoms of WHMS first began. Afraid of Alzheimer's disease because it existed in two aunts and her mother but also afraid of estrogen because of what she had heard about its risks over the years, she worried considerably about her WHMS symptoms. Maria probably fit the "Worried Well" category. However, with the rush of life she had kept no notes over time about which WHMS symptoms she had and had no clear sense how they had been when she was fifty-four or fifty. She didn't have an accurate sense of how she was then. Her personal time line sense of history was not all that she would have wished. However, as she grew older she worried more and more about developing Alzheimer's disease and imagined each WHMS episode was a harbinger of the disease. She couldn't tell if her symptoms had actually progressed, if she had gotten used to them, or if she was just worrying more because of age. Had she recorded her symptoms on the WHMSSI she would have had a more objective basis for not worrying or making a decision about whether to consider taking estrogen or another treatment.

THE PERIMENOPAUSAL OR MENOPAUSAL SYMPTOM "CIRCUS" CHART

The Perimenopausal or Menopausal Symptom "Circus" Chart ("Circus" Chart for short) below is a snapshot way of describing to yourself or your doctors the kind of perimenopause or menopause you are experiencing at the moment. Are you experiencing only one kind of symptom possible during this stage in life or more than one? Are you experiencing what I call a one-ring circus of symptoms, a two-ring circus, or a three-ring circus? "Only WHMS symptoms" is a **one-ring circus**; "two different sets of symptoms" such as WHMS plus mood/emotional symptoms is a **two-ring circus**; WHMS plus body symptoms is also a **two-ring circus**; all three sets of symptoms possible during this stage, WHMS plus mood/emotional plus body symptoms, is a **three-ring circus**. You get the idea. I emphasize that the chart is for communication purposes with others for making objective what is inside you in a convenient simple form. The "Circus" Chart will not tell *you* anything you don't already know. Refer to Appendix I for possible body or mood/emotional symptoms.

Mark the following circle to communicate to a doctor which kinds of perimenopause- or menopause-associated symptoms are bothering you most right now. Use **W** to indicate WHMS symptoms, **B** for body symptoms, **M** for mood or emotional symptoms. If you have only one kind of symptom write that letter in the center. If you have two or more kinds, create *slices*. The slices of the pie need not be even. Use bigger slices to indicate which symptoms bother you most.

You could also use this to take a "snapshot" record of where things stand with you at the moment for later comparisons. Carolyn P., for example, a fifty-three-year-old children's book writer, never had a hot flash before or since becoming menopausal at age fifty or any other physical symptoms associated with menopause. She experienced only WHMS symptoms from the age of forty-nine onward. But at age fifty-two she found herself suddenly irritated by many things. Her flare-ups with her teenage children were appropriate in content but in retrospect sometimes seemed emotionally excessive. One day she realized that her overreactions emotionally were becoming a pattern and probably were related to menopause. She had assumed that whatever happened in menopause happened all at once and didn't continue as an evolving process as seemed to be the case with her. In Carolyn's case, at age fifty, she would have marked the circle below with only a *W* (for WHMS symptoms). However, three years later she would have marked the circle with both a *W* and an *M* (for mood/emotional symptoms).

The Perimenopausal or Menopausal Symptom "Circus Chart"

W= WHMS Cognitive/memory/speech/behavior/attention symptoms that affect my life

B = Body symptoms such as hot flashes, sleep disruption, vaginal dryness, fatigue, bladder leakage, and new headaches that affect my life

M = Mood or emotional symptoms such as irritability, anger, unexpected crying or tearfulness, rapid mood shifts, emotional flatness or depression, and anxiety that affect my life

The diagram above describes which kinds of symptoms are affecting my life now and in what relative proportions.

The specific symptoms that bother me most specifically are:

WHMS	Mood	Body
_____	_____	_____
_____	_____	_____
_____	_____	_____
_____	_____	_____
_____	_____	_____
_____	_____	_____

*Date:*_____

*Current treatments I am taking*_____

_____

*I have been taking this since*_____

The "Circus" Chart is a communication tool intended to be used for helping those you might consult get the "picture" of what you are experiencing during perimenopause or menopause in relation to the three categories of symptoms that are possible at this time or for your own record-keeping purposes. It is more like handing someone a video of yourself than a diagnostic tool that will tell *you* what you "are." You *know already* what you are experiencing. The "Circus" Chart will help make that clearer to others. Fill it out and show it to your doctor as a record of what is bothering you most when you visit him or her. Also fill one out after getting treatment with possibly hormones, or antidepressants, or other medications that may be used to control symptoms around menopause as a record for the doctor's files to reflect whether the treatment is having an impact. You might also use it if you use over-the-counter treatments for any of the symptoms possible around menopause.

Carolyn S., 53, a friend, started using my "Circus" Chart with its list of symptoms as a way of remembering what was happening to her over time—as snapshots so she could remember what was bothering her most at a particular time interval. But she also started bringing her "Circus" Charts to her psychiatrist, a psychopharmacologist, when she decided her mood symptoms were affecting her marriage to a dangerous degree. She felt she was *inexplicably* too angry, tearful, and depressed at times and wanted to be able to control herself better. Her psychiatrist was trying different medications sequentially and Carolyn used the "Circus" Chart as a form of recording over the course of months her response to different treatments, which she would then show to her doctor. They helped as a shorthand tool for tracking changes over time.

THE WHMS GOLF-COUNTER SYMPTOM FREQUENCY TECHNIQUE

I suggest you use this simple handy technique *to measure at once all WHMS symptoms* you may have and to find out if you are staying stable, getting better, or getting worse with time or to decide if a particular treatment, doctor-recommended or self-recommended, is helping you or not over time.

Go to a sporting goods store and buy two or more two-inch-long plastic counters on a key chain, known as a "golf-score caddy." Wilson Sports makes one. I bought them in an Anaconda sporting goods store. The counters are available in white or red and can count from 1–99 events. You turn a knob with your thumb to advance the score by one and the score appears in a little window. They cost under three dollars. I suggest you buy at least two, one white and one red. In the Notes you will find a number you can call to find out where these are available.

You will be using these counters over a two-week period to measure *any and all* WHMS symptoms that occur. (Two weeks is better, but if you can't, then do one week.) You will be using one counter—*the red one*—to record any symptoms during the day that bother, or embarrass, or cause you difficulty a lot—that you consider *major*. Use the red counter to measure symptoms you find somewhat alarming. You will be using *the white counter* to measure any WHMS symptoms that occur that are *not major,* that you notice but that don't distress you much.

I suggest that you record your "major" and "not major" scores at the end of each of the two weeks. Having scores for each of two weeks will give you a sense of how much your symptoms can vary in frequency from week to week at a given time period. Use the scores for the two weeks as an upper and lower range of your score.

WHMS "Golf" Score of Symptom Frequency

Date	Week 1	Week 2
# Major symptoms		
# Not major symptoms		
Total # of symptoms		

Treatments I have been on: (List since when) _____

_____

If you have more than ninety-nine symptoms in a week, scratch or write with a pen "1" in front of the window on the counter and use the counter to start again so that your score is 100 plus whatever is in the window.

What is most important to the success of this method is to try to keep these counters near you *at all times*. You might choose to keep the counters in a pocket, or a handbag, or on a long ribbon or string or chain around your neck under whatever you are wearing. The idea is to have the counter present the moment a WHMS symptom occurs, so you can't forget about it.

At the end of each week, fill in the above chart or make up your own. Enter the scores on your red counter next to "# Major symptoms" and the score on your white counter next to "# Not major symptoms." Also add both of these up to get the total number of symptoms. Use the numbers for each of the two weeks as a range. Try also to include weekends, because WHMS symptoms may occur more in your personal life when you are more likely to just "be" and aren't as likely to be working with directed attention. If you decide not to use any treatment you might want to use this technique every year to see if things are fairly stable or are changing for the better or worse. You can also use this technique before starting a new treatment regimen and again after several months. Copy or enter these scores onto a sheet and staple them into your loose-leaf binder in the section marked "Golf Scores." As you test yourself at sequential times you can see if your range of total symptoms is shifting up or down (worse or better) or if you have more major than minor symptoms than before, or vice versa.

SYMPTOM DIARY

I suggest that when you use any of the instruments above you also write a paragraph or two as a symptom diary to give a gestalt—an overall picture—of how you are affected by the symptoms you have and your state of mind and mood in relating to them. Also note whether anything unusual or stressful or wonderful is happening in your life. Keep the sheets of this symptom diary together in the divider with your WHMSSI results and "Circus" Chart. This will give you a "picture" of yourself for later recall and comparisons.

If you choose, you can describe any and all of the following: the contexts in which symptoms seem to occur—do you detect a pattern? Do symptoms occur more on weekends than weekdays, more when you are tired, or does it matter? Are you coping well with symptoms overall? If so, how? Describe the symptom(s) that bother(s) you most at the moment. Note which have gotten better, or worse. If you are perimenopausal keep track of your periods here. Note if they are longer than usual, shorter, heavier, lighter, when you recall you last had one, etc. (Highlight this information so you can find it later.) Write down what you have tried that either helps or doesn't help, or that you are planning to try (some self-management approaches).

You may think to yourself "What can I gain from writing this down now when I already know what's going to be in the diary?" For one thing you will know in a year from now how you felt this year. Further, I can only say that in working with patients, symptom diaries have been a useful way for patients to focus in on their symptoms and to become actively curious about them. Something about shining a beacon of attention and directing motivation toward a goal can lead to helpful revelations and some solutions down the road. If nothing else, you will have a way of remembering in the future what a certain time in your life felt like from the inside. You can even, if you choose, leave this diary as a distinctive life-cycle legacy to younger women in your family, so your experiences may help them in some potential way, perhaps to let them know that women once had to go through this and, because of directed research efforts, no longer need to anymore.

IV

WHAT TO DO IF YOU HAVE WHMS

9

Doctors, Women, and
WHMS Symptoms

So you have WHMS symptoms and need to find a doctor who can help. How can you set things up before your appointment to determine if your doctor will take the time to answer your questions? What questions can you ask that will clue you in to the state of awareness of the ob/gyn you are talking to about the potential effects of estrogen loss on your symptoms? What criteria can you use to assess your satisfaction with your visit? What can you expect to find in the average ob/gyn regarding menopause in general and awareness of WHMS symptoms specifically. (My comments in this chapter will refer primarily, though not always, to ob/gyns.)

How do you set up your visit to assure you get the time you need with a new or familiar ob/gyn or to quickly learn that you will be unlikely to get what you need from this particular doctor when you need it?

Women with WHMS symptoms as well as women first encountering perimenopause and menopause often need time to talk with their doctor beyond the usual annual physical inspection to get information and to have things explained. Here is how you can discover quickly if you are likely to get that time: When you call for an appointment tell the person scheduling appointments that you are coming in to discuss symptoms you think may be related to perimenopause or menopause and will need time to discuss them, be informed about the realities of menopause or perimenopause, and possible treatment options. Indicate that you are willing to wait for an appointment at a future time when the doctor will be able to have time to talk.

In this way when you see the doctor she or he will have had sufficient advance notice to work around *your* time demands for talk. If you have set it up in this way you can get an impression of how much your needs are likely to be accommodated in future interactions.

USEFUL QUESTIONS TO ASK YOUR OB/GYN TO DETERMINE IF HE OR SHE IS KNOWLEDGEABLE ABOUT MENOPAUSAL MEDICINE AND ESTROGEN-AND-THE-MIND RESEARCH

There is little point in going to a doctor for help if he or she won't know how to help you. So plan to invest some time screening for a doctor who can meet your needs. When you have a recommended name (see below) you might schedule a regular visit or alternatively call to say you are considering switching ob/gyns and would to like schedule an appointment *simply to meet and talk with the new doctor.* (I have done this to discover a doctor was "not for me.") At the visit, ask some or all of the following questions. Remember this doctor could potentially be of considerable help to you over time or stand in the way of your getting help by virtue of inexperience or ignorance about women with your needs. Don't be too passive in being your own health advocate.

You can respectfully ask:

- What have women told you over the years about how menopause (or perimenopause) affects thinking or speech or behavior? (Has this person been listening and crediting what at least some women have been reporting?)

- Are you familiar with the research of Barbara Sherwin (regarding effects of estrogen loss on verbal memory and new learning)? What do you think of it?
- Are you a member of the North American Menopause Society?
- Do you subscribe to the medical journal *Maturitas* or *Menopausal Medicine*? (The first is the journal of the International Menopause Society; the second is a quarterly newsletter of the American Society for Reproductive Medicine.)
- Have you had the opportunity of taking any continuing medical education credits or courses in recent years about menopause medicine? What are some of the issues in the field right now?
- Are you familiar with the research about estrogen's roles in the brain?
- What symptoms do you believe are hormone-related during menopause (or perimenopause)? (How short is this list? Does it include any of the symptoms women with WHMS have described in this book?)

More Questions to Ask

Here are some added considerations and questions suggested by Pam Boggs, Director of Education of the North American Menopause Society (NAMS), for women trying to find a doctor knowledgeable about treating women in the years surrounding menopause:

1. Ask the doctor "What percent of your practice is devoted to menopausal women or post-reproduction-age women?"

2. An indirect indicator is to look and see if all the magazines in the office have to do with babies. If so, you know this doctor isn't being sensitive to your needs.

3. Ask "What are your recommended regimens for menopause-related disturbances?" Does he or she have only one universal regimen or different choices? A physician experienced in menopause medicine will have more than one.

4. Ask "Do you offer any other non-hormone regimens for treating menopausal symptoms such as hot flashes?" If your doctor is "into" this field he or she will know that (1) a high dose of 800–1200 international units of vitamin E will work for hot flashes or that (2) eating daily servings of soy food products can be helpful in controlling hot flashes and vaginal dryness. We don't yet know what an effective or too high a dose is, so NAMS doesn't recommend [soy-derived] powders or pills at this point. We do know, however, that small doses can be helpful.

5. A good question to ask is "If I come to you and you do prescribe a hormone when will you want to see me again?" A less competent doctor will say in one year. I'd like my doctor to say "In three months." A doctor trying to individualize treatment for you specifically would want to see how you, the individual patient, are responding to it. Women vary enormously in symptoms and responses to treatment.

Pam Boggs adds: "Women are often [unduly] loyal to doctors who gave them their babies. You do have permission to switch doctors even if [your ob/gyn] was good for your children's delivery. You have to interview doctors to find one who is good for your needs at this time. Refer to our [NAMS'] list of doctors, use the yellow pages, or ask those around you [to find a suitable doctor.]"

TO IDENTIFY A DOCTOR WHO MAY BE KNOWLEDGEABLE ABOUT MENOPAUSE AND PERIMENOPAUSE

- Call the North American Menopause Society for their list of menopause *clinics* around the country. (See Appendix II for information.)
- Call the North American Menopause Society for their list of *physician members.* Though NAMS does not do any credentialing of the doctors who are their members, at the least "they have demonstrated an interest in menopausal women" according to Pam Boggs.
- Join a menopause support group in your area even for only a few sessions to meet with women who may know a good responsive ob/gyn or nurse practitioner knowledgeable about treating WHMS

symptoms or perimenopause and menopause in general. The leader of the support group too may have cumulative experience with women about good doctors in your area. Contact the American Menopause Foundation (see Appendix II) for referral to such groups around the country.

• Contact the American Menopause Foundation for a list of its member physicians. Remember though that not all physicians who are on such lists are guaranteed experts about menopause.

To Assess Your Satisfaction after a Visit Ask Yourself

• Did I feel rushed?
• Was I given a chance to talk without being interrupted continually?
• Did the doctor take a thorough history?
• Were my questions responded to?
• Were my concerns pooh-poohed as nothing to worry about without being addressed respectfully?
• Did the doctor or nurse practitioner ask about my family or health history risk factors before prescribing a hormone replacement treatment (if this applies to you)?
• Did this doctor strike me as knowledgeable about the questions I needed answers to?
• Did I feel I was being talked down to or pushed into trying a treatment I expressed doubts about?
• If I requested it, was I given supportive research information to help me make any specific decisions about prospective treatments?

Keep in mind that ob/gyns are experiencing a demographic shift in their practices as baby boomer women "age out" of fertility and delivery needs. You may be in a buyer's market and your questions may help to influence the educational interests of ob/gyns. According to Pam Boggs, "Fewer women are coming to them [ob/gyns] for fertility-related needs. To survive, the American Fertility Society recently changed its name. Ob/gyns are seeing this shift already. If doctors want to keep patients they will have to keep up educationally with the changing needs of patients."

Keep in Mind

With respect to the results of your doctor visits keep in mind the following advice from Gillian Ford, a hormonal educator at the Center for Hormonal Health in Roseville, California, in her excellent book *Listening to Your Hormones*. "Remember that normal blood test results . . . do not guarantee that you are free of hormone imbalance. Not everyone who has hormone deficiency knows about it." This is not a call for you to dismiss all medical test results but rather to emphasize that much yet remains to be known factually about the "science" of what changes when during the transition from premenopause to menopause. Just as symptoms of hypothryoidism can often manifest without objective test indicators at first—and be "subclinical" initially—so too it appears that the WHMS symptoms of ovarian hormonal changes can possibly occur before present tests indicate anything clinically is occurring.

Overview: What Can You Expect to Find

There are thousands and thousands of ob/gyns in practice today. What can you expect to find if you wander into the offices of one at random:

- You can expect to find that not all ob/gyns are menopause experts—an assumption I surely had when I began to study menopause. My thought as I discovered this was "If ob/gyns aren't menopause experts then *who in the world is there to turn to?*" "Ob/gyns are women's health specialists but [they] are not necessarily menopause experts," in the words of ob/gyn and menopause expert and researcher Dr. Robert Greene, Polly Van Benthusen's physician, a doctor, you may recall, who untypically sought out specifically extra training in menopause medicine.

  In some highly reputable ob/gyn residency programs ob/gyn residents receive a scant two hours of *directly targeted formal instruction* on the treatment of menopausal issues. (My assumption and hope is that they learn more incidentally about perimenopause and menopause in the course of hands-on training, but I don't bet on my assumptions in this area anymore.) A clinical endocrinologist who chose not to be quoted directly told me that "Ob/gyns are basically trained to be surgeons and have needs for action and motor behavior. They aren't diagnosticians or people who like to sit and talk. You can tell the first year in medical school," he says, "who is going to be a surgeon and who is not. You can spot them even by the way they walk."

Dr. Eileen Hoffman, an internist and women's health advocate affiliated with Mount Sinai Medical Center in New York and author of *Our Health, Our Lives,* writes: "Currently there is no way to know if a doctor [speaking of doctors in general] is truly skilled in women's health. There are no certificates or diplomas to signal competency. Doctors only gain up-to-date knowledge about women's health by learning it on their own. It's certainly not taught in medical schools yet . . . although this is beginning to change."

For many doctors trained in the past and now in practice, menopause and perimenopause were considered *stages in development,* not stages involving potential health consequences and treatment. Judging by the lecture sessions that exist at ob/gyn professional conferences, ob/gyns seem to be "up" on the needs for treating osteoporosis and heart disease with hormone replacement therapy—they've had years to master this now relatively long-known information—but the profession hasn't yet caught up to the new research on estrogen's roles in the brain and the need for educating women, diagnosing, and if necessary treating cognitive/behavioral symptoms associated with hormonal changes.

• You can expect to find ob/gyns who don't have much time to talk to you about menopause when you need a lot of time to ask questions and discuss answers. The wife of a major ob/gyn leader in the menopause field, confided in me. She said "Most ob/gyns are just too hassled and don't have the time or energy to work with menopausal women. They don't have spare time for talk between the unpredictability of delivering babies, executing specially timed procedures for infertile women, and their office schedules. And most menopausal women need that time to understand what's happening to them—you know, what options they have or about [taking] hormone replacement therapy. [The relationship] doesn't usually work out too well, is what I hear from my friends. Most women I know

217

get their information [about menopause] from television or magazines, not their doctors." In this regard, menopause expert Dr. Lila Nachtigall, who has trained many ob/gyn residents as a professor of obstetrics and gynecology at New York University's School of Medicine and who is also a leading researcher on estrogen's effects, told me this story about "talking" and the added time constraints imposed by the realities of practice in HMOs. She said, "I recently ran into one of the [ob/gyn] residents who I helped train a number of years ago. She now works for a major HMO and asked me a very sophisticated question that related to menopause. I said, 'You seem to have a good grasp of this topic. Do you want me to refer patients to you who I can't take on?' She said, 'Oh no! Menopausal women need too much time to talk!' With HMOs ob/gyns now have much higher caseloads and less time per patient." Dr. Nachtigall said. Other experts I spoke with confirmed the "no time to talk" and HMO picture.

- You mainly can expect to find physicians (ob/gyns, internists, neurologists, psychiatrists, etc.) who are *not* yet familiar with the research on estrogen and the brain and therefore who may not be willing to treat *only* your WHMS symptoms alone with hormone replacement therapy unless you are also interested in taking it to treat established perimenopausal and menopausal symptoms such as hot flashes and vaginal dryness or for preventive purposes, i.e., to prevent osteoporosis or heart disease.

- You can expect to find ob/gyns who are *not* aware of the range of cognitive/behavioral symptoms that can accompany perimenopause and menopause and may suddenly look at you quite skeptically from a new psychic distance as though you were having psychotic delusions. You may lose credibility for full sanity in describing your symptoms in accurate detail not unlike Quiana Mortier and find your symptoms glossed over.

- You can expect to find ob/gyns who may incorrectly interpret your symptoms as mainly due to the secondary effects of (1) hot flashes and nighttime awakenings; (2) the side effects of depression, which can result from the biochemical changes associated with perimenopause and menopause (estrogen loss); or both and refer you for psychotherapy for the latter. Such physicians won't realize that your symptoms likely *are* potentially treatable with hormone replacement therapy and may not consider this option for the symptoms you describe.

- You can, though, expect to find physicians who *are* aware of recent research indicating an association between taking estrogen and a reduced risk of Alzheimer's disease. The multiple studies that showed this association were given considerable coverage in newspapers and on TV over the last several years. So ob/gyns may be willing to treat you with hormone replacement therapy if you indicate that that is your expressed interest—reducing the risk of Alzheimer's disease.

- You can expect to find some physicians—particularly some women physicians—who may have a preset political agenda that involves categorically not wanting to "medicalize the natural state of menopause." They want it to be a "normal" stage for *everyone* even when it doesn't lead to a normal life for everyone. Such doctors don't recognize the variability of responses possible during perimenopause and menopause among women losing estrogen and may not be sensitive or receptive to hearing what you are telling them. They may be averse to recognizing that for some women estrogen loss can produce the equivalent of a hormone deficiency-disease disorder not dissimilar to hypothyroidism. At a May 11, 1998, conference on women's health, for example, at Ulster County Community College in upstate New York, a well-known women's health advocate and internist, trying, I assume, to make women unfearful of menopause, declared with categorical fervor and no proviso: "Menopause is not a disease. . . . Depression is more the result of women's lives than hormones." While this may be true for some or even many women, it appears not to be true for all women.

What if You Have Trouble Finding an Ob/Gyn Who Is Ideal

If you can't find your ideal doctor, here is what you can settle for at the minimum:

- You need an ob/gyn who is educable: one who is willing to "hear you out" about your symptoms without dismissing them, who may be willing to hear what you have learned about estrogen and the brain and cognition, and is willing to read what you may give him or her, i.e., this book or articles that discuss this topic.

- If you think you might need or want to try hormone replacement therapy, at the minimum you need an ob/gyn or ob/gyn nurse practitioner who doesn't just have one universal hormone replacement form of treatment but who feels comfortable trying different combinations of estrogen treatments and/or different forms of progesterone treatments to meet your individual needs and responses to treatment (see next chapter). If that doctor or nurse practitioner knows how to treat hot flashes or vaginal dryness or how to administer treatments to prevent osteoporosis or heart disease, it is possible that the same kind of treatment may help your WHMS symptoms.

- If you are interested in taking non-hormonal treatments you may have to find an ob/gyn or nurse practitioner interested in holistic health or alternative treatments, who may be "up" on the literature on plant-based estrogens (phytoestrogens) such as those in soy products, cloverleaf, etc., and on other non-hormonal, plant-based or vitamin-based forms of treating perimenopausal and menopausal symptoms. Networking with other women or speaking with a neighborhood pharmacist may clue you in to such a person. Bear in mind, however, that even plant-based estrogens and other plant-based treatments for menopause can have estrogen-mimicking (agonist) effects or, on the contrary, *anti*-estrogenic (antagonistic) effects on your brain's estrogen receptors and *you may not know which is happening*. Not enough is known yet about the biological action of each of these many agents. Moreover, our reproductive hormone systems are full of complex negative feedback loops and complexly interacting mechanisms. So while it may appear safe to try every and any nonprescription treatment, be aware that you may possibly be producing opposite biological effects than the ones you intended. My suggestion, therefore, based on what I have learned to date is not to go overboard dosing yourself with any non-hormonal treatment. (If you try hormonal replacement therapy my guess is your doctor won't let you go overboard on these since she or he will be writing the prescriptions.)

Before seeing a doctor I suggest you assess your WHMS symptoms on the measurement and communication tools I described in chapter 8, ideally two weeks before you go to see any health practitioner so you will have "baseline" measures to report. Bring them or your whole binder with you to your visit and show and explain the tools to your doctor. Indicate to her or him that rather than guessing about what is happening over time with respect to your WHMS symptoms or in reaction to any forms of treatment, you would like to use these tools in partnership as a way of objectively recording changes and as a concise time-saving way of communicating those changes. (Your doctor might be delighted to have something that gives her or him a sense of what you and other patients like you might really be talking about with respect to symptoms.) Indicate that you would like to use the tools at the start of visits as an aid for reviewing specifically how things have been going for you between visits. Then go over the symptoms you've marked on each instrument and review what changes have occurred on these tools over time if you have been using them for a while. Indicate what you have tried that's helped or not helped. Your doctor will see that you "mean business" about these symptoms. And if he or she can't be bothered with the tools altogether there may be a message there for you. This doctor may not have the available time to problem solve around *your* specific needs.

CONCLUSIONS

If you begin looking for a good doctor, asking around, chances are much better that you will eventually find someone to meet your new specific needs than if you keep going to someone who isn't right for you at this time of your life.

While there are many more women now in the practice of obstetrics and gynecology, my own limited personal experience with about five women ob/gyns has been that they are not necessarily more informed about estrogen/brain research or clinically tuned in to women's WHMS symptoms from intimate doctor/patient contacts than their male counterparts. I wish I could report it were not so. Perhaps many are too young to have yet gone through menopause, though I believe many are certainly of perimenopausal age. Perhaps they have been deferring to what their profession has taught them, rather than as well to what women could teach them. You can help matters along by educating doctors of both genders about estrogen and the brain research and about WHMS symptoms.

I suggest that in addition to getting your information from physicians you help yourself with bibliotherapy—book therapy. Read books about perimenopause and menopause and become informed yourself. You might consider writing to the authors of books in this field to inquire if they know of a knowledgeable menopause expert in your area. Consider subscribing to menopause newsletters (see Appendix) to gain information about menopause experts or writing to the editors of these publications for any help they can offer you in terms of referrals. If you hear about a great doctor you might even consider making a longer-distance trip than you usually would. I have heard of several women who fly out to San Francisco from the East Coast to see Dr. John Arpels, another ob/gyn menopause expert whose knowledge and insights in this area I much respect. Good luck hunting.

10

If You Choose Estrogen and Progesterone to Treat WHMS

If estrogen loss has produced the WHMS symptoms you have at menopause then estrogen/progesterone replacement therapy may well be the answer to your cognitive problems—when it isn't contraindicated—just as it is for those who suffer from hot flashes, vaginal dryness, or osteoporosis. For perimenopausal women with WHMS symptoms for whom it's not contraindicated, low-dose birth-control pills, with estrogen and a form of progesterone, may be the answer.

The decision to try hormone replacement treatments remains, however, as individual as one's personal or family history and as complicated as ever. First, that decision might involve whether to try estrogen for a *three-month diagnostic trial period* to see if it helps. If it does then estrogen loss likely *has* been producing the WHMS symptoms. (Such a trial could potentially be used to discriminate whether the symptoms are due to stress or estrogen loss, before a woman decides, for example, to leave a desirable though stressful job or situation.) Second, estrogen might be used for *a few years* to quell changes that are significantly affecting your quality of life at this pressing, possibly inflexible, interval of your life or, third, for *more than a few years* long-term for preventive and protective effects on the brain, heart, and bones.

What the new research on estrogen's relation to Alzheimer's, the brain, and women's memory has done is simply added more plusses to one side of the equation. But it has not taken away the approach avoidance, damned if I do/damned if I don't, "what if" fears of many women surrounding the decision. "The equation for taking estrogen now has changed," aging expert Dr. John Rowe said at an "Estrogen and the Brain" conference in New York City in 1997. "We know now that women taking estrogen after menopause reduce their chances of getting cognitive impairments." He didn't, though, say how to "figure" that equation if your sister has had breast cancer, but your mother (or father) is showing signs of Alzheimer's disease; or if you are the older mother of a young child and don't know which you fear most—being senile at your child's wedding or being dead and not present at all from the currently estimated 1/100 added chance of getting breast cancer from hormone replacement therapy. (See below.)

I empathize with the unfairness inherent in being told "It's an individual decision." Whenever I hear this or read this I want to shout "*You're* the medical doctor," or "You're the medical expert, *you* know better than most of us how to size up and weigh or judge these different factors and risks. Don't slough this risky integration-demanding job off on those not used to juggling fourteen or forty balls in this complex area at one time, or who haven't had life experience to see how subjectively often in life a one in a hundred risk can materialize in a pool of real patients." Ideally, what a resourceful and knowledgeable person needs to do for women with this quandary is develop, together with experts in this field, a computer program decision-tree questionnaire that "asks" you all the relevant family history and lifestyle and life values questions pertinent to your individual prospective decision about taking hormone replacement therapy. Then factor in those variables with *all* the relevant updated knowledge from research studies and the life experience-based judgments of the best clinical experts in this field and spew out an intricately and methodically figured, comprehensive, rational answer based on known risks, on whether you should take the stuff or not (which you then might choose to ignore anyhow). But at least you could say to yourself, "Given what's known, the weight of the evidence stacks up this way or that for me personally."

Let me emphasize again that virtually no one is yet aware of the scope of symptoms that comprise Warga's Hormonal Misconnection Syndrome. There are thus no officially sanctioned recommended guidelines at present for treating, per se, the range of symptoms in WHMS by the North American Menopause Society (NAMS) or the American College of Obstetrics and Gynecology (ACOG). Physicians can't prescribe for or treat what they don't know about. In this chapter I do, however, offer the treatment guidelines of menopause experts, ob/gyns I respect who are aware of possible verbal memory and learning change aspects of WHMS symptoms, based in part on the research of Barbara Sherwin, and from their own years of experience treating women with such symptoms. (See below.)

I am also now in a position to tell you, to my great surprise, that as of May 1998, the American College of Obstetrics and Gynecology, for the first time, recognized in a newly released publication the possibility of treating cognitive symptoms with estrogen replacement therapy, not only in menopausal women but in perimenopausal women too—another step forward. (The leaders of this organization, however, are not yet aware of the broader scope of WHMS symptoms; they are mainly familiar with the verbal memory changes reported in Barbara Sherwin's research.) As I sat down to write this chapter, in the mail I received—I had requested it—the latest ACOG Educational Bulletin advisory on *Hormone Replacement Therapy* (HRT) addressed to its member "obstetricians and gynecologists," replacing an earlier 1992 bulletin. When I first requested in the winter of 1996 this organization's educational material for women patients (to be dispensed in doctors' offices) there had been no mention in any of the material sent to me of possible cognitive symptoms associated with perimenopause or menopause that women might experience. Yet now in a section titled "Indications" for giving HRT, listed *first,* ahead of indications for treating changes in other potential symptoms of perimenopause and menopause such as sexual function, cardiovascular symptoms, osteoporosis, and genitourinary symptoms, it said "Central Nervous System Symptoms" (meaning the brain here) as a category for which hormone replacement therapy could be helpful. Here is what that educational bulletin specifically says:

> Changes in neurologic function such as increased irritability, mood disorders, mild depression, hot flushes, and sleep disturbances may arise during the perimenopausal transition even before the onset of menopause. *Decreases in memory and other cognitive changes have also been reported* in some menopausal women and younger women in whom menopause has been surgically induced. . . . *[T]reatment with 1.25 mg per day of conjugated equine estrogens [Premarin] was found to be significantly more effective than placebo in reducing central nervous system symptoms* (i.e., hot flushes, insomnia, irritability, *poor memory,* anxiety, and headaches). *Hormone replacement with adequate doses of estrogen can in many cases effectively reverse cognitive changes and improve function* [emphasis added].

Under a heading titled "Therapeutic Options" the bulletin says:

> Hormone replacement therapy should be considered to relieve vasomotor symptoms, genital urinary tract atrophy, and mood and *cognitive disturbances* as well as to prevent osteoporosis and cardiovascular disease. It also may be considered to help prevent colon cancer, Alzheimer's disease, and adult tooth loss [emphasis added].

On the front page of the bulletin, a disclaimer of sorts says:

> This document is not to be construed as establishing a standard of practice or dictating an exclusive course of treatment. Rather it is intended as an educational tool. . . .

Despite the disclaimer this bulletin represents a giant step forward in recognizing that cognitive symptoms in women can exist with estrogen decline and can be frequently reversed with estrogen replacement. ACOG is to be commended for taking this step (even if some of the data they cite to support estrogen improving cognition, i.e., a 1977 English study that is twenty-two years old, and could have been helping women for twenty-two years longer had this and other similar studies at the time been followed up with more confirming studies). The question now of course is whether this information will be read and incorporated into medical practice. To this end, I urge you to show the ACOG quotes in this book to your ob/gyn and other physicians. If not for your benefit then to benefit women who may be in greater need of such help.

Before moving past the above ACOG quote, it may be useful at this juncture to point out that the treatment dose of 1.25 milligrams per day of conjugated equine estrogen (Premarin) ACOG cites as effective in relieving memory and other menopause-associated symptoms is higher than the typical starting dose of 0.625 milligrams. That higher-than-minimal levels of hormone replacement therapy may be necessary to improve cognitive symptoms is also the professed view of Dr. Uriel Halbreich, an estrogen/behavior/cognition researcher who has done research with menopausal women at the State University of New York at Buffalo. So keep these views in mind as an option to pursue if you no longer have periods and decide to take hormone replacement therapy.

In this chapter I will initially be offering you information on who estrogen therapy is generally *not* indicated for and information on assessing the risks in taking hormone replacement therapy. As a non-physician, a research and health psychologist, I will share with you some personal considerations I would take into account in weighing a decision to take hormone replacement therapy. I will provide you with recent research evidence, and the results of my interviews with experts that suggests that all the major types of estrogen now available on the market appear to "work" in the brain in offering protection of brain neurons against multiple forms of potential damage though some appear to differ in their sites of specific action. On the basis of interviews with women and from readings, I also want to caution you up front that due to the variability inherent in women discussed earlier, and the variability of known actions of different forms of estrogen, some estrogen brands and types may work less well for you specifically than other brands or types, and that it may take a number of months of sequentially trying different variations of estrogen/progesterone combinations or regimens (three months on a brand is a reasonable trial I have been told) to find a hormonal treatment format that maximally "does it" for your WHMS symptoms. Such variability among women is to be expected. Be aware too that WHMS is a new syndrome and that the subtleties of its treatment need still to be explored and defined.

To date, insightful sensitive ob/gyns aware of cognitive symptoms have not been in a position to use tests or assessment tools with which to objectively name symptoms and measure changes after hormone treatment has begun. They have mainly had to "wing it" and rely on their own and their patients' communication skills and ability to discuss difficult-to-characterize symptoms in trying to determine if there have been any improvements with treatment. Sensitive assessment tools and change-measurement tests have been sorely needed to know whether hormonal treatments are working or not, so the treatment process is not merely a hit-or-miss effort, but more systematic. I hope the description-and-assessment tools I presented in chapter 8 will begin to correct this problem. Using these tools and techniques will help you know more specifically what you are trying to treat and if you are getting detectable improvement.

Below you will find the treatment guidelines of two excellent menopause experts I respect considerably, Dr. William Andrews and Dr. Maurice Cohen. I have found both to be aware in overview that women during perimenopause and menopause can experience distressing changes in cognition. Both have had experience treating such symptoms with hormone replacement therapy. Dr. Andrews, in his capacity as a menopause expert and former president of the American College of Obstetrics and Gynecology, is playing a significant role politically in helping to disseminate within his profession knowledge about research on estrogen and the thinking-remembering parts of the brain and the potential effects of estrogen loss on memory and thinking in women.

Dr. Cohen, one of the founding members of the North American Menopause Society, actively disseminates his knowledge at NAMS workshops and at professional lectures throughout the year. I have spoken with more than a few of his patients and know that he takes both the time and interest to meet his patients' individual needs. I know that Dr. Cohen and Dr. Andrews are eager to see objective assessment tools used for measuring cognitive changes in women.

Last of all I will offer you some treatment option tips that I have culled from readings and interviews with experts and advice on what to do before and after starting treatment to more subtly assess whether hormone treatment is benefiting you.

WHO SHOULDN'T TAKE ESTROGEN?

According to the North American Menopause Society (NAMS) estrogen replacement therapy is not indicated for those with the following conditions:

- Presence of breast cancer
- Abnormal uterine bleeding of an unknown cause
- Liver disease
- A history of blood clotting disorders
- Very high levels of triglycerides (NAMS)

The American College of Obstetrics and Gynecology Lists as meaningful "Risk Factors" for taking HRT the following in its recent (1998) educational bulletin on Hormone Replacement Therapy:

- Thromboembolic disease [a history or family history of blood clotting disease]
- Endometrial hyperplasia [abnormal tissue changes] and endometrial cancer
- Endometriosis
- Breast cancer

BREAST AND ENDOMETRIAL CANCER RISK WITH ESTROGEN USE

Since fear of breast and/or endometrial cancer remains a major road block standing on the decision-making road to considering possible treatment with hormone replacement therapy for many women, let me begin by offering you one expert's way of thinking about such a decision. I heard it presented at a meeting of the 1997 North American Menopause Society, a relatively conservative organization with members from different disciplines that has more than a few officers and members very much against the "medicalizing of the natural state of menopause" with long-term drug treatments. I offer this not as a rec-ommendation to take estrogen but as a tool for decision making, ideally together with an informed physician.

Discussing a "practical strategy for decision making regarding estro-gen therapy," Dr. Richard J. Santen, Professor of Medicine and Associ-ate Director of the Cancer Center at the University of Virginia Health Sciences Center in Charlottesville, Virginia, said: "Our approach [in as-sessing the risks of breast cancer from taking estrogen replacement ther-apy] is to interpret existing data in the most conservative fashion and assume the worst case." Analyzing data on the relative risks of develop-ing breast cancer from a then-recent nurses' health study, together with collective data from many other relevant studies (meta-analyses), and the data on the incidence of breast cancer in the population, Dr. Santen came up with the following "absolute risk" assessment of the potential "price" of taking estrogen with regard to breast cancer. Here is what he concluded:

> Absolute risk—From the patient's perspective, the critical issue is the ab-solute risk of developing breast cancer. *Using a worst-case scenario, the ab-solute risk for a patient is a one in one hundred chance of developing a breast cancer over a ten-year period that would not have developed without hormone replacement therapy* [emphasis added]. This estimate would be slightly higher (i.e., 1.5 in a hundred chance) for a woman over sixty-five years of age.

Dr. Santen went on to add that even when breast cancer occurs dur-ing use of hormone replacement therapy, the likelihood of dying from it is reduced by 10 percent since the type of breast cancer likely to occur tends to be a slower growing, lazier kind of tumor, one less likely to spread quickly. He also noted that women on hormone replacement therapy tend to have a 15 percent greater rate of compliance in going for yearly mammograms than do women not receiving hormones. So women on HRT are more likely to get early detection of breast cancer, which tends to reduce the risk of a patient dying if it is diagnosed. He noted that one-third of patients with breast cancer die of that disease and fewer if diagnosed early as a result of mammography screening, but taking estrogen replacement therapy reduces by as much as 50 percent the risk of dying of a disease that is much more often lethal in women—heart disease. "Taken together" he said:

> . . . *the absolute chance of dying from breast cancer as a result of taking estrogen for over ten years is only one in 300. This figure derives from the worst case analysis* [emphasis added] and is probably an overestimate. At the same time, these women have a much reduced chance of dying from heart disease because of estrogen administration.

With respect to fears of developing endometrial cancer from taking estrogen replacement therapy Dr. Santen noted that although there is a slightly elevated risk, the risk can be virtually eliminated by taking a suitable dose of progesterone daily for fourteen days rather than for twelve or ten days as is more routinely recommended. He said, "It is helpful to explain [to your patients] that estrogens do not cause endometrial cancer provided that [a progesterone is] administered *at a dose of at least 5 milligrams of medroxyprogesterone for fourteen days per month or 2.5 milligrams daily*" [emphasis added].

In addition to Dr. Santen's assessment, here are some additional factors that place women at elevated risks of breast cancer:

- Having one or more first-degree relations—a sister, mother, or daughter—who have had breast cancer; the vast majority of breast cancers, however, appear not to be familial or hereditary.
- Having an inherited variation in the BRCA1 and BRCA2 genes, which are associated with inherited breast cancer (tests exist to check for these mutated genes).
- Breast cancer risk also increases with the following factors: age—older women are at greater risk than younger; having no children or children after age thirty; and either early onset of menstruation—before age fourteen, or menopause onset after age fifty-five.

Dr. Nancy E. Davidson, who holds the Breast Cancer Research Chair in Oncology at the Johns Hopkins School of Medicine, writing in *Scientific American* notes:

[T]he connection between breast cancer and hormonal therapy is not clear. Several dozen studies of various types have yielded mixed results. In aggregate, they suggest that less than five years of estrogen therapy has no impact on breast cancer.

These then are factors you can plug in to you deliberations equation. However, for some women even Dr. Santen's assessed 1/100 extra absolute risk of breast cancer over ten years may be *one* extra risk too many. You may recall that Polly Van Benthusen first felt this way when she was offered hormone replacement therapy. In this regard I pass on to you a Yiddish proverb my mother has used through the years: *"Vey (as in 'Oy vey') tse deym vus se bafalt"* which roughly translated means "It's woe to you, if you're the one singled out by fate to be 'it.'"

I know that many women have taken estrogen for years without incident. In response to my *New York* magazine article, for example, a woman wrote a letter to the editor stating: "As a seventy-one-year old woman who has taken estrogen for thirty-one years, I find myself healthy . . . and indeed, fairly smart (I think . . .)." At the same time I fear that the honest information I present in this book may imprudently drive women to rush to take estrogen treatment, which for them may have dire consequences.

So weigh your options carefully and pay heed to the contraindications. WHMS symptoms might be temporary in your case—hot flashes often are—and may not necessarily progress. "Can you live with the symptoms?" is one relevant question you might also be considering.

POSSIBLE REASONS FOR CONSIDERING TAKING HORMONE REPLACEMENT THERAPY

If there were *no* contraindications to taking hormone replacement therapy I would consider doing so in relation to WHMS symptoms:

1. If the *quality of my life* was being *significantly* affected by WHMS symptoms in an ongoing manner so that my daily functioning at work, or in my personal life, was significantly altered

2. If my economic survival depended on it or if I was in serious danger of losing my "significant other" because of WHMS' ongoing presence

3. If I planned to have a long active professional life, and that profession necessitated being cognitively in tip-top shape on a rigid ongo-

ing basis; if it didn't allow *any* margin for occasional distracted attention, or flash "glitches" in performance

4. If I saw in my family history a strong tendency toward Alzheimer's disease

5. If the WHMS symptoms I detected in myself, even without significantly changing my work or personal life, began to significantly *erode my sense of self* so that I started retrenching and self-protectively circumscribing my life, changing the essence of who I had long been, for the protective purposes of not exposing any unpredictable WHMS symptoms.

6. If "living in my head" and limberly "spinning the wheels" of my brain and communicating my ideas constituted the essence of me and seemed imperiled by WHMS changes over a span of more than a year

7. Lastly, it would be easy to take hormone replacement therapy for WHMS symptoms if I had already made the decision that I needed to take the same treatment long-term because I was at significant risk of cardiovascular disease or osteoporosis, by either family history or documented medical evidence (and was unwilling to alternatively engage in diet and exercise behaviors known to moderate those risks).

Given the above, if I arrived at the conclusion that my WHMS symptoms were probably caused by estrogen loss I might consider taking hormone replacement therapy for up to five years and then reevaluate my decision down the road. It would be my hope that in the interim new designer estrogens—hormones synthetically designed to do only good things and not bad ones at estrogen-receptor target organs in the body—would come out and make my decisions about longer-term treatment moot. These would be designer estrogens specifically engineered to keep active estrogen receptor pathways *in my brain* and hopefully also other *nonreceptor* estrogen pathways in my brain in working order. Such designer estrogens for the brain, also known as SERMs, for selective estrogen-receptor modulators, are currently on the drawing boards of many major pharmaceutical houses.

Two existing designer estrogens now on the market are *not* targeted for action in the brain, and since they reinitiate brain-centered hot flashes in some women who have taken them, they may not do all that estrogen does in the brain. They are raloxifene (marketed as Evista), for the prevention of osteoporosis, and tamoxifen (marketed as Nolvadex), for preventing breast cancer. According to Florida brain researcher Dr. James Simpkins the designer estrogen tamoxifen unlike most estrogens "is not neuroprotective in the brain with respect to estrogen receptors alpha and beta."

While no available designer estrogens yet exist *that specifically stimulate the brain,* my belief is that present technology, coupled with a world wide baby boomer market for such a formulation, will drive companies and researchers into double-time overtime to develop them. I suspect that this will become even more the case when the high prevalence of WHMS is recognized as creating an even younger potential market for such drugs.

WHICH ESTROGEN/PROGESTERONE TREATMENTS WORK BEST?

Which kinds of estrogen work best for cognitive symptoms? From my interviews with women it seemed evident that all the different kinds of estrogen most commonly used by women in the United States worked well for at least some of them. The most common forms used in the United States are (1) conjugated equine estrogen (a stew of different kinds of horse estrogens available only as a pill and only in one brand, Premarin, the most common form of estrogen presently in use) and (2) 17 beta-estradiol (an estrogen equivalent to the body's main and strongest estrogen), available as a pill or in different brands of skin patches.

When I asked researchers in the field, informally, what they thought of the different kinds of estrogen, over the course of several weeks' interviews I heard widely divergent views. One leading researcher told me that when she needs to she will only take Premarin. Yet another leading researcher railed disparagingly against Premarin as "horse piss" since it is made from the urine of female horses. Another told me that 17 beta-estradiol was much better in her experience as a researcher and as a woman and in Europe was much more commonly in use than in the United States.

It turns out that recent research evidence about estrogen's effects on the brain supports the view that *all* the forms of estrogen in major use now can be helpful in the brain. Neuroscientists Pattie Green, Katherine Gordon, and James Simpkins of the Center for the Neurobiology of Aging in Gainesville, Florida (and similar confirming research from Germany) have found that all the estrogen formulations now on the market, even very weak estrogen formulations, offer multiple forms of neuroprotection—brain-nerve-sparing effects—as long as they have a distinctive chemical hallmark—a phenolic A ring in their structure. (If you don't have a grasp of chemistry don't even try to understand this.) They have also found that more than a few of the relatively weak estrogens in plants, known as phytoestrogens, have this same nerve-protecting structure and can confer an array of protections for brain neurons from different kinds of toxic harm or deprivation that can occur, including some of those associated with Alzheimer's changes.

Across the country on the West Coast Dr. Roberta Brinton, a professor within the Department of Molecular Pharmacology and Toxicology of the University of Southern California's Pharmaceutical Sciences Center, has also studied the structure and action of many of the existing estrogens on the market. She has found that the major estrogens in use today can have dramatic effects in promoting structural changes in brain neurons in different thinking-related parts of the cerebral cortex, potentially increasing the apparent complexity of nerves via "neuronal outgrowths." But she has also found that the different estrogens appear to produce somewhat different effects in different regions of the cortex and with complicated patterns of response to different doses. This overall optimistic but complicated picture suggests that there are likely to be subtleties of treatment necessary for ob/gyns to ultimately master in treating specific WHMS symptoms with estrogens (perhaps different estrogens for different symptoms) and reasons for women to try different estrogens if they are not ideally being helped by one. But this picture also suggests that researchers trying to formulate ideal estrogens for maintaining the complexity of the different thinking parts of the brain will have many "building blocks" to play with in ultimately creating an ideal estrogen or designer estrogen for brain and cognitive maintenance.

Recent research also suggests that using an antioxidant, Vitamin E or C, together with estrogen can boost "the neuroprotective potency [strength] of estrogen by an average of 400-fold." Researchers from the lab of Dr. James Simpkins have found that "a combination of estrogen therapy with antioxidant therapy may prove more effective than either alone" [in protecting the nerve cells of the brain.] The antioxidant/estrogen combination seems to help stimulate the body's own antioxidant damage-protection defense system, boosting what scientists call a person's host resistance.

Dr. Simpkins in an interview said to me, "We know from the autopsy studies of Haiko Braak, a German researcher, that the neuropathological events [abnormal brain changes] that lead to a seventy-five-year-old brain with the features characteristic of Alzheimer's disease can start in the thirties [e.g., are evident in the autopsied brains of thirty-year-olds]. Estrogen deprivation, I believe, can have consequences for women. I believe the goal is *prevention* or *arrest* of [such] disease. Estrogen deprivation is a disease condition or a pre-disease condition. We are doing women a disservice if we don't inform them of the risks involved in not taking estrogen replacement—the added risk of Alzheimer's disease, more negative outcomes from possible strokes, the added risks of bone disease, heart disease and mood change. Only one in five women now decides to use estrogen. Either physicians aren't giving women the correct balance of information or they are underestimating the possible [beneficial] effects we now know of."

Dr. Brinton too sees merit in the use of hormone replacement therapy in menopausal women. The bigger picture, she says, is that "There will be 43 million post-menopausal women in the United States by the year 2000. In years past most women worked inside the home. By the time they were menopausal they did not usually have high-demand lives. Today in our culture women don't have the same opportunity of kicking back. We have to stay forever young in terms of our brain. The demands of our jobs can change literally every day. The marketplace is competitive for men and women. Before now, women didn't have to face these kinds of challenges. As a scientist I, like many women, have to learn new information every day. This is the reality of many women's lives today."

However, not all medical experts concur with this view, at least not yet, and perhaps never. Breast cancer surgeon Dr. Susan Love does not. Nor does former director of the National Institute of Aging Dr. Robert Butler. Both in interviews told me they are not quite ready for women to sign on long-term for estrogen replacement therapy to prevent cognitive decline. It's way too soon, they suggest. They want to see more clinical research evidence—research with women and, ideally, double-blind placebo-controlled trials—that shows clear-cut advantages of doing this long-term. Dr. Love told me "It's interesting stuff [the estrogen/brain research], but I still remain unconvinced that estrogen is the answer to all of life's problems. You do pay a price for using it long-term. There may be other ways of dealing with these cognitive symptoms at less of a price. Women were not designed," she says, "to have estrogen in the same supplies all their life."

Dr. Butler in an interview said to me, "The history of medicine is the history of one [sensational] hypothesis after another tumbling away. It's all very interesting [the present estrogen-preserves-cognition hypothesis and research]. It's a worthwhile hypothesis. We'll see if something comes of it in ten years. It is too soon to be recommending that all older women begin to take estrogen to improve cognition or to prevent Alzheimer's disease. There are people," he said, "who jump on anything [new]. There are not yet enough studies to characterize how important or significant estrogen really is [in maintaining the cognitive functioning of women.]"

IF YOU DECIDE TO TAKE ESTROGEN/PROGESTERONE THERAPY

If you do decide to take hormone replacement therapy—estrogen together with a progesterone if you have a uterus—know that some women experience dramatic relief within a week as in the case I present below, but for many women it commonly takes up to three months to see results for symptoms related to estrogen loss. And for some, as you've seen, it takes months longer or switching treatments. It is also a possibility that estrogen may not help all women with WHMS. Too much yet remains to be known.

I suggest that you first measure your WHMS symptoms for a baseline interval of two weeks before starting treatment to note how frequently the most bothersome symptoms occur as well as how much they bother you. You can use the WHMS Screening Instrument and the other tools I presented in chapter 8 for this purpose. Make several photocopies of the original and fill it out before treatment, and then three months after treatment test yourself again and compare the scores of the two assessment instruments to see if there are meaningful changes taking place. You should have a sense of whether you are better or not, though the screening instrument will help you remember how you felt three months ago. If there are no meaningful changes follow the suggestions I offer below.

Try to find a good ob/gyn or a nurse practitioner in the ob/gyn field. Ask your medical expert if he or she is familiar with treating cognitive symptoms. Ask for a description of the possible ways he or she would treat these symptoms. Show her or him the WHMS Screening Instrument and other tools you have filled out before coming for a visit. Show him or her the treatment suggestions below and ask if he or she prefers any particular alternative or would have any objections to using those in this book by Drs. Andrews and Cohen.

I suggest that you also read books in the library or in bookstores that describe the pros and cons of taking estrogen/progesterone treatments, and even estrogen/testosterone/progesterone forms of treatment, so you understand the basis for various treatment options. (Just as estrogen is not only a female hormone, testosterone is not only a male hormone but is present and has effects in women, sometimes different effects in different women. For some women it has effects on sexual drive, energy, and cognition. But it can produce undesired side effects and should not be taken without the adequate discussion of risks with a physician.) You might read up on these topics in books on menopause, perimenopause, hormone replacement therapy, women's health, etc. You'll feel less like a guinea pig and more in control of the situation if you become aware of different options, and the opinions of different experts.

IS IT TIME NOW TO TREAT PERIMENOPAUSAL AND MENOPAUSAL WOMEN WITH COGNITIVE CHANGES WITH ESTROGEN AND IF SO WHAT'S USEFUL TO KNOW?

When I asked Dr. William Andrews if he thought it was time for ob/gyns to start treating women with hormone replacement therapy in light of what's presently known from the research evidence, he said, "I do think there is enough evidence to consider treating postmenopausal women for cognitive symptoms with hormone replacement therapy. I think the woman has to be willing to take it. If she is going to be miserable worrying about breast cancer then maybe it's not for her. Each woman has got to make that decision. If she doesn't feel capable of making it herself and wants me to, then I would advise her. It has to be a mutual thing but it also has to be what a woman is comfortable with.

"I think that estrogen can be very important for the maximal functioning of women," he says. "A certain number of women say that menopause is natural and you ought to just let everything run its course. I think death is natural too, but you would rather have it later than sooner. I think the former view is a nihilistic view. I think you want a good quality of life as long as you can have it. That's really the critical variable. As long as you've got good mobility and good cognition, live well as long as you can. Lose those things and the quality of life goes down." He says, "As a result of the Alzheimer's research literature and Barbara Sherwin's work more doctors now may be willing to treat [women with HRT] when they hear cognitive symptoms being reported by them. In my practical experience," he says, "I have found that if women get control of symptoms at a higher dosage level then you can go down afterwards to a lower dosage and it often keeps working." The mechanism? "I think that women just don't need as much as time goes on. It's biologically plausible that you could need decreasing levels." Regarding the efficacy of treatment for specific cognitive symptoms he says, "I can't say I've had enough experience with the cognitive symptoms to say for sure what works best for treating specific cognitive ones. Studies like those of Barbara Sherwin [who has looked at multiple-dose levels] would have to be done to determine that."

Dr. Cohen in our many interviews concurred with much of Dr. Andrews's thoughts in this area. Discussing menopausal women in particular he said, "I don't hold to waiting the standard twelve months before I decide to treat a women with HRT complaining of cognitive and/or emotional symptoms. [The official definition of menopause within the field of ob/gyn is twelve months without a period.] Some women," he says, "are just suffering too much." Dr. Cohen, as does Dr. Andrews, provides different forms of treatment to women who are still having periods and to those who aren't: low-dose estrogen/progesterone birth-control pills for women who are still having periods (perimenopausal) and lower-doses of estrogen together with progesterone HRT for women without periods any longer (menopausal women) though some knowledgeable physicians sometimes treat perimenopausal and menopausal women similarly.

Dr. Cohen believes it's very important to screen not only for common systemic conditions such as diabetes and hypertension, but very specifically for different kinds of *thyroid dysfunction* in both perimenopausal and menopausal women. "If you don't rule these potential thyroid changes out you can miss what's happening. I believe that changes in ovarian function can act as a physiological stressor to the system, and if you have a genetic predisposition to either hypothryoidism [too little] or hyperthyroidism [too much] then the change in ovarian function can tip the balance and trigger thyroid disfunction. Both the thyroid and estrogen changes have to be treated. It's a common mistake for this not to be diagnosed. I know because I did it myself till I learned otherwise."

He also favors using a *patch* of 17 beta-estradiol for women with many cognitive or emotional symptoms. He says, "My sense is that the patch offers a more continuous form of administration than conjugated equine estrogen pills (Premarin). Pills gets broken down in the liver first—this is known as the 'first-pass effect.' The patch bypasses the liver where breakdown products known as metabolites can dilute the amount of estrogen that gets *directly* to the brain. You also can't measure directly how much estrogen is being absorbed in the blood when there are all these breakdown products and you can with a patch of 17 beta-estradiol."

He says, "I don't always start [treating] at the lowest level [of estrogen] depending on the severity of a patient's symptoms. If women don't have many emotional and cognitive symptoms I may alternatively give them Premarin."

If a menopausal woman's uterine lining isn't thick, as assessed sometimes with a sonogram, Dr. Cohen deems it safe and desirable only at first to give her estrogen alone for six weeks without progesterone. The reason for this he says is that "I want the patient to memorize and be cognizant of the estrogen response. I want them to be a barometer of what estrogen feels like in their body. I also ask them to monitor changes in mood and cognitive dimensions. I do this also because in some women progesterone produces some negative side effects and I want to see what estrogen is doing before I confound the picture [with the regular administration of progesterone]."

He says, "Some women without periods any longer or irregular periods have no detectable cognitive or behavioral changes and some behave as if they have a disease process caused by absence of a hormone—an endocrinopathy [a hormonal abnormality]." Based on his experience with perimenopausal and menopausal women experiencing strange physical or mind symptoms and subsequently taking estrogen and seeing them resolve, he has come to believe "that atypical symptoms in the body that show up during this five- to ten-year time-window before and around menopause have to be considered as possibly relating to the hormone changes."

Pointing to what's not known he says, "We don't know anything yet about maximizing a woman's cognitive response. Normally during the years of menstruation women's estrogen levels vary from a mid- [menstrual] cycle level high of 400 picograms in the blood [this can vary markedly over the course of a normal month] to under 20 picograms after the last period—when menopause begins. We don't know enough about what blood levels of estrogen correlate with cognitive improvements with most women now. Work needs to be done in this area to determine such things. Should we be aiming at getting higher blood levels of estrogen by giving higher doses in women to get a better level of improvement in the cognitive symptoms? We don't know."

Some women with serious mood or cognitive symptoms, he suspects based on his experience, "may well have to be on estrogen replacement therapy forever." The ultimate solution he believes "will be a SERM [a designer estrogen] that works on the brain but that doesn't stimulate the breast and uterus."

HOW I TREAT COGNITIVE SYMPTOMS (WHMS)

I asked both Drs. Andrews and Cohen, "If a perimenopausal woman, or a woman in the menopause age range, who hasn't had a period for twelve months, comes to you saying things like 'I'm losing it' and reports uncharacteristically missing appointments, having word-finding difficulties, being absentminded and other cognitive symptoms, how would you treat her?"

Dr. William Andrews

Dr. Andrews is past president of the American College of Obstetrics and Gynecology and Professor Emeritus of Obstetrics and Gynecology at the Eastern Virginia Medical School. He would start out with both kinds of women "taking a thorough history, doing a physical exam, and obtaining appropriate lab screening to see if there are any other problems going on."

Treating Women Who Are Menopausal

1. If nothing else was found to be at the heart of her symptoms I would advise estrogen.

2. I would start her at the equivalent of .625 milligram conjugated equine estrogen (CEE) [Premarin] or 0.05 milligram of a patch of 17 beta-estradiol or the equivalent dose of another estrogen. I don't think the data on starting at higher doses is convincing and I think there could be negatives to it.

3. If she was still having hot flashes or significant symptoms I would go up to the 1.25 level of Premarin or, in terms of the estrogen patch, to 0.1 milligram of 17 beta-estradiol.

4. For continuous regimens I'd prescribe 2.5 milligrams of

medroxyprogesteroneacetate (MPA) daily or 100 milligrams of micronized progesterone daily.

5. For sequential (cyclical) regimens I'd prescribe 5 milligrams of MPA or 200 milligrams micronized progesterone for twelve to fourteen days per month.

6. I'd do this for six months or so to see if it was working.

7. If it was I'd then go back down again to the next lower [dose] level. For women who have had a hysterectomy a progestin is not needed.

Treating Perimenopausal Women

1. To determine if a woman is in perimenopause I'd find out if she is still menstruating, and if cycles are irregular do an FSH [follicle-stimulating hormone] test on the third to fifth day of her menstrual cycle [three to five days after bleeding begins]. If her FSH is greater than twenty, that is an indication of perimenopause. Also a lower maturation index on a Pap smear is suggestive of decreased estrogen. Obtaining a serum estrogen blood test incurs additional expense and I don't believe it is necessary in most cases.

2. If a woman is not perimenopausal, if she has good ovarian function, a serum estrogen blood level test taken in the middle of her cycle [around day fourteen] should be above one hundred. If it is less than that she may well be perimenopausal.

3. I'd give a woman who was perimenopausal with cognitive symptoms estrogen in the form of a low-dose birth-control pill, specifically 20 micrograms [as in Loestrin 1-20 or Alese] daily. This contains both estrogen and progesterone. The estrogen in this is low.

4. I would try that for six months. If that wasn't helping I think we'd start looking further into other possible causes for her symptoms.

Dr. Maurice Cohen

Dr. Cohen is co-Director of the Women's Health Program at Northshore Diabetes and Endocrine Associates, New Hyde Park, New York; Staff Gynecologist; founding member of the North American Menopause Society; Assistant Professor of Clinical Gynecology and Obstetrics, Albert Einstein College of Medicine, New York. For all women Dr. Cohen takes "a detailed history. I want to hear in detail about any symptoms women are experiencing. I do a physical exam, and a lab screening to see if there are any other problems."

Treating Menopausal Women Who Appear To Have Had Their Last Period

1.   If they are symptomatic the goal in these women is to replace estrogen that isn't there now in sufficient supplies to eliminate symptoms.

2.   If a woman's FSH levels are high [greater than 50] and her estrogen levels have dropped [under 25 picograms], I treat with hormone replacement therapy.

3.   Depending on different factors I give women a sonogram before treating them with hormones to see how thick the lining of their uterus is.

4.   If a woman had many cognitive symptoms I'd start her on a patch of 17 beta-estradiol, of .05 milligram or .1 milligram depending on what she told me.

5.   To make sure they are absorbing the estrogen [on a blood test] I want their blood levels of estrogen to be in the 50 to 100 picogram range. Overall there is a wide margin of safety in the HRT levels we use.

6.   After the first round of estrogen alone typically I want women to start on micronized progesterone at the beginning of every month. Many women have a negative mood reaction to progesterones, even the natural yam-based micronized progesterone I prefer, which you have to order from special pharmacies. [See Appendix II for listings of pharmacies.] I ask women to take the progestereone at bedtime so that the sedating side effects some women experience with it can be sidestepped. I suggest that women take 100 milligrams of micronized progesterone twice a day for the first twelve days of the month if they choose a cyclic regimen (which produces a monthly period). Or if they choose not to have a period, I have them take 100 milligrams every night. This is called a continuous regimen.

7.   If they chose a cyclic regimen I ask women to compare how they feel on the days when they are on progesterone and not on it because in some women the estrogen can help and then the progesterone can reverse the effect.

8.   If women are in the early stages of menopause and have been on

a 2-milligram dose of estradiol for a year, then after one year of good symptom control I cut back from 2 milligrams daily to 1 milligram.

Treating Perimenopausal Women

1.   I check their blood counts and screen for anemia from heavy periods or bleeding from fibroids, which can produce thinking problems, fatigue, and other changes. Sometimes patients don't mention this to the doctor.

2.   I also look at diet and will suggest reducing excessive amounts of caffeine or sugar.

3.   If women are still having their periods and there aren't contraindications I will give them low-dose birth-control pills. There are two that have a lower dose than all the others. They have 20 micrograms of ethinyl estradiol. These are Loestrin 1/20 made by Parke-Davis and Alesse by Wyeth-Ayerst.

4.   By treating these women with the lowest dose of the combined estrogen/progesterone birth-control pill you override their own fluctuating ovarian function. The vast majority will respond to this.

5.   Within one to two months there will be a demonstrable improvement or I consider that this avenue of intervention is not working.

IF YOU ARE NOT GETTING GOOD RESULTS AFTER THREE MONTHS, HOW TO SWITCH

If you are experiencing some improvement in your WHMS symptoms but not a whole lot you might consider staying on the same treatment longer to see if the symptoms gradually improve over time, or decide to switch depending on how badly you need relief. In one of the studies I described earlier women who were seventy-five years old and given estrogen replacement therapy kept on improving on cognitive tests for eighteen months before they stopped improving and reached a plateau. It took Polly Van Benthusen seven months to see appreciable improvement. Wait perhaps for several months longer if you've seen evidence of some change. But first be sure to have your doctor check via a blood test that you are absorbing the estrogen you are taking. Your blood level of estrogen should be in the 50 to 100 picogram range, in the view of Dr. Maurice Cohen.

If you are not experiencing *any* meaningful change in your WHMS symptoms after three months consider doing something different. Dr. Elizabeth G. (alias) did this. A forty-nine-year-old research scientist/physician with a twelve-year-old son, she found she suddenly had no energy though as a former tomboy she loved regularly playing sports with her son. "I found that as I walked from my lab to my office I would forget as many as eight times a day what I went in to get. It was becoming increasingly frustrating. I couldn't think of the words I needed when I needed them." Having read my *New York* magazine article she recognized herself in the symptoms I described. She brought the article to her ob/gyn and was put on one form of continuous estrogen/progesterone therapy. When she didn't experience much relief, after several months, she switched from a pill to a patch form of 17 beta-estradiol and after two months found her memory and verbal symptoms had improved remarkably. But her energy was still lower than she deemed desirable. So her doctor recommended an estrogen formulation that also contained a small amount of testosterone [Estratest]. She took this along with the progesterone she was using, and within several weeks her energy returned. She was delighted with her improvement when I last met her. So don't be too passive about switching or suggesting you want to try something different or worry about "insulting" your doctor's treatment recommendations. You are the one in need. This is not a recommendation, however, to be cavalier about ingesting hormones.

How to Switch

Discuss different options with your doctor. This might mean:

1. Switch from an estrogen stick-on/leave-on patch (several brands exist) to estrogen pills (several kinds of estrogen exist in pill form, as well as different brands for some kinds of estrogen) or switch from a pill to a "transdermal" patch form of administration. Estrogen pills get broken down in the liver and this can lead to variable levels of estrogen "dosing" over the course of the day. Estrogen patches don't involve the liver and could give you more consistent levels of estrogen over a time period. You could, for example, switch from a 17 beta-estradiol pill to a 17 beta-estradiol patch or vice versa.

2. Switch to a different brand of a patch or different brands of a pill. (There's only one kind of conjugated equine estrogen [CEE], so if you are taking Premarin you can't switch to another kind.)

3. Try different *progesterone* formulations. Micronized progesterone made from yams is believed by more than a few of the physicians I spoke to to produce fewer negative mood effects in some women. It has to be special ordered by mail from a pharmacy (see Appendix II). This kind of progesterone is different from the rub-on cream also made of yams, which can be bought over the counter. The micronized progesterone contains pharmaceutically standardized doses, i.e., you are getting biologically equivalent doses in each pill.

4. Try different amounts of progesterone in relation to the amount of estrogen you are taking. Some believe, and research by Barbara Sherwin has shown, that the balance between the two hormones can affect mood symptoms; perhaps it may affect WHMS symptoms too.

Regimens: Different Ways to Take Hormone Replacement Therapy

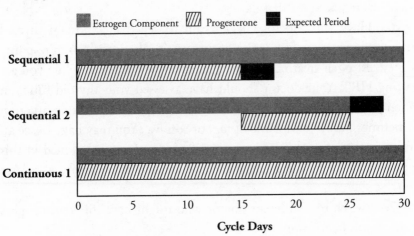

Common types of estrogen-progesterone hormone replacement regimens. The shaded bars represent the duration of estrogen therapy, the diagonal-patterned bars represent duration of progesterone administration, and the solid bars indicate when vaginal bleeding is expected.

Figure 4

5. Try different timing sequences or regimens of medication. If you've been taking estrogen and progesterone *continuously* every day (you won't have a period with this regimen), then try switching to one of several possible *sequential regimens,* e.g., estrogen and progesterone taken together some days but not every day. (Sequential regimens lead to having periods again, but mimic more your body's natural prior cycle.) Have your doctor spell out very specifically what days you will be taking each hormone if you go on a sequential regimen (see Figure 4). Then make a calendar chart for several months that spells out which days you take which medication and which days you take no medication. Don't leave this to your memory, if you are having memory problems. You will feel frustrated if you aren't sure what you need to do on different days and may end up feeling you are "playing with hormones" and with potential danger. So plan ahead so you know what you need to do on a particular date. One researcher I interviewed in this field who was on a sequential regimen of hormone replacement therapy had her husband program into her computer a medication-taking calendar chart, indicating what medication she had to take on which days for a whole year, so she never had to think about it or try to remember what she had to do. She looked in the appropriate file in her computer to see what was required for that day.

6. Have your doctor check again to see that abnormal thyroid function in your case is not also occurring simultaneously or in response to new estrogen treatment. It may need to be addressed while you are getting HRT. Your doctor should have assessed your thyroid function when you initially went to see him or her. Thyroid and ovarian function sometimes play a joint game of tag, or seesaw. (You may have to see an endocrinologist or thyroid specialist if your ob/gyn isn't skilled in this type of treatment. I've been told some are and some aren't. Ask: "Are you . . . ?")

7. Switch to a different doctor who might have different insights into what is happening.

8. Join a menopause support group to get some ideas from women who may have gone through the same thing or know of skilled ob/gyns in this topic area. The American Menopause Foundation offers such groups around the country. Their number is listed in Appendix II.

While you are waiting to detect improvement you might console yourself with the possibilities that by taking estrogen you may be helping to protect your brain's neurons from various forms of toxic damage; forestalling new cognitive erosion, possibly reducing your risk from later Alzheimer's disease or a delay in its onset if you are destined to have it; or helping to prevent osteoporosis, heart disease, colon cancer, tooth loss, urinary problems, painful intercourse, etc. But don't persist too long if you see *no* indications of help after a reasonable amount of time.

Case #6: Cheryl Calhoun

Cheryl Calhoun (her actual name) is an energetic fifty-two-year-old commercial bank vice president in northern California who loves her job and can scarcely imagine life without it. Married and the mother of a grown son, she has been taking estrogen since she was forty-eight. Over that span of time she has changed her estrogen medications and/or regimen of medications a total of seven times, in order to control physical symptoms associated with the years around menopause or to maintain an intellectual status quo she hadn't initially been aware was slipping. Her case illustrates that over the span of perimenopause or menopause, at least in some women, changing dosages and regimens of medication may be required to maintain a status quo on "well-being and sharpness." Cheryl is another one of Dr. Robert Greene's patients.

Reproductive Status: Perimenopausal when she started taking hormones. Since she is on estrogen and progesterone, she can't tell if she has become menopausal. Her need for higher doses over time, however, may reflect underlying biological changes in reproductive status.

I had minimal information about menopause and no poignant signals that anything was beginning when I went to my old ob/gyn Dr. D. I was forty-seven then. My periods were fairly regular though lighter than they used to be. I had no complaints, but Dr. D. suggested I was at the age when I should start to consider taking hormones. It was surprising to me because I had no symptoms. I said thanks but no thanks. One year later I had blood tests that showed that my hormones were getting low and I had started to have night sweats but no hot flashes. They didn't bother me at all. I went right back to sleep. I wasn't opposed to hormones because there is a history of heart disease in my family, and estrogen is supposed to protect against heart disease, so I started taking Premarin and Provera at the lowest level, I think, everyday at age forty-eight. At first my night sweats went away and then they came back.

I changed ob/gyns around then and my new doctor gave me a higher dose of estrogen. I suddenly started noticing that I was feeling so much better mentally than I had before. I hadn't been aware that I *wasn't* feeling well but the difference when I took the higher dose was quite noticeable to me. It gave me back mental sharpness that had apparently been slipping away. I love my job, I truly do, and I'm good at it. I needed to stay very good at what I did. I found that my communication skills improved at the higher dose. I wouldn't lose my train of thought as much. My writing skills and my ability to read and retain improved. I read a lot for work. And my concentration and retention weren't as good as they had been in the past especially in reading complicated things that were difficult to absorb.

Details didn't stick. I would try to have a conversation with an associate about current events—things I knew I knew and they were back there somewhere but I just couldn't pull them up and bring them forward. I was disgusted several times when I briefly forgot my social security number, after knowing it for a lifetime. Another time I forgot my ATM code. I use it for my voice mail and I couldn't call in. I was so pissed. I'd walk right by a store I intended to stop in. One time at a Hospital Auxiliary meeting I had some ideas for a lake project and they loved my idea; but I couldn't think of the names of all the twelve resorts on that lake and couldn't discuss the idea. I was mortified that I couldn't name them and said I had them back at the office. One time I simply forgot to put the car in "park" when I got out. I'd never done that before and haven't again. It's always been so automatic with me. I also stopped making appointments for Monday mornings because I would miss them. I would forget to look at my appointment book over the weekend.

When my new doctor increased my estrogen to correct the night sweats I saw a very meaningful difference in my memory. I remember being so pleased by this. My ability to come up with words or phrases I wanted at the time got better, though it's still not 100 percent. Before, nothing would come to me in the split second that I needed it. You start looking for words and shuffling for other words. When this happened I'd become afraid that I'd end up without a job, staying in a bathrobe and chewing bonbons all day. Others apparently didn't notice. I continued to get promotions, and raises; my accounts grew.

I am a person who goes 110 mph all day and I like that. That's the way I want it to be. When I can't do that I'm very disappointed. I found that estrogen took away feelings of fatigue that I started to have for no reason.

Altogether over the four years I've been on estrogen I've changed what I've been taking about seven times. I've changed from taking estrogen and progesterone together to not taking them together and then back again. I've never gone down to a lower dose. I've changed medications when I didn't have a sense of well-being anymore or felt a sharpness was waning. Whether it makes sense or not I don't know but within days I've felt sharper.

As of four months ago I readjusted my medications. Now I'm on 5 milligrams daily of progesterone and I take two pills of .9 milligrams of Premarin [estrogen], so it's 1.8 milligrams daily.

It seems to me that the effects of menopause are gradual and you get used to the effects. I think you can change drastically over a period of a year and not notice because the changes are so gradual. I thought memory problems began at seventy-five or eighty for those it occurs in at all, and when I saw what was happening to me I thought it was aging. I was really disappointed that I was one of the ones it would affect. I didn't discuss these changes with anyone. I think there's a tremendous need for educating women about what hormone changes can do to you, how they can change you. People don't know about this. It hasn't been taken seriously. Look how long it took them to nail PMS. It was a joke before to people—they didn't believe it or take it seriously. People are not treating it as a joke anymore. I hope that's what happens here.

Obviously many questions remain unanswered in taking estrogen for WHMS symptoms. Do certain regimens work better than others for different biological subtypes of women? Are certain WHMS symptoms more resistant to improvement than others? Is there a critical period for getting maximal return of function after symptoms begin or after a woman's last period, when estrogen levels plummet? Do short, acute bursts of treatment help more than long-term ongoing treatment? Would alternating types of estrogens monthly maximize improvements? Are there different kinds of effects with estrogen taken continuously versus sequentially? What happens to receptors with continuous treatment? Do more receptors "turn on"? Do they stay "turned on" over time or turn themselves off in the circular feedback loops that are characteristic of hormone signals in the body? Do they get deformed with constant stimulation? Research will have to answer these questions.

Remember for what it's worth that you have lots of company whatever you decide to do. Millions of baby boomer women approaching or entering menopause today are pioneers on a frontier of new scientific discoveries. They are weighing the same decisions you are. Remember if you are *really* in a quandary that many women have survived into old age without making this decision and without becoming demented or basket cases. You have the option open to you that they did: doing nothing. Or you may choose to try one of the non-hormonal forms of treatment or behaviors I discuss in the next two chapters.

In a letter to the editor in response to my *New York* magazine article, Marie C. Wilson, president of the Ms. Foundation for Women, aptly summarized the present state of affairs for women with WHMS, with respect to taking estrogen. She wrote:

> Women have had to navigate through menopause by becoming "texts" for one another . . . . As a result of the sparse attention to women's health research until the last decade, each of us makes a decision about hormone-replacement therapy knowing the facts aren't in and that *we* are the experiment. It's unfair to look at those of us who take it and say we are avoiding aging. What so many of us are avoiding was made clear in this article—the potential loss of our ability to continue to financially support ourselves and our families through menopause and beyond.

11

Non-hormonal Approaches for Working with WHMS

F or some women, taking estrogen and progesterone is simply not an alternative they would consider. Fears about taking it daily would outweigh any possible benefits. And even though some women decide to take estrogen and progesterone initially for their WHMS symptoms they sometimes later choose, for reasons of family health history or other reasons, not to stay on them indefinitely but to explore other forms of treatment. This was the decision Dr. Fredericka Xerov made.

Case # 7: Dr. Fredericka Xerov

A fifty-three-year-old former radiologist, who now holds a Ph.D. in genetics counseling, Dr. Xerov is married to a physician and the mother of three children, one still young. She was referred to me by a menopause support group leader. Her case illustrates the approach/avoidance relationship many women

have with respect to taking hormones and the need for other safe forms of
treatment for the symptoms associated with the years surrounding menopause.
   Reproductive Status: Perimenopausal when her WHMS symptoms began
at age forty-eight.

After being a successful radiologist for fifteen years I decided at age
forty-four that I wanted to change careers. I had stopped enjoying what
I was doing. I had only twenty years left of a working life and the question was, did I want to keep doing this for another twenty years. I had a
young child who was in nursery school and I thought "What now? I
wanted to do something that would hold my interest. I decided to get a
Ph.D. in genetics counseling. I wanted to help people and to interact
with them.

   I entered graduate school in the fall and for three years I did real
well. In my fourth year I had an internship and started for the first time
seeing patients in a hospital. I had finished my thesis, which had gone
well, obtained my Ph.D., and was preparing for my boards—the written exam part and the state licensing exam—when I noticed that I had
difficulties studying for it, concentrating, retaining information. I also
felt a little depressed. I tried exercising every day because I was suddenly
lacking in energy; and it didn't make sense, because I wasn't working. I
was just devoting myself to studying. My older kids were in school and
I had someone taking care of my youngest child. The exercising didn't
seem to be helping.

   A year before, at forty-seven, I had decided I no longer needed to be
on birth-control pills. Soon after that the only indication I had that I
was perimenopausal was that my husband, who is also a physician, told
me I was becoming very dry when we made love. I was still menstruating normally. On the advice of an ob/gyn I started taking Premarin
(conjugated estrogen) for the dryness and it went away. I felt like a new
person. I got a burst of energy. It was very dramatic. I could sit down
and get something done. But then I also started to get irregular bleeding. I went to the doctor and he tried changing the dose and put me on
a different kind of progesterone; but it felt like he didn't have or know
too many options in terms of treatment. His uncertainties about what
to do didn't inspire me with confidence. I didn't go back to him but I

stayed on the estrogen and progesterone. I prescribed them for myself. But then things started to change. That whole internship year my sleep was irregular and I also started to get hot flashes at night. I found when I was studying for the written exam I had to really concentrate to get things done.

Then my mind started behaving even more strangely. I would try to write notes after a session with a patient and try to think how to put into words things that had just happened and I would draw a blank. No thoughts would come. It would take me so long. I felt like I had to dredge it out of myself. I couldn't put precise thoughts together. It was hard to get coherence and relevancy. I thought I should have stuff to say but it wasn't coming to mind. I didn't catastrophize. I said it must be because I'm not sleeping well or because I was adjusting to a new situation but that didn't add up. I just knew I was struggling. I was feeling slow in responding to patients, slow in generating ideas. It was the feeling of not being with it, being out of it, like a not-well-oiled machine. And with time it didn't get easier. I was struggling more rather than less. It felt like the neuronal pathways in my mind were not getting carved out—were not forming.

I felt like this most of the time. And only slightly better with sleep. It felt like I was going uphill the whole time.

I don't think other people noticed. If I was at a seminar I'd participate. I think I did my job well and at work I wasn't that impaired. I tried ginseng and ginger tea because I felt so sluggish mentally and drinking the ginger tea cleared my head. I think from what I know now that the perspiring from drinking it helped somehow.

I was taking the estrogen and progesterone daily but my mind problems got worse. Whenever I'd use my brain in my daily life it wasn't functioning. I'd go to the grocery store and would draw a blank on what I came to get. Things wouldn't come to me the way they would have in the past. Even reading. I couldn't figure out what I was reading. I wasn't absorbing. I found myself reading less. I could go to a movie and forget what I saw in a minute. I had a hard time getting words out correctly. I'd walk into a room and wonder "What am I here for?" I'd also forget things I'd known forever: One day I looked at the geraniums in our window box and couldn't think what their name was. I'd forget to turn off the stove and pots would burn. I put a timer on the stove now. I found that my math skills got slower but I didn't need to use them much. Possibly as a reaction to all this I found that I had much less tolerance for complexity. I didn't want to do anything too complex. I also had total blackouts on where I put something or that I had done certain things. I would find evidence that I had done something and have absolutely no recall of having done it. "Did I do that?" I would think to myself. Also my memory retrieval skills were way off.

Even though my life was generally disjointed in this way the things that happened weren't a huge problem. They were more like annoyances and petty frustrations. The worst part was that I was aware of what was happening to me even though others weren't and I didn't know what it meant and what would happen next.

At the end of my post-doc year I developed severe fatigue for perhaps a year and half. All I really had to do at that time was drop my stepdaughter off at school and pick her up later. But I was just so tired all the time I could barely get myself up the stairs or put away dishes. I was really dragging myself around. I had to take my oral licensing exam at this time and for a couple of months before I rested up and did practically nothing. I found it hard to focus in. Some days I felt like my brain really wasn't working. But I joined a study group and amazingly I passed the test.

Around this time I started to write everything down—all the little chores and errands I had to do—and I carried the list with me. It was the only way I could be sure I didn't slip up.

If something took three or four steps I had a hard time planning out sequentially what had to be done in what order, the logistics of it. Before it was just natural for me to attack it without a thought; now I really had to work at it and could do it, but with much greater effort. I would think to myself "This is not the way I used to be. I used to juggle all these responsibilities." I had been director of my own private radiology operation. I had hospital responsibilities, social responsibilities, my husband, the children. Now I had a much simpler life and fewer responsibilities and I was functioning only marginally. After the experiences with the last gynecologist I went to I was wary of going to another one with all these symptoms I had never heard of before. I knew they had arrived with the sexual dryness and later the hot flashes. But I know that doctors think women who tell them these things are crazy, that we must be nuts. I know how they think. I've worked with them a long time.

All I know is that I began to suspect all this had to do with my gradually losing estrogen.

Finally I was sick of feeling the way I did. I just wasn't going to live life like that, feeling tired, old, and that I couldn't function. It may sound silly but I looked in the telephone book for help because I couldn't think of where else to look. I saw Dr. B.'s name. He's an ob/gyn and a menopause researcher and it said his office ran menopause support groups. I went to one of those on my birthday as a present to myself and then went to Dr. B. [a California menopause expert I cite in this book] a month later. From the group I learned it wasn't just me, that there were other women experiencing what I was. It was a relief to find I wasn't alone in this, the fatigue, the mind fog, the memory problems.

Dr. B. said that I'd been doing everything wrong. He said, "Here's a brand new estrogen patch, Climara. The patch means that you'll be getting more consistent blood levels of estrogen than with the pill." He had me slowly taper off from the other estrogen and he very, very slowly had me work up to a full patch of Climara in very small increments, every three weeks. We cut the patch into pieces. He said, "Your body needs time to get used to that level." He said something about the brain's receptors needing this gradual increase to get activated again. He also figured out from what I told him that I was retaining water and this explained in part why after I perspired from drinking hot tea and lost water I felt clearer in my head. I went on a low-salt diet and I noticed an improvement from this regimen.

Dr. B. said we would manipulate three things: the estrogen over a matter of months and the addition of progesterone afterward, and we would try out a little testosterone.

All I know is that I have definitely improved a lot since I went on this regimen. I can now write and put my thoughts together comfortably. I can compose a letter and read professional material. I had also developed shoulder and hip stiffness after dinner when I would stand up that took four or five steps before it went away. This cleared up within a short time when I went on the estrogen. I could get right up.

I also tried a little of the testosterone. It was great. It gave me an extra boost pretty quickly. My energy got much better, my focus, even my muscular strength. It was noticeable, the change. I think that certain women need these hormones during this period. The question is what to do after the worst is over.

I tried both the oral form [of the testosterone] and the cream. The cream was great for [sexual] arousal but I'm off of it now. In fact I want to get off of all the hormones. I have a strong history of cancer in my family but not of heart disease, and I want to taper off slowly to see if I can go off of them without getting a lot of symptoms back. I'm also thinking of trying soy products because they have the weak plant-based phytoestrogens.

One of the theories, Dr. B. said, is that the symptoms women get at this time come from abrupt *fluctuations of the hormones,* not from a deficiency of them. He says that the ovaries produce radically different amounts of hormones from month to month during the years around menopause and that that's what may cause the negative symptoms; and that in older women the shifts from month to month are much less dramatic and the symptoms get milder.

I often think to myself "Isn't it amazing that no one has picked up on this in all these years. That this has been ignored the way it has!"

In follow-up Dr. Xerov sent me a copy of something she had written about the societal context of her experience and on the likely origin of many of the folk medicines that are now becoming so prevalent for self-healing. She wrote:

> There are those who do not want menopause to become a "disease." They say we should weather this period naturally, as women did in the past. Women should not have to consult a physician and take "medicine" because our ancestors did not. The medical establishment is blamed for "medicalizing" menopause, which is a natural state. Women who resist hormone replacement therapy can afford to do so because their quality of life is still acceptable. But because I was having such a difficult time, I was grateful that estrogen and testosterone were available.

We shouldn't assume that our ancestors breezed right through menopause. I doubt that they just sat by as they felt themselves feeling less vital and productive. All the "natural" remedies that exist for menopause today, I suspect, were found because women in the past had the same need to feel better that I did. Many women in the past probably suffered in silence just as many suffer in silence today. I sometimes think to myself, how many professional or career women had to slow down or retire early because of these symptoms because they couldn't be competitive in the marketplace any longer and didn't trust telling anyone, or had any doctors who knew what they were talking about? I think many women resist playing around with Mother Nature until they lose their sense of well-being and feel their quality of life plummeting. Going *au naturel* may be fine for women who are lucky enough not to have these symptoms. But those of us who have had a more difficult transition appreciate the efforts being made to increase our knowledge about menopause. Because of my medical background I feel we should not embrace herbs and "natural methods" while rejecting modern medicine to help us navigate through what can be a choppy transition.

The question is what can you do if you are experiencing WHMS symptoms and can't or won't take estrogen replacement therapy or rather, hormone replacement therapy?

Given all that scientists now know about the many biological functions estrogen plays in the brain, it is plausible that substituting for some of these functions with scientifically established safe non-hormonal agents and behaviors, known to mimic some of the functions of estrogen, may be one avenue for attempting to manage the estrogen-loss basis of WHMS symptoms.

What kinds of estrogen mimics am I talking about? Agents and behaviors that individually mimic one or more of estrogen's known glucose fuel-supplying, memory-enhancing, neuroprotective, antioxidant, anti-inflammatory, neurotransmitter-enhancing, attention-enhancing, vascular support-enhancing, brain oxygen-boosting, nerve-growth-factor promoting, or other functions.

THE VITAMIN ANALOGY

Let me offer you an analogy: We now accept in large measure that taking in pill form specific vitamins and minerals can be a useful—if not ideal—substitute means for obtaining the vitamins and minerals a body needs to function well and that normally would be obtained in a healthy diet.

I am proposing that a substitution for some of the *functions* normally fulfilled by estrogen in the body with estrogen mimics may also prove beneficial as an alternative. Yes, it is true that whole foods probably offer the added benefits of pinball interactions among the naturally occurring vitamins and minerals and trace elements we know and don't yet know about as they intermix in whole foods. And yes, obtaining estrogen naturally from within the body or getting it externally in the form of hormone replacement therapy may similarly produce maximizing biological effects that the piecemeal estrogen-mimic route I propose may not. But we know that supplemental vitamins and minerals in those lacking them can do considerable good alone (i.e., a less well-known example: treating vitamin deficiencies before surgery can significantly reduce the risk of postsurgical complications). And it is plausible that although piecemeal estrogen mimics may not do *all* that estrogen can do, they may nonetheless prove helpful.

Let me not misinform you. Since WHMS has never been identified or researched before, I can't tell you that this approach has *proven* value. It has plausible value. It has the backing of a rationale based on available research evidence. And as you will see, at least some of the suggestions I propose have been recommended already for overall health or preventive purposes in the past. Some, as you will see, may delight the appetite of the child in you if not entirely please your friendly nutritionist.

THE ESTROGEN-MIMIC PLAN FOR ADDRESSING WHMS SYMPTOMS

I propose the following plan as a plausible method of substituting for some of estrogen's known functions in the brain, based on available research evidence. I can't tell you how long it may take to experience any change or for certain that you will experience definite changes. But I believe this is worth trying. So that you are not merely "flying blind" indefinitely I suggest you monitor the frequency and intensity of all your WHMS symptoms, or your most distressing WHMS symptom, for one to two weeks before starting this plan in the ways I suggested in chapter 8 and then again after you have been trying this plan for one to three months. Later in this chapter I will discuss the amounts to consider in implementing this plan. It involves:

The Estrogen-Mimic Plan

1. *Developing a "grazing" pattern of eating glucose at regular intervals* throughout the day (preferably in the form of complex carbohydrate foods, which end up as glucose. Or for quick but short-term action, glucose in the form of sugar) to boost and provide a steady supply of the brain's major fuel, which is known to enhance memory functioning, verbal and spatial retrieval fluency skills, attention, and acetylcholine synthesis (a neurotransmitter), all of which can diminish with estrogen loss.

2. *Using glucose* after *learning* something important, as a *highlighter* to enhance memory retention.

3. *Ingesting phytoestrogens such as genistein* with a phenolic A-ring chemical structure from soy products (as well as other plant-based products). These weaker plant-based forms of estrogen are now believed by some to provide brain neurons with the same protection and resilience against various biological assaults in the brain that natural body estrogens offer: protection against beta-amyloid deposition (the kind found in Alzheimer's patients), against oxygen starvation, against nutrient starvation, against oxidative free-radical damage.

4. *Using an antioxidant such as Vitamin E regularly,* plus, if desired, other antioxidant foods or substances such as blueberries, vitamin C, genistein, caffeine, (yes, caffeine) etc., to compensate for the free-radical damage-protection estrogen offers as an antioxidant.

5. *Using an anti-inflammatory agent* such as ibuprofen to mimic estrogen's role as an anti-inflammatory agent and to guard against potential Alzheimer's-like induced changes.

6. *Eating acetylcholine synthesis–boosting foods* such as *(a)* glucose (or complex carbohydrates) and *(b)* choline-rich foods to boost the synthesis of the neurotransmitter acetylcholine, which is indirectly diminished by estrogen decline through estrogen's direct regulation of the acetylcholine-stimulating enzyme choline acetyltransferase (CHAT).

7. *Taking in serotonin-boosting agents or foods* to replace estrogen's potential serotonin-diminishing functions in those experiencing unaccountable low-grade to higher-grade forms of "flattened" emotions or depression, or PMS-like mood alterations: Saint-John's-wort; or Prozax, Paxil, or Zoloft obtained under the supervision of a physician.

8. *Using attention focusing/enhancing agents* such as caffeine (as needed) or Ritalin (as prescribed) if the quality of your life is seriously being affected by inattention, poor concentration, reading and writing problems, and if both are not contraindicated for your particular health risks. To assess this, I suggest you decide to use either under a doctor's supervision, preferably a psychopharmacologist's supervision, on a trial empirical basis to see if it makes a difference.

9. *Doing aerobic exercise on a regular basis* to *(a)* increase the brain and body's vascular support system (it can boost blood vessel size and complexity), *(b)* enhance the brain's oxygen supply, and *(c)* boost nerve-growth-factor release—all functions associated with or related to estrogen.

About Glucose: The Glucose Facilitation Effect

Surprise! The old placebo sugar pill wasn't really an inert inactive placebo after all. (And uh-oh about all the research that's relied on such placebos as "control" inactive substances.) It sounds practically too simple and too good to be true, but glucose, it has been found, is a potent memory agent apart from being the brain's only nonstorable source of fuel. (In case you don't know, sugar's sucrose becomes glucose in the body as do complex carbohydrates such as potatoes and pasta.) If you were to do a computer search of the research literature today in a medical library on glucose and memory, out would pour at least an inch and a half of published reports and reviews on this form of brain "gold."

Here's what some of them would say:

Extensive evidence indicates that relatively modest increases in circulating glucose concentrations enhance learning and memory processes in rodents and humans . . . Recent evidence suggests that glucose may [boost the "memory ink" neurotransmitter] acetylcholine release in the hippocampus. The relative safety of glucose has permitted tests of glucose effects on cognitive functions in humans. Glucose also enhances learning and memory in healthy aged humans and enhances several other cognitive functions in subjects with several cognitive pathologies, including individuals with Alzheimer's disease and Down's syndrome. Thus, increases in circulating glucose concentrations have robust and broad influences on brain functions that span many neural [nerve] and behavioral measures . . .

Here's another quick "take" on what glucose can do: "Dementia of the Alzheimer type (DAT) is accompanied by disruption in glucose regulation and utilization that may contribute to its characteristic memory impairment. Increasing glucose availability by raising plasma glucose improves memory in [such] patients . . ." *and by a rather startling 100 percent in test scores* in some studies of Alzheimer's patients, according to major glucose researcher Paul Gold. The authors of the earlier quote go on to point out that "potential mechanisms for such improvement may well be the presence of glucose-related insulin receptors in the brain's major memory processing center—the hippocampus—and increases in glucose utilization in parts of the cortex also involved in memory and typically damaged in Alzheimer's patients." Thus the memory centers of the brain have sticky "fingers" already built in and waiting to snag and make use of glucose.

And guess what else improved in *normal* healthy *elderly* subjects given just 3½ tablespoons of glucose, i.e., sugar? Skills that form the basis of major WHMS symptoms: memory, retrieval of memory, the ability to verbally generate and pull out information (verbal fluency), attention, and the ability to pull out or generate from memory spatial information (figural fluency). In a study of twenty-eight healthy elderly subjects with a mean age of seventy-three, researchers tested subjects under two conditions, on either 50 grams of glucose, equal to about 3½ tablespoons of sugar, or 27.3 milligrams of saccharin (not sugar), on various memory and nonmemory measures. They later switched treatments and tested the subjects again on equivalent test measures. Those given glucose showed *"an enhancement effect on both the recall of the [test figures] as well as verbal fluency and figural fluency . . . and [enhanced] performance on a test of divided attention . . .* These findings," the authors wrote, "suggest that a specific *facilitation of retrieval mechanisms* may account for enhancement of both memory and fluency performance." [Emphasis added.]

And glucose doesn't just help elderly healthy subjects. It's been found to help subjects of all ages. Neuroscientist Dr. Donna Korol, a research associate in the psychology department at the University of Virginia at Charlottesville, has been researching neurological mechanisms of aging, changes in neurocognitive functioning in rodents and humans with age, and with Dr. Paul Gold and others what has come to be known as "the glucose facilitation effect." She says, "With glucose if baseline levels are low, like in an overnight fast, glucose for breakfast increases performance on tests, particularly verbal tests, such as recalling prose passages and some paired words tests of learning and memory. There's a 30–40% improvement," she says. "This is a very consistent finding [across many studies]. You also see the same type but even greater facilitation [improvement] when cognitive deficits are greater, as with Alzheimer's patients and with Down's syndrome adults. There's a larger percent increase in performance, for example, a doubling of scores on paragraph recall." Dr. Korol also notes that caffeine acts to enhance memory as well.

Dr. Korol and her colleagues have studied glucose enhancement in college students. "We used a hard task," she says, "because we didn't see the effect initially with easier tasks. We used memory for a prose passage three times as long as the ones typically used and more complicated as well. We also used an attention test. *We found a 30% increase [in performance with glucose] in women and men relative to their performance on saccharine. They could remember 30% better a long prose passage on the glucose."* [Emphasis added.] The improvement in memory, she notes, lasted "through the testing period for 40–45 minutes and it stays up longer than that." The improvement, she notes, "stays up longer in healthy elderly subjects than in young adults however." The same effects, she notes, have also been reported in children and young adults by Claudia Messier at the University of Ottowa in Canada, and David Benton at the University of Swansee in England.

Moreover, for women suffering fatigue during perimenopause and menopause Dr. Korol notes that "There's a huge literature on work from Europe and Germany on glucose, fatigue, performance and athletes." Glucose, she says, has been found to help "maintain performance" and reduce "fatigue at extremes of performance," i.e., when demands for performance are fairly low or relatively high, but less so when demands are intermediate.

Glucose research also indicates that *glucose taken after a learning experience* can retroactively stamp in or imprint better experience or learning into memory. In one study, for example, animals were given either an injection of glucose, or salt, or nothing one hour after prior exposure to new objects. The last day of the study animals who had received glucose spent more time than the other treatment groups exploring a new object rather than a previously experienced one, suggesting to the researcher that "glucose retroactively improved the memory for the previously observed object." That is why I propose that you try glucose after experiencing something you particularly want to remember.

For perimenopausal or menopausal women experiencing estrogen fluctuations or loss, however, glucose shortages may occur not just after a long night's fast but throughout the day, since estrogen loss reduces the brain's ability to use glucose. In a recent report of research Dr. James Simpkins, for example, writes: "Ovariectomized (OVX) female rats show significantly lower capability of brain glucose ultilization, whereas estrogen replacement of [ovariectomized] rats causes a 20–30% higher capability for glucose utilization in all regions of the brain except the median eminence. Additionally we have demonstrated that treatment of [ovariectomized] rats with 17 beta-estradiol [estrogen] increases [glucose] extraction across the blood-brain barrier [supplies coming from the body to the brain]. This enhancement of glucose extraction by the blood-brain barrier may contribute to the widespread increase in glucose uptake in the central nervous system following estrogen treatment." Estrogen replacement, Simpkins has additionally found, boosts by 40 percent expression in ovariectomized rats of a major protein that is the first step in transporting glucose from the body to the brain across the blood-brain barrier—a glucose transporter 1.

(As a side note you might want to be aware that fructose, the kind of glucose that comes from fruits, does not as readily cross the blood-brain barrier as do other forms of sugar. So eating fruit isn't the ideal route for getting the glucose facilitation effect on memory and cognition.)

What this research suggests, therefore, is that by providing your body with greater and more regular supplies of glucose (in whatever forms you choose) you can in one fell swoop increase the synthesis of the memory neurotransmitter acetylcholine; improve your short- and longer-term memory; possibly improve your attention, verbal retrieval fluency, spatial memory retrieval fluency; and counter fatigue! And you get to indulge in what some think of as sinful food.

Furthermore in both women and rats Simpkins has experimentally shown that at least some intermittent symptoms associated with peri-menopause and menopause in women—hot flashes—are associated with declining levels of glucose. In a 1990 study he and a colleague re-ported that in postmenopausal women intervals of the day when blood glucose is elevated are "free of hot flashes while the subsequent decline in glucose is associated with the reappearance of flushing episodes."

Similarly in animals, Simpkins found that tail-skin temperature "flushing" episodes in rats were associated with glucose deprivation. Per-haps then, other intermittent symptoms associated with estrogen loss, such as WHMS, might also be related to glucose supplies.

Dosages Used for Glucose Facilitation Effect

Dr. Korol says, "We use 50 grams of glucose in our studies. That's equiv-alent to about 3½ tablespoons of sugar, or 1½ servings [½ cup = one serv-ing] of unsweetened cereal (carbohydrates) or a Snickers bar. We put the 50 grams of glucose in a lemonade; 50 grams is pretty sweet," she says. "Normal orange juice has 25–30 grams of sugar."

Senior research nutritionist Lea Antzis of New York Hospital-Cornell Medical Center's General Clinical Research Center informs me that 50 grams of sugar is equivalent to 50 grams or 3½ tablespoons of a potato (a complex carbohydrate that ultimately becomes glucose). A potato, incidentally, has been found to also boost serotonin levels and provide stable availability of the neurotransmitter, as opposed to fast rise-and-fall levels of the neurotransmitter. I refer you to the book *Potatoes not Prozac* by Kathleen DesMaisons for information on how to substitute complex carbohydrates for each other, in this case in relation to the glucose facilitation effect, and also in relation to boosting serotonin levels via diet.

Antzis notes that after consuming glucose it takes between fifteen minutes and half an hour for it to be released into the bloodstream, and between half an hour and an hour for complex carbohydrates such as cereal or a potato to be released into the blood stream. Memory and glucose researcher Dr. Donna Korol notes that "If you add fat to simple sugar [as in a Snickers bar] it slows down absorption of glucose."

I suggest a "grazing" pattern of regular intake during the day of one of the above sources of glucose to facilitate maintaining a steady state of glucose availability in your body to see what impact this has on your WHMS symptoms. Since the glucose enhancement effect in young people lasts at least forty-five to fifty minutes, according to Korol, you might consider using this as the upper limit of how often to "feed" your brain when you need to be especially sharp. You might also evaluate your memory before and after this plan of treatment, by dealing yourself a "hand" of seven cards at regular intervals and see how many cards you correctly remember as a check to note if your memory is being affected for the better.

For using the glucose facilitation effect to "stamp in" the memory of a particular experience you might prefer to use glucose instead of a complex carboyhdrate because of its quicker rate of absorption into the bloodstream. Take it within an hour of the experience.

Let me add that I am by no means recommending an all-glucose diet, but rather a diet in which glucose is obtained from various sources and in conjunction with other foods required for a balanced diet.

About Phytoestrogens

I propose using genistein as part of the estrogen-mimic plan because, as noted in an earlier chapter, estrogen has multiple neuroprotective effects and often acts as a chemical shield guarding neurons from *"Star Wars"* attacks from different internal and external sources of danger. Weak plant-based estrogens, or phytoestrogens, such as genistein found in soy products and many other plant materials have also been found to confer the same neuroprotective effects as the most frequently used forms of estrogen replacement therapy by virtue of the presence of the unique chemical structure known as a phenolic A ring.

How can you obtain the phytoestrogen genistein? You can obtain it in multiple ways: by eating soy-based foods such as tofu, tempeh, soy hot dogs, soy butter, a GeniSoy protein bar; via soy-based protein powders with isoflavones you mix with juice or milk; and via prepared soy drinks. You can obtain it in pills, such as Nature's Plus Ultra Isoflavone or Solaray Genistein PhytoEstrogen or Source Naturals Genistein or Solgar Genistein. An extensive listing of the reported (though possibly not actual) amounts of isoflavones (genistein is one of several kinds of isoflavones) in these different soy-based products and pills can be found in an article by Bonnie Liebman, "The Soy Story," in the September 1998 issue of the *Nutrition Action Healthletter,* published by the Center for Science in the Public Interest. (I list some of these in Appendix I.)

Things to watch out for: *Diet* soy-based products are often lacking the "goodies" you may want. So are soy products processed using alcohols, which destroy the isoflavones. *Water-processed* soy protein powders are the ones you want. Not all soy foods list their isoflavone content, so it's not always clear what you are getting. Soy sauce has little or no isoflavone content. Plant-based estrogens can compete with regular estrogens in estrogen receptor sites in your body, so if you are taking estrogen already you might be getting the weaker substitute if you decide to use both. If you are taking tamoxifen, which is often prescribed for women with breast cancer, plant-based estrogens *may not be advisable* because they can interfere with the anti-estrogen effects of this designer estrogen.

How much genistein should you take? There's not yet one answer when it comes to helping the brain and mind in women with perimenopause and menopause. And even in areas of health where soy has been found to be effective, e.g., in reducing cholesterol, improving the elasticity of women's arteries, and preserving bone density in the spine, more knowledge is making the picture more complicated rather than always simpler. Even in reducing cholesterol the amounts of soy-based isoflavones (62 milligrams per day) that proved effective in one group depended on the initial cholesterol level of those taking it in a study reported in 1998. So the answers may vary depending on individual starting factors.

There are also seemingly paradoxical effects or bimodal response effects. In a 1994 study, for example, in which a *high* and a *low* dose of the soybean estrogen genistein were used in rats who had had their ovaries and hence estrogen supplies removed (to study the effects on their bones, i.e., osteoporosis), it was found that a *low dose* of genistein had positive bone effects equal to those of the estrogen in Premarin (conjugated equine estrogen) but *a high dose did not.* So go figure!

Dosage: How much then should you take? I suggest to play it safe that you aim for no more than, and possibly the low end of, the ballpark amounts that the Japanese presently consume. (We can't be sure that the Japanese and Asians over the centuries haven't become uniquely adapted to their diet, in a way we might not be to ours at present.) According to soy expert Mark Messina of Loma Linda University this amounts to between 30 and 50 milligrams of isoflavones per day or the equivalent of 7 to 10 grams of soy protein a day. (The genistein is in the isoflavones.) Appendix I lists different soy-based products and foods and their approximate isoflavone and soy protein content. You might be getting other health benefits in doing this. Asians, including the Japanese, tend to have fewer hip fractures and heart attacks, less prostate and breast cancer, and much fewer hot flashes. Is consuming soy the only reason? Probably not, but it seems that it may be at least part of the picture.

Antioxidant: Vitamin E: Estrogen has been found to be a potent antioxidant capable of soaking or mopping up highly interactive molecules known as free radicals. These have the ability to kill off cells, including brain neurons, by fracturing DNA and other cell parts or destroying cell membranes as the result of the process known as oxidation or oxidative stress. Aging alone and many disease states associated with aging are thought to be associated with increased oxidative damage. In recent years it has been shown that estrogen can eliminate most of the oxidation in cells that can arise from exposure to beta-amyloid, a distinctive protein known to collect to an abnormal degree in the brains of Alzheimer's patients and which some suspect to be a major contributor to the cause of the degeneration of brain neurons affecting memory in Alzheimer's patients.

Estrogen has also been shown to reduce free-radical damage arising from other potential agents toxic to brain neurons. As a well-known antioxidant, vitamin E as noted in a prior chapter has been shown to boost mightily estrogen's neuroprotective effects and to stimulate the body's own native repair mechanisms. Vitamin E, like estrogen, has also been found to delay the progression of Alzheimer's disease in those who already show evidence of it. In a large multicenter National Institute of Aging–funded study conducted at twenty-three U.S. research centers it was found that vitamin E delayed the effects of Alzheimer's in moderately advanced cases by seven months and permitted those with the disease to handle self-care functions longer.

Moreover, a 1998 study found that use of both vitamins E and C, another antioxidant, were associated with a reduced risk of developing Alzheimer's disease. The study examined the use of vitamins E and C in 633 people sixty-five years and older with no Alzheimer's disease. It then tracked the frequency of newly arising cases of Alzheimer's disease over an average span of 4.3 years. The study initially evaluated by directly examining the number of all vitamin supplements the subjects took in the two weeks before beginning the study. After an average follow-up of 4.3 years ninety-one of the subjects had developed diagnosable Alzheimer's disease. However, none of the twenty-seven vitamin E users had the disease *when 3.9 persons were expected on statistical grounds to develop it.* And none of the twenty-three vitamin C users developed Alzheimer's disease *when statistical estimates predicted 3.2 would*—both statistically significant findings.

Interestingly, the study found no association between developing Alzheimer's disease and the use of multivitamins in general. The study concluded: "These data suggest that the use of higher-dose vitamin E and vitamin C supplements may lower the risk of Alzheimer's disease."

These findings of reduced risk of Alzheimer's with vitamin E parallel findings reported for estrogen. Antioxidants therefore, like estrogens, may be viable preventive substitutes for reducing the risk of Alzheimer's, perhaps by preventing the gradual oxidative cell damage that estrogen before menopause guards against and by maintaining longer a larger brain reserve capacity for a longer span of years.

In addition to vitamins E and C, antioxidants are plentiful in fruits and vegetables. And recently a study at Tufts University School of Medicine revealed that blueberries were found to rank among the highest in fruits in antioxidant properties.

Dosages and Foods: Studies indicate that higher than minimal levels of vitamins E and C are associated with the reduced risks of, or delay in, progression of Alzheimer's disease. According to Dr. Barrie Cassileth, a relatively conservative authority, writing in *The Alternative Medicine Handbook,* "Excess [vitamin E] does no harm except in extreme amounts (above 1080 International Units)." Based on prior Alzheimer's-related studies you might consider using 800 IU daily. Natural food sources for vitamin E include wheat germ and whole grains, green leafy vegetables, vegetable oils, nuts, seafood, and eggs.

Although 200 to 400 milligrams per day is the recommended daily dose of vitamin C still in effect, according to Dr. Cassileth "[E]xcess vitamin C is excreted in urine, and side effects are uncommon," she says. You could theoretically take higher amounts with relative impunity if you determined that to be prudent.

You might choose to follow the practice of Harvard-trained Dr. Andrew Weil, the fifty-five-year-old author of *Spontaneous Healing* and a recognized expert on natural alternative treatments. He recommends for others the same "antioxidant cocktail" he takes every morning: vitamin C (1,000 milligrams), vitamin E (800 IU), mixed carotenes (one capsule), selenium (200 IU), and coenzyme Q10 (100 milligrams). He also suggests omega-3 fatty acids (as in fish and flaxseeds or flaxseed oil) and green tea.

Alternatively you might consider getting vitamin C, and the other antioxidants as well, from whole food sources: oranges, grapefruits, broccoli, carrots, fish, etc.

Take note that genistein, ginkgo biloba (from the ginkgo tree), and caffeine are also antioxidants. Caffeine, Dr. Cassileth notes (probably a coffee lover as I am), "contains antioxidants comparable to those found in fruits and vegetables." A note of caution: Those who take anticoagulants need to consult a doctor before taking vitamin E since it can alter blood-clotting functions.

Anti-inflammatory Agents

I include an anti-inflammatory agent, such as ibuprofen, in the estrogen-mimic plan because estrogen has known neuroprotective properties, which appear to include moderating or tempering the inflammatory process that some researchers believe is involved in the development of the distinctive beta-amyloid plaques that are found at autopsy in those with Alzheimer's disease. These can act to gum up the neuronal "works" and appear to lead to the massive nerve-cell death observed in memory and thinking regions in Alzheimer's patients. Estradiol (an estrogen) has been found in the test tube to break down the precursor protein fragments that can lead to clumps of beta-amyloid deposits. And with estrogen loss, these precursor protein fragments may not get broken down just as before and may lead to less preventive maintenance with regard to preventing beta-amyloid toxicity.

An anti-inflammatory agent may offer a form of protection against the inflammation-suspected risks associated with beta-amyloid buildup after the decline or loss of estrogen during perimenopause or menopause. And as noted earlier, autopsy studies of healthy individuals suggest that such beta-amyloid buildups can begin even in one's thirties without any evidence of behavioral symptoms.

I also suggest use of an anti-inflammatory agent because of the findings from a National Institute of Aging and Johns Hopkins University study that lasted fifteen years and involved 2,300 people. It was found that use of over-the-counter anti-inflammatory drugs such as ibuprofen for two years or more (used for treating arthritis, or other pains) was associated with a lowered risk of developing Alzheimer's disease. In this study neither use of aspirin, which is also an anti-inflammatory drug, nor Tylenol (acetaminophen), which isn't an anti-inflammatory drug, was associated with a reduced risk of Alzheimer's disease. This study showed *an association* between the two factors, but was not designed to detect a causal connection. Studies are now ongoing to determine whether use of the ibuprofen and other anti-inflammatory agents actually can cause such results and in what dosages.

Dosage: No *known* dosages are as yet recommended, even by the Alzheimer's Association.

So it's best to discuss taking ibuprofen or possibly other over-the-counter nonsteroidal anti-inflammatory drugs, more commonly known as NSAIDs, with a doctor first. Although over-the-counter NSAIDs are now frequently used, if used chronically they can lead to gastric side effects such as peptic ulcers and impaired kidney function. They are useful but not to be "popped" necessarily daily or casually. Remember that aspirin, which is now recommended for regular use in preventing heart disease and other ailments, can also cause gastric consequences such as gastric bleeding. To play it safe, until recommended guidelines are issued, you might consider taking ibuprofen twice a week (if your doctor deems that prudent for your specific situation).

Acetylcholine Synthesis–Boosting Foods

I suggest using acetylcholine-synthesizing foods in the estrogen-mimic plan because acetylcholine is a major neurotransmitter—a "memory ink"—that neurons involved in memory and throughout the brain use to communicate with each other. It has been established in research that estrogen loss directly diminishes the enzyme that leads to the production of acetylcholine, so with menopause, supplies of the neurotransmitter are likely to be reduced. Boosting availability of acetylcholine via foods may help substitute for such losses.

The glucose facilitation effect, which boosts memory, is known to prompt synthesis of acetylcholine. This makes sense since memory-improvement findings apply not just to young people but to Alzheimer's patients who are known to be highly deprived of acetylcholine-producing cells. The glucose may be improving memory by boosting deficient supplies of acetylcholine. Even the proportionally greater improvement in memory scores in AD patients than in younger subjects suggests that the glucose-acetylcholine-synthesis effect on memory may be at work.

As noted above glucose and complex carbohydrates (which end up as glucose) are known to produce acetylcholine synthesis. So by following the first two steps of the estrogen-mimic plan you will already be fulfilling the "boosting acetylcholine" goal.

You might also include in your diet choline-rich foods. Choline is a precursor of acetylcholine synthesis and can be found in such natural foods as grains, beans, lettuce, and cauliflower. As the essential ingredient of lecithin, choline is also present and listed in the ingredients of many baked goods, instant foods, and chocolate candy.

Serotonin-Boosting Agents or Foods

I include serotonin-boosting substances or foods because it is known that estrogen loss can affect, through different routes, supplies of the neurotransmitter serotonin. Based on my interviews flattened affect or varying degrees of depression seem to be a common feature of perimenopause and menopause in women, apart from life-event factors.

Since ongoing depression is known to independently be capable of affecting memory, and since long-term depression is even known to compromise the integrity of the functioning of the memory center known as the hippocampus, I think it is prudent to substitute for the potential serotonin-diminishing effects of estrogen decline or loss, with foods or substances known to elevate serotonin levels, if you experience *unaccountable* bouts of depression or emotional flatness in association with perimenopause or menopause, or estrogen loss for other reasons.

If you plan to go the "whole foods" route I suggest you consider relying on the readily available low-calorie (if not drenched with fattening toppings) potato for (1) its serotonin-promoting benefits, (2) its glucose-promoting benefits (the complex carbohydrate will ultimately break down into glucose), and (3) for its known hunger-quenching potential. To develop skill in maneuvering serotonin supplies from whole foods I recommend you read *Potatoes not Prozac* by Kathleen Des-Maisons for her information on this and about food guidelines relative to serotonin.

Alternatively, consider getting your serotonin supplies, under a doctor's supervision, from Saint-John's-wort or one of the selective serotonin-reuptake inhibitor (SSRI) drugs used for treating depression such as Prozac, Paxil, Zoloft, and a new entry into this category, Celexa.

Saint-John's-wort, or hypericum, is a flower-derived herbal substance that has long been popular in Europe as a treatment for mild to moderate depression. Research in the United States at present is aimed at documenting its effectiveness for depression. (Note: Saint-John's-wort should not to be used together with drugs such as Prozac, Zoloft, Paxil, or Celexa. Also Prozac requires some five weeks to "wash out" of the body. So do not use Saint-John's-wort after Prozac use for some five weeks.) Furthermore, according to Dr. Donald Klein, director of research at the New York State Psychiatric Institute, Prozac "has not always been effective with people on either end of the scale, the ones who are barely impaired and those who are very ill." Prozac, he says, "is very effective with people in the middle."

Dosage: For Saint-John's-wort and any of the SSRIs I urge you first to consult a doctor regarding recommended dosages for your specific emotional needs and physical requirements.

Attention-Focusing/Enhancing Agents

Research by Dr. Marylou Voytko, Associate Professsor of Pathology and Comparative Medicine in the Department of Neurobiology and Anatomy at the Wake Forest School of Medicine in North Carolina, documenting the compromising effects on attention of estrogen loss in monkeys, together with the experiences of women I have interviewed with WHMS with attention, concentration, and reading problems, lead me to see the need for agents that can boost attention and concentration, in an estrogen-mimic plan to combat WHMS symptoms.

What has the potential for doing this? Caffeine and Ritalin.

If it is not inadvisable in view of your unique health history and risks, I suggest you consider asking your doctor about the safety for you of using caffeine for this end, when you need to be particularly sharp. Caffeine is known to boost attention and, according to memory and aging researcher Dr. Donna Korol, "to boost memory" (perhaps by boosting attention first). As noted earlier it is also an acceptable antioxidant according to Dr. Barrie Cassileth. So you would be getting double and possible triple duty from using it. Moreover, given our long familiarity with it, it has the added benefit of relative safety with ordinary use. And in fact the "jumpiness" it evokes in some may alternatively be viewed in this context as a potential "readiness to attend," react, and "take in" sensitizer.

Ritalin, as you may know, is a drug commonly prescribed by physicians for use with children experiencing attention deficit hyperactivity disorder, who are having difficulty concentrating, focusing, sitting still, and for those experiencing narcolepsy. It is considered a stimulant but is considered to have paradoxical effects in children, getting them more focused. I took it when I was involved in sleep research years ago at what is now the State University of New York's Health Sciences Center in Brooklyn under the supervision of a physician who was the principal investigator of the research we were engaged in. It kept me awake as I watched other people's brain waves during sleep.

I don't at this time recommend its use generally for WHMS symptoms, but if your situation is dire—if attention and concentration problems are threatening to undermine important facets of your life—you might seek out a psychopharmacologist. Call a medical school psychiatry department for a referral to one, explain your situation, and try it on an empirical basis to see if it helps. It helped at least one woman I interviewed who was given an attention deficit diagnosis by a physician who was not aware of WHMS symptoms in relation to estrogen loss. One of Ritalin's suspected roles is in preventing the reuptake of the neurotransmitter dopamine, one of the neurotransmitters likely to decline in women with estrogen loss. So Ritalin may compensate for estrogen loss and in part mimic its effects. More research on this first needs to be done, however.

Aerobic Exercise on a Regular Basis

I include aerobic exercise on a regular basis as a way of mimicking estrogen's abilities (1) to maintain the blood vessel health and elasticity of the body's vascular support system, (2) to enhance the brain's oxygen supply, and (3) to boost nerve-growth factor release, all functions associated with estrogen as discussed in chapter 3. In the next chapter, on behaviors that can boost your mind and brain function, I discuss the supportive research evidence indicating that exercise can mimic at least portions of these estrogen functions.

Dosage: How much exercise is up to you, but my sense, wrong or right, is that straining somewhat to exceed one's level of performance over time in the short run and aiming with advancing years to maintain one's level of performance are goals that would sufficiently "tax" a body to keep "growing" in the ways that would mimic estrogen's nerve-growth-stimulating and vascular support–enhancing functions.

What Else?

Are there other things that might help WHMS symptoms that are not hormones? There may be—such as ginkgo biloba, DHA, or DMAE, over-the-counter substances reputedly beneficial for memory that are available in health food stores. From my perspective, their basis of action, the efficacy of the extracts available in the United States and/or the insufficient knowledge about them leads me to not include them as recommended for memory or related symptoms here at the present time. I suggest you read up on them in the many books now available on alternative health care.

So to recap, the estrogen-mimic plan for addressing WHMS symptoms entails using the following foods or substances as a plausible but not yet proven approach to compensating for the potential loss of biological functions or neurotransmitters associated with estrogen's known roles in the brain, which may be affected with the loss of estrogen during perimenopause and menopause:

- Glucose (in the form of complex carbohydrates or glucose)
- The soy-based phytoestrogen genistein
- Antioxidants such as vitamin E plus other antioxidants, if desired
- An anti-inflammatory agent such as ibuprofen
- Acetylcholine-synthesizing foods such as glucose, complex carbohydrates, or choline-rich foods
- Serotonin-boosting foods or substances such as Saint-John's-wort, Prozac, Paxil, Zoloft, etc.
- Attention-focusing/enhancing substances when in dire need, such as caffeine or Ritalin after a doctor's approval of both for your unique health restrictions
- Aerobic exercise for boosting nerve-growth factor release and the fuel supplies network in the brain and body via an enhanced vascular support system

Potential solutions to life's problems can come from many directions. This plan is a feasible one and a plausible one. Since WHMS is entirely new this plan has simply never been tried before. See if it helps you and any WHMS symptoms you may have and let me know what happened. (See Appendix II for where to send the information.) It's not inconceivable that together we may make what is plausible, possible.

12

Behaviors That Can Boost Your Mind or Brain Power

Phyllis V., a forty-nine-year-old, single, child psychologist, had been experiencing WHMS symptoms for several years when she read my *New York* magazine article. She recognized herself in some of the symptoms I described and wrote to ask me what she could possibly do to help her "hang on to her mind." Though no one in her family had had it, she too had been fearing early Alzheimer's disease. She wrote that as a psychologist her verbal dexterity and mental acumen were the major tools of her profession. What could she do that could make a difference? She wrote that she was not a candidate for hormone replacement therapy. There was too much of a history of breast cancer in her family to risk it. And she was averse to "playing" with "alternative stuff." What could she do?

The information in this chapter is for people like Phyllis. It is also for those who want to do whatever they can in addition to using either hormonal or non-hormonal treatments to facilitate improving or maximally retaining their cognitive skills over time.

———————

The revolution in thinking about the brain that helped revamp science's ways of understanding what estrogen does and how plastic the brain continues to be into adulthood has also produced other payoffs in knowledge that, interestingly, dovetail with the needs of women who can't take estrogen. Based on a large bounty of research evidence it appears that *engaging in specific behaviors* can meaningfully affect for the better the brain's structure and biological functioning during adulthood—even into late adulthood. Still other research shows that simply by challenging wrong defeatist assumptions and thoughts you may have about what declining memory implies, you can improve your memory. Last of all, practicing preventive health maintenance in the face of common mind-compromising health conditions can help you prevent needless erosion of cognitive skills.

Let me list for you behaviors you can engage in that science suggests can have important cognitive consequences

CHALLENGE YOURSELF WITH NEW LEARNING

Rather than giving in to an undemanding, cognitively safe life, research indicates that challenging yourself with new learning can potentially *enhance your brain's connectivity* and ability to handle complexity over time. New research shows the brain has plasticity not only in response to the stimulus of estrogen long into adulthood, but has ongoing remodeling ability into adulthood, in response to the stimulus of behavior.

Research from the University of Illinois laboratory of neuroscientist William Greenough and that of his colleagues, spanning two decades, has repeatedly confirmed in animal models that actively participating in and engaging complex enriched environments can actually change, even in elderly animals, the structure and function of the brain not unlike the ways that estrogen can, in leading to more richly "branched," varied, connected, and sprouting neuronal connections. Engaging in complex experiences (behavior) and attempting mastery, it has been found, can actually turn on the functioning of genes! (So say good-bye to the "old hat" and overly simplistic "environment versus nature" or "genes versus behavior" dichotomy of yesteryear since (1) it's now known behavior can actually turn on genes and since (2) genes never exist independent of a specific environment in which they are expressed!)

What the work of Greenough and his colleagues suggests is that by keeping cognitive complexity and challenge in your life, you make it possible for complexity to keep up with you over the long run. "Pushing the envelope" in this way may well keep it open and unstuck. You may recall that when Dr. Fredericka Xerov felt foggy and cloudy she nonetheless kept studying for her licensing exam and was able to pass it. Her "pushing" despite the fog may well have been a factor in her passing. I have heard similar accounts from other women experiencing WHMS, where volition and directed effort overcame WHMS' apparent roadblocks. To keep cognitive complexity in your life consider taking a continuing education course or learning a new complex skill despite any fears you may have—don't worry about how you will do in it, just plan to try.

You might consider learning how to search the "information highway," for example, or how to join an online chat group; attend weekend seminars at a museum or educational center; or pick some new area that interests you and read as much about it as you can, pushing the envelope if the going gets rough at times. Create or join a monthly reading group. Join or create an investment club. If you really want a complex challenge plug away at deciphering the instructions for programming your VCR to tape what you want (if you haven't yet) or attempt to master the subtleties of another piece of equipment in your life you have resisted engaging so far. Set your expectations so that you don't even necessarily have to succeed. Choose to define success as merely attempting to grapple with whatever you decide to do. (But whatever you undertake, also reward yourself for taking on challenging ventures. You'll tend to persist longer if you do. And remember that studies of learning show that work-rest cycles rather than endless drilling effort often leads to better retention and learning).

Apart from boosting your brain's connectivity and ability to handle complexity, education early on and throughout life can apparently buffer your brain from erosion later in life. Research indicates that both high levels of educational attainment and early exposure to complex experiences may offer you some protection against cognitive erosion later in life. Research has shown that high educational attainment seems to play a role in protecting against the development of Alzheimer's disease and reducing disability in old age. Neuroscientists speak of education as building up "an increased threshold to damage against the losses of normal and abnormal aging." And early exposure to complex experiences "may offer some protection from 'wear and tear' degradation" of the brain according to Greenough and his colleagues J. Black and K. Isaacs. Mechanisms invoked in this protective effect include learning at an early age how to master stress-coping skills in the face of complexity, and developing more complex blood vessel support networks in the brain, among other factors.

If you are still in the middle of your life you may have plenty of time left to add density or resilience to that educational protective "cushion" as a hedge against what may occur in the future. And even in old age, apparently that kind of "growth," scientists are now telling us, is still possible: "Exposure to complex experience in old age can also generate new synapses in the cerebral cortex and cerebellum," Greenough and his researchers declare in their work. So don't give up a cognitive "life" at the first signs of WHMS. Keep guard against a dumbing, downward spiral of expectations of yourself.

CHALLENGE YOUR COORDINATION SKILLS

Research from the same lab—that of William Greenough and his many collaborators and students—also indicates that physically enriched and challenging environments can lead to greater physical coordination and brain changes for the better, in adult rats. If you've got the WHMS "dropsies," or other aspects of your coordination have somewhat changed, you may be able to compensate with a relevant form of practice to regain or improve on prior skills, at the same time keeping fine-tuned neuronally your brain's ability to execute specific movements with precision and grace. Leading neuroscientist Michael Merzenich has shown in research with adult monkeys that when a monkey was trained to repetitively use its middle finger, the part of the brain that was devoted primarily to getting input from that finger expanded in size. The behavior had the consequence of altering the physical organization of the brain. The brain is "a network that is continually remodeling itself," Merzenich said in the journal *Science* in an article with the informative subtitle: "A striking body of recent work suggests that the adult brain can reorganize itself in areas that were long thought to be completely hard-wired [unresponsive to change]."

Keep in mind that pianists, violinists, and conductors often maintain manual, physical, and memory precision and mastery well into old age despite whatever depredations age may wreak. The demands of the work they do may keep them as fit as they stay. For maintaining overall coordination and balance consider taking up the balance, coordination, and self-centering exercises known as Tai Chi, which even elderly Chinese frequently practice daily outdoors. Yoga contains many exercises that increase balance and coordination as ballet certainly does. If the dropsies affect you, consider taking up fine finger–coordination crafts such as cloisonné, mosaics, jewelry making, beading, or playing pickup sticks. If you have never played an instrument or haven't played one for a while consider doing so.

EXERCISE

If exercising for a trim figure or physical health hasn't motivated you, consider whether physical exercise might be worth it to you for keeping your brain in shape. Again research from William Greenough's lab with adult female rats indicates that exercise can increase the number and branching complexity of the *blood supply routes to the brain*. This expanded vascular network can bring greater amounts of brain-food/fuel deliveries (glucose) to a brain that may have had reductions in such deliveries because of diminished estrogen supplies. "There is considerable evidence," says William Greenough, "that physical exercise enhances vascular blood perfusion and provides greater amounts of 'fuel' for the brain. The brain," he notes, "can't store anything in the way of fuel. It doesn't store fat or carbohydrates. The brain is dependent from moment to moment on its blood supply for the delivery of that fuel. We have seen in animal studies that exercise can increase the number of capillaries and the extent of capillary branching in the brain."

In their 1998 book *Successful Aging* Dr. John Rowe and Dr. Robert L. Kahn point out that "older men and women who engaged in strenuous physical activity in and around the home were more likely to maintain . . . high cognitive function." In explanation the authors note that research with adult rats found that exercise was associated with enhanced production of nerve-growth factor, a substance that "promotes growth of new brain cells." And remember what estrogen does—enhance production of nerve-growth factor. So here again you can compensate for potential changes due to estrogen loss with a behavior that may pinch-hit for the same function.

EAT BREAKFAST

Speaking of the brain and its fuel supply, old-fashioned moms had it right. There's brain value in eating a good breakfast, not skipping meals, and eating on time. After a night's fast your brain may be low on glucose. If your estrogen supplies are low or highly variable your brain may be getting fewer or less regular fuel delivery(ies) than it used to. So compensate for estrogen loss with greater regularity in fuel delivery. Studies in children, young adults, and the elderly have shown that skipping breakfast takes its toll in impaired memory and mental performance. Studies have shown that verbal fluency, recall ability, and attention (WHMS symptoms) are hurt by hunger.

LEARN STRESS-MANAGEMENT TECHNIQUES

Choose to actively diffuse stress. Learn to control the potentially compromising effects of stress on the brain's leading memory and attention structure, the hippocampus. Canadian neuroscientist Sonia Lupien, a former student of Bruce McEwen, found in a study of sixty-three- to eighty-year-olds that high levels of the major human stress hormone (cortisol) lead to shrinkage of the hippocampus and to worse performance on memory tasks over time than was the case with age-matched individuals with moderate levels of the stress hormone.

Exercise is one way to diffuse stress, but consider learning several of the stress-moderating self-regulation techniques used in the practice of health psychology and behavioral medicine to give you control over moderating stress. You might give yourself a buffer against cognitive decline in this way.

You can easily learn these techniques yourself from a good tape cassette, or video or a book that explains the rationales for doing what you are doing. (In Appendix II I offer a relaxation tape that teaches several techniques, which I developed for use with patients who came to me for learning stress management.)

Learning several of these will give you choices of tools to pick from during stressful times. And having choices available provides you with more of a sense of control in a situation, another way to mitigate stress—offering yourself options. You might consider learning (Jacobson's) Progressive Relaxation Training, one of my favorite techniques, which when learned well can be compressed into a virtually instant relaxation aid, or Visual Imagery relaxation exercises, or breathing exercises, different meditation exercises, or self-hypnosis for relaxation.

Then actually work on using them during stressful times. I suggest you practice at least two or three long enough so that you can actually feel the unwinding or letting go of tension in your body and mind. If you can't experience the physical feeling of letting go in your body (your mind will follow) you likely haven't practiced long enough or haven't been tuning in to what you are experiencing as you do the exercises. Or you may be trying a technique that is simply too alien for your individual temperament. You might then consider trying several sessions of biofeedback with a trained practitioner to help you better see or hear or "tune in" to what is happening to your body or to reassure yourself that these techniques actually can affect your body. I also suggest you depend not only on physical exercise for stress management because you won't always be in places where you can do it (an airplane or a meeting). However, you usually can use the above relaxation techniques anywhere once you have learned them well enough.

DRILL AND SKILL

As the mother of a school-age child I have witnessed in adulthood the specific steps in at least one child's acquiring pronunciation skills; reading mastery; and spelling, math, and writing skills. Conscious attention to details, effort, and repetition or practice are key ingredients (assuming a developmental readiness). With mastery, however, by adulthood these skills usually have become virtually reflex, automatic behavior that no longer require conscious attention to detail. We just read. We don't think about how to do it. We write the letters of words without thinking about it. I suggest that if WHMS "glitches" in spelling, writing, calculation, speech/pronunciation, or other acquired skills such as driving pose any true problem for you it is quite likely that bringing the same kind of conscious attention, effort, and practice to these skills that you brought to them when you first acquired them may well help get them back to "automatic" fitness again. (And relearning usually takes much less time than totally new learning so you are likely to get up to speed much faster than the first time around.)

I see WHMS symptoms as predominantly reflecting changes in non-conscious "automatic pilot" behaviors that a person need not think about anymore or in terms of their subcomponent parts. Or they reflect changes in instinctual behavior, such as the near-perpetual awareness of one's self or "I" in one's environment (except perhaps during sneezing or the heights of orgasmic pleasure).

As human beings, however, we have volition and can bring a conscious "Maglite" beam of attention, directed effort, and will to situations. It is my suspicion that many of the skills that become less fine-tuned in the WHM Syndrome can be fine-tuned again with such renewed learning and conscious attention to details. I base this in part on having seen what it is possible to accomplish in terms of cognitive retraining from working with traumatically brain-injured individuals who have had to relearn virtually everything—from how to tie a shoe lace to counting to reading again. I base it also on the ability I have seen in older motivated women and men—immigrants from the Soviet Union among others—to learn to speak, read, and write in new languages, with new alphabets. The plasticity of the brain is something you should learn to count on.

To bone up on basic skills again I suggest you go to a teacher's supply store or a large book store and get workbooks that include math or math reasoning skills or lists of spelling words. To learn to focus buy workbooks that have "comprehension" paragraphs and questions and check to see how many you get right over a span of several weeks. Ask for SAT (Scholastic Aptitude Test) or GRE (Graduate Record Examination) workbooks or even easier ones. Also consider drilling yourself regularly in whatever areas your "glitches" happen to be in. Consider doing what Katherine Kennedy and others have done: working anagrams or crossword puzzles to flex their verbal and spelling "muscles." Play Scrabble or Boggle to jiggle your verbal recall skills. Leave a pocket dictionary in the bathroom if your spelling skills have declined and surf the pages at your leisure as a way of upgrading these skills or compensating for the kinds of feelings of diminishment that Katherine Kennedy felt. Carry a deck of cards like Sherry Strumph and practice remembering the cards you deal yourself in a hand one minute, five minutes, and fifteen minutes later. I believe that the *motivation* to do better at whatever skill it is constitutes half the battle, since motivation, as I see it, acts somewhat like a sensitizing spotlight to focus attention on something that interests you.

LEARN SELF-HYPNOSIS TO FOCUS YOUR ATTENTION

Consider also learning self-hypnosis as a potential aid to focusing your attention discretely on what you want to. Hypnosis represents focused, directed attention, and *self-hypnosis* represents self-directed focused attention. It's a way of talking to your "self"—perhaps that errant "I" if you have WHMS. Since it's been found to be able to control other usually nonvolitional aspects of mind such as pain perception, and in stage hypnotist performances to control what one "sees" or doesn't "see," it may conceivably be useful in "upping" attention and memory volitionally or accessing dimensions of mind involved in producing WHMS symptoms. It would be useful as well for managing stress. You can get referrals to appropriate hypnotists from the Society for Clinical and Experimental Hypnosis or from the American Society of Clinical Hypnosis. (See Appendix II.)

YOUR ASSUMPTIONS ABOUT MEMORY LOSS MAY BE LIMITING YOUR POTENTIAL

Aside from whatever the specific facts about your memory are, research indicates that *what you say to yourself about your memory*—your attributions, assumptions, and beliefs about it—can have real and negative implications. "If you get into the mind-set of expecting yourself to forget, you often do," says Margie Lachman, a professor of psychology and director of the Life Span Development Psychology Laboratory at Brandeis University. Negative expectations, she says, can lead to a downward spiral in outlook and effort. *"When you are preoccupied with forgetting,"* she says, *"you don't focus on the skills needed to remember information."*

Dr. Lachman has been researching the effects of beliefs about memory controllability and ability in young, middle-aged, and older people with respect to memory functioning. She has also been examining strategies for improving memory in members of different age groups. "[N]egative beliefs about memory competence and controllability can have far-reaching consequences," she and her colleagues write. "These consequences may include increased dependency on others, avoidance of memory challenges, seeking unnecessary medical attention, reliance on medication, depression, anxiety, reduced effort, and decreased motivation to use one's memory [i.e., "dumbing yourself down"]. She says there is [research] evidence that those who have lower confidence in their abilities and those who believe they have little control over their memory show poorer performance.

Many people, says Lachman, hold maladaptive beliefs about memory in general that don't help and even harm them. These can include "the rigid idea that aging leads to memory deficits that are inevitable and uncontrollable. People," she says, "attribute memory problems to a lost capacity to remember, with the belief that effort won't help at all." This outlook, she says, leads to lowered expectations about one's ability to be successful in remembering and to a sense of despair.

A more productive set of beliefs likely to lead to better memory performance she says is recognizing that *one can have control over memory functioning* and do something about bad memory. "It's much more helpful to hold the view that memory involves a set of skills that can be acquired and maintained with effort. It's also true. Viewing it this way leads people to persist longer in developing different ways to cope with memory problems, and leads them to encourage themselves with positive thoughts when they do run into difficulties so they don't get beaten down and give up. Viewing memory this way can improve performance by creating a "can-do" sense of self and fostering effective problem solving."

In this regard think of Polly Van Benthusen's positive "can-do" attitude toward her WHMS memory and scheduling symptoms: her determination to become a "technoweenie," keeping calendars at work and at home, and asking her boss to check her work. Her overall adaptive belief that there was something to be done about her situation counteracted what could have been a state of demoralization and helped her persist in coping with her life at a difficult time.

The National Center on Women and Aging, in a booklet titled *Your Memory: What Changes and What You Can Do About It,* written by Dr. Lachman [see Appendix II], offers the following advice about memory that may help your recall skills and change defeatist assumptions you may have:

- A good deal of research shows that adults over sixty and into their eighties and nineties can improve their memories significantly with practice. [If they can you likely can too.]
- Memory can improve by just using it.
- Practice and repetition with memory skills can improve performance.
- Write things down. A 1996 study by Dr. Lachman found that "writing things down in a list form helps remembering even when the list is not used for recall."
- Create triggers for your memory: put your umbrella on the doorknob immediately after hearing of a rainy weather forecast. [Leave

Post-it notes to yourself on the door of things you need to do that day so you see them before you leave. Transfer them to your appointment book as you walk out the door.]

Plan to notice more than in the past distinctive features or aspects of people, places, or things you want to remember as a way of sharpening your attention and memory skills.

TO PREVENT COGNITIVE EROSION, CONTROL MIND-LIMITING CHRONIC HEALTH CONDITIONS

Lastly, practice preventive health maintenance to guard your cognitive skills from unnecessary erosions brought on by chronic disease states that are known to have the potential for compromising cognitive skills over the long run.

- Monitor and reduce ongoing high blood pressure with diet or drug treatment. It can lead to mini-strokes over time and multi-infarct dementia. Uncontrolled high blood pressure on an ongoing basis has also been associated with declines over time in scores on intelligence tests.
- Control diabetes with diet, medications, or self-regulation behavioral techniques.Uncontrolled diabetes on an ongoing basis is also associated with memory and cognitive impairments—through glucose disregulation.

I eventually met with psychologist Phyllis V. In the course of talking "psychologist talk" she told me that she had long been looking forward to attending a summer training seminar in her field held on Cape Cod in August. She wanted to learn new treatment techniques she had heard were effective with children but she didn't know whether she should go or not. The seminar involved engaging in interactive exercises, and Phyllis was concerned that her intermittent bouts of WHMS fogginess and occasional verbal difficulties in marshaling questions concisely might get in the way and make her look foolish. She wondered as we talked should she expose herself in a less than ideal light to colleagues who might be there? Her symptoms had left her with a diminished sense of herself. She also wasn't sure if she would be able to absorb the material that would be coming at her in one fell swoop during the week, and she wasn't sure she wanted to find out in case she couldn't. Phyllis decided she would probably not go and would take another watercoloring course in Provincetown instead.

Assuming she did that—I don't know in actuality what she ultimately decided—what do you think of her decision in light of what you've read in this chapter? What options did Phyllis have open to her that she wasn't aware of? What could Phyllis have said to herself to warrant going to the seminar? What could she have done to work around her specific fears, to accommodate their reality for her? No one can crawl into your skin and decide what's best for you, obviously. But I ask you to think about these questions as a way of beginning to be reflective about your own situation. Are you circumscribing your life in ways that may not be adaptive over the long run? Are you giving up on yourself in any way—your dreams and hopes and plans—because of WHMS symptoms? How *have they* affected you if at all? Do you have the equivalent of Polly Van Benthusen's "can-do" attitude? Take the time now to reflect on where *you* are. And plan to be creative in problem solving around any situations that come up that involve WHMS or your concerns about WHMS.

13

Coping with WHMS

For many women with WHMS there isn't much of a need to cope altogether with symptoms since they don't much get in the way but are more surprising distractions in the usual pattern of things. However, for women who have more frequent or intense WHMS symptoms, or whose lives leave little room for occasional glitches, or who can't escape experiencing alarm reactions whenever WHMS symptoms occur, different forms of coping strategies are possible.

WAYS OF COPING

Interviews with women and my experiences as a health psychologist suggest to me that there are many ways to cope with WHMS symptoms. These can include:

- Working on your attitude or outlook
- Becoming better organized and methodical
- Becoming a "technoweenie" with electronic or mechanical aids
- Compensating for the effects of WHMS in different ways
- Developing contingency plans and options to keep hope alive and fight despair
- Garnering social support for what you are going through
- Reassuring yourself with self-talk
- Developing "cover" statements to use when WHMS glitches occur
- Becoming aware of where your mind is: bringing directed attention to what was automatic

Before examining these different forms of coping let me offer you some quick "takes" on how some women with WHMS have coped:

Deborah D., a gifted fifty-eight-year-old writer and Yale graduate who had been menopausal for some three years, didn't know what to make of her WHMS symptoms before we spoke and had been chastising herself as "stupid" as a result of the symptoms. When she felt especially stupid, she said, she would compensate and show off her intellectual skills by spouting insights and facts in discussions with friends to show *herself* she still merited being a Yale graduate. (I'm not recommending *you* do this, but illustrating a coping strategy.)

Marilyn E., a forty-eight-year-old account executive at a public relations company, now perimenopausal and experiencing many WHMS symptoms, uses a "week-at-a-glance" calendar to take a mental snapshot of her week's upcoming appointments. She highlights her appointments and the boxes they appear in with a Day-Glo marker and then refers to the "snapshot" in her mind's eye. This works for her.

Pattie S., the editor of a menopause newsletter, knows WHMS symptoms are common in women and copes with her own by telling herself her "glitches" don't matter. She accepts and works around her glitches, has no interest in taking estrogen, and takes heart from the bigger picture of her overall knowledge, competence, and attainments.

Sarah V., a forty-eight-year-old menopausal stay-at-home mother of two young children in New York City with WHMS symptoms was continually forgetting where her husband had most recently parked the car on the city's streets the night before or that morning. She would typically ask him on his way out the door and he would shout out the answer. But she often was preoccupied with the children and didn't take the time to write down what he said. By the time she needed the car to take the children for a doctor's appointment or to visit a friend she had forgotten what he had said. She bought herself a small inexpensive voice recorder on a key chain on which she kept one set of car keys. She kept it attached to a magnetic hook on the side of the refrigerator. When her husband called out where the car was parked in the morning she dropped everything and recorded where the car was that day, hanging the keys back on the side of the fridge. She also recorded on it memos of what she had to buy when she went out. When she left the house she listened to the taped message or messages. (See Appendix II.)

Evelyn V., a fifty-two-year-old antiques store owner, now menopausal and with many WHMS symptoms, keeps small Post-it pads and pens all around her at work, at home, and in her pocket at all times. She writes "to do" messages to herself and stuffs them in her pocket. After dinner each day she goes through the notes from the day and posts them on the fridge, in her weekly organizer, in the bathroom, and on the inner side of her entry door to cue herself as a way of compensating for her erratic memory.

Polly Van Benthusen began to use an erasable pen as a way to manage the reversed letters she often found in her writing.

Cynthia K., forty-eight and perimenopausal, a high school history teacher, with flickering math skills, at least for now, never leaves home without a thin wallet calculator she uses for computing dinner bills with friends. Even when she doesn't feel the need to use it, knowing she has it handy relieves her of anticipatory anxiety.

These women and others I interviewed came up with their own coping strategies for addressing WHMS symptoms. WHMS doesn't have to be a bar to problem solving, and as the mother of invention, necessity, I suspect, will lead you to solutions specific to your own situation. You will have to get yourself into a problem-solving mode, however, and out of a mode of possibly downplaying or putting down your thinking skills. Remember that WHMS symptoms are intermittent. Your cognitive/behavioral skills are still there for you to draw on, particularly if you apply yourself to them with directed effort. Don't be harsh with yourself or devalue your abilities. Be your own good mother and offer yourself the support and understanding you would give to a child or good friend you loved. Make use of the suggestions below if they fit your style and use them to trigger coping solutions of your own. "One of the real pitfalls of experiencing many of these symptoms," feminist writer Letty Cottin Pogrebin told me, "is that women going through this begin to side-line themselves and think they aren't entitled to be center stage anymore."

WORKING ON YOUR ATTITUDE OR OUTLOOK (OR KEEPING THE BIGGER PICTURE IN MIND)

Working on your attitude or outlook when it comes to WHMS is probably one of the most important coping tools you can draw on since it affects so much else. It requires first accepting that the way you are looking at your situation now need not be the only one that is possible; that a different outlook, through a differently colored lens, on your situation *is a possibility* and may have a better payoff in how you view or react to your situation. When the college music instructor I mentioned earlier didn't understand what was happening to her, her attitude toward herself and her WHMS symptoms was a harsh and punitive one. She loathed herself every time a WHMS glitch occurred. Her self-hate created radiating waves of feeling that didn't simply limit her glitches to when they were occurring but let them ripple and spill, affecting her far longer than was absolutely necessary. When she understood why she was behaving as she did she had a much more tolerant attitude toward herself. The symptoms were now "understandable, forgivable, and excusable." She moved on when they occurred or did what she had to, to manage them, but didn't wallow in feelings around them.

Theoretically, she could have chosen to be forgiving of herself even without understanding the basis for WHMS symptoms.

Sherry Strumph in effect did this in an attitude switch that worked for her particular life. She did a turnaround practically by fiat, from being a person who always felt she had to be right, or in control, to one who decided to accept herself the forgetful way she was *for now*. "It's not the way I was but it's the way I am now," she would counter when her husband expressed dismay at not being able to count on her reliability as he always had. Sherry recognized that she wasn't *only her symptom*. She was more than it and deserved her own self-regard, even if she was occasionally fallible.

The woman I cited earlier, who was experiencing different tones of "fog" among many WHMS symptoms, even while taking on a new job, opted for a tolerant outlook by acknowledging the likelihood that getting into a "state" over each WHMS episode would only make her anxious and make things worse. She decided that her approach or attitude would be "I'll do the best I can and try not to worry too much about the rest because that won't help." Developing this kind of self-tolerance made it possible for her to brainstorm and devise self-management tools that were working well when I last spoke to her. She wrote everything down that she had to do the next day or in the future in a book before she left work and brought the book home with her. She managed life at home too with an organizing book.

The editor of the menopause newsletter I cited who declared to herself that her WHMS symptoms "didn't matter" created a coping attitude by stepping back and asking "What's the bigger picture here?" a technique I suggest you try. She recognized that her public "glitches" and her private ones weren't the most important things about her, respectively, professionally and personally. The "bigger picture" as she saw it was that she had considerable knowledge to impart, competence in carrying out what she wanted to overall despite any glitches, and attainments she was proud of and believed she would be able to continue despite her symptoms.

You may be wondering how is it possible to change your attitude or outlook or belief if you see things one way or believe in what you believe? It is possible. Attitudes and outlooks and beliefs can change quickly in a radical turnaround. Chances are you once believed in tooth fairies or Santa Claus and then one day stopped holding those beliefs. Attitudes and outlooks can turn around that way too, particularly if you see an example of someone you can respect who models a different attitude or outlook.

See if you can figure out what your outlook is on WHMS symptoms. Ask yourself if this outlook is adaptive and helps you cope or persist in the things that are important for you in your life, or if this outlook undermines you and makes things worse. If you can't figure out how to overcome an unadaptive attitude on your own I suggest you follow my suggestions below for getting social support and see if you can expose yourself to those with similar concerns who model a more adaptive outlook.

Becoming Better Organized and Methodical

It has been rewarding for me to see how some women with WHMS have managed "to keep it all together" in both their professional and personal lives despite more-than-mild WHMS symptoms by getting effectively organized with self-management techniques they dreamed up. One woman, a forty-two-year-old perimenopausal nurse who works in a nursing home and is the single parent of two children, told me that developing WHMS symptoms has made her a much more methodical and organized person than she was before she developed any symptoms. She now takes the time to stay on top of everything methodically. She writes down everything she needs to do, when it needs to be done by, and then checks everything off. She has become a creature of fixed *volitionally controlled* habits when it comes to things of importance that depend on attention and memory and retrieval. She's become more voluntarily obsessive you might say. She takes little for granted in these areas and doesn't let herself "just be" or coast through routine jobs. And writing things down, as we learned from Dr. Lachman, probably facilitates her recall.

However, it can take trial and error behavior to work out the kinks of managing in this way. Sherry Strumph, for example, found that she wrote things down "religiously" but would forget to read what she had written. Cuing yourself, thus, to read what you write may be one of the steps you might have to work out. You could use behaviors you engage in every day, such as mealtimes, as naturally occurring daily "prompts" or triggers to look at your calendar for what you have to do. You could use washing your face, or brushing your teeth, or visits to the bathroom to cue you to look at your calendar/organizer, or list of things to do.

Here are some ideas on how to become better organized and methodical:

- If you have been in the habit of continually doing two things at
  once *don't any longer* if memory and attention are your WHMS
  symptoms. Practice bringing your attention to bear down like a drill
  press on things that are of importance to you.
- Become a creature of fixed habits. Put things in the same place every
  time. Cue yourself to not "mindlessly" put things down that you
  will need in the near future. Cue yourself to be mindful at distinct
  times: when you walk in the door, before you leave the house, before you leave work, etc. Being methodical helps considerably in reducing the load on your memory.
- Go to a stationery store and get appointment book/calendars—one
  for work, one for home, and one for your bag. Explore the different
  kinds—week-at-a-glance, monthly, etc., before you decide. Consider having in each one columns or sections marked with the same
  headings (1) Re: Work, (2) Re: Personal, (3) Re: Family or whatever
  headings work for you so it's all mapped out in one place.
- Order a personal organizer's catalog of calendars or a specific Filofax
  product or refill (see Appendix II).
- Consider writing everything down on small Post-it pads and trans-
  ferring them to your calendars so you make your notes portable as
  cues, from your pocket-book calendar to the bathroom mirror as a
  cue for a morning task you need to get done the next day.
- Leave small Post-it notes on the doorknob of the door from which
  you exit the house in the morning, the bathroom mirror, the refrigerator, etc., to remind yourself of things you need to do before leaving the house, office, etc.
- Don't leave things to chance with the thought "I'll probably remember it."
- Ask someone you trust to check your work if you are concerned that
  WHMS symptoms may be affecting it.
- If you need help getting started or prioritizing a task, ask for help,
  call a friend or someone you have considerable trust in. Say "I value

your input" or hint that you didn't get a lot of sleep the night before if you think being covert is wisest in the situation.

- If you are really concerned about your ability to rely on your memory for important personal data buy an accordion folder and alphabetically organize it. Keep in it your Social Security number, your ATM bank code, other important numbers, the birthdays of people important to you, their telephone numbers and addresses. List the names of your cousins or the children's names of family members, etc. Keep your insurance policies in the same folder. Keep it all in a metal box in a place in the closet you are likely to see and not forget about. (*USA Today* writer Anita Manning in an article on baby boomer forgetfulness described a woman with WHMS-like memory blackouts who hid her jewelry before leaving on vacation and had no idea where it was when she returned.)

- In your telephone books write the names of the spouses of people listed, their children's names and ages at a specific year, their birthdays, etc.

- Keep a timer by the stove so you don't burn out pots and kettles.

- Develop a nighttime regimen and stick to it ritually: of locking doors, shutting off coffeemakers, computers, etc.

Becoming a "Technoweenie" with Electronic or Mechanical Aids

Devices to assist memory or to help with organizing a life are plentiful in office supply, "gadget," or electronic stores such as Staples, OfficeMax, The Sharper Image, Hammacher-Schlemmer, Brookstone, Radio Shack, and the catalogs of these and other stores. I suggest you make it a habit to inquire about "personal organizer" devices or to look around in sections in stores that contain personal organizers. Also you might order catalogs from the above stores to see what's new. New gadgets come out every month it seems, though not all the ones in stores are always listed in the catalog. Here are some you might consider investing in for helping you with WHMS symptoms:

- The Day-Timer Appointment Reminder Multi Alarm system is a low-cost, low-tech, highly useful inconspicuous 5" x 1½" gadget that lets you schedule up to thirty-one alarms at half-hour intervals from morning till night by moving a little switch from left to right and then beeps you discretely at the right time or times. It looks a little like a black miniature vegetable grater and weighs a little over an ounce. It can be slipped or clipped into a binder, appointment calendar, pocket, or purse; it has an LCD clock on it, a built-in stand, and a clip. It costs at this writing $14.99 with batteries included if you order it from Day-Timer by phone directly. Or you may be able to find it in some Staples stores. When the alarm goes off you can look in your appointment calendar to see what it is you have to do, whether it's calling or meeting with someone, taking a pill, or reminding yourself to set the house alarm or shut off the coffeemaker at night. (See Appendix II for product information.)

- Many stores have several useful devices: a new digital voice-memory recording alarm device lets you prerecord your own reminders to yourself at up to four preset times with up to four messages. It costs about $30, can fit in your palm, and has up to 116 seconds of recording time. You can use it to remind yourself before an appointment what to bring with you, what you need to take with you before leaving work, what you need to pick up before getting home, etc. It also has a built-in talking clock function. It can tell you how much remaining memory you have left on it. (See Appendix II for product information.)

- Many stores sell a four-minute tapeless digital personal recorder that lets you record memos throughout the day. It's 4½ inches tall with a clip and stand and costs under $40. It lets you skip messages or play only the last message. (See Appendix II for product information.)

- I suggest for days when you are not feeling entirely yourself you keep on hand and take with you a small lightweight microcassette tape recorder to tape meetings as a backup to memory, or to tape what follow-up things you need to do right after a meeting. The advantage of microcassettes is that the tapes are small and easy to file. Many stores offer inexpensive microcassette tape recorders with fast playback that let you record on one ninety-minute tape up to three hours of information for about $40. Be sure to keep a supply of tapes on hand and to mark what's on them methodically or they are worthless when you need them. (See Appendix II for product information.)

- Friends who use electronic personal organizers such as a palmtop to record appointments, memos, telephones, addresses, etc. swear by them. But you have to be willing to overcome the inertia of learning how to use one. They offer the advantage of being able to record virtually all the details of your life in one small package, but the disadvantage is that they are sealed black boxes that can potentially frustrate you in times of need and don't offer the reassurance that an appointment book can. Polly Van Benthusen, who used both, ultimately reverted to her nonelectronic gadget. I would try both and start with the paper appointment calendar as a quick and ready coping tool and then at my leisure explore the electronic organizer to see which fits my needs better, ultimately. There are lots of different brands of electronic personal organizers, which cost different amounts. Ask friends who use them what they like or don't like about theirs. If you want a list of different kinds and their relative advantages as well as a guide to other memory aids gadgets, self-help books, cassettes, CDs, etc., you might want to order The Memory Catalog. (See Appendix II for information.)

Compensating for the Effects of WHMS in Different Ways

Yale graduate Deborah D. compensated for her sense of low self-regard as a result of experiencing WHMS symptoms (she didn't understand why they were occurring), by showing off her insights or command of facts, but compensating could take many different forms. It might mean specifically practicing facial recognition skills if changes in facial recognition in particular are affecting you. You could learn to focus on distinctive features more in new faces you meet and pay attention more to "taking in" a new face. You could even develop for yourself "new-face cards" using magazine photos stapled on index cards and testing yourself on names you print on the back of each one, playing a game of match the face to a name written on the back.

Compensating could mean taking a continuing education course in a topic that you have long meant to study. It might mean developing a skill that you have long meant to develop, whether doing Irish step dancing, or learning how to prepare subtle sauces for vegetarian meals, or learning about landscaping, or studying an exotic South American Indian culture.

The idea behind compensating is to build up your self-esteem by focusing on what you are good at or enjoy or by challenging your own self-perceived limitations with effort. Keep in mind that some researchers suspect that the memory-for-details glitches that frequently accompany aging and that can be a feature of WHMS for some may have the payoff of permitting a person to better "see the forest for the trees," to abstract and synthesize better. See if you can detect any positive "take" on your symptoms you may not have considered before. One women said to me that the upside to her symptom was "that everything old is new again."

Developing Contingency Plans and Options to Keep Hope Alive and Fight Despair

If the occurrence of a spate of WHMS symptoms on certain days convinces you that your life will soon be in ruins, or if estrogen loss–based depression leads you to despair without any explanations for why you are feeling so bad, I suggest that you give yourself a ready-and-waiting "out" from feeling despair over the sense that there is nothing you can do and that you are helpless.

I suggest that when you are feeling well you devise a step-wise contingency plan of action that you might pursue to buck you up when you are feeling low. This might mean locating a menopause support group in your city and finding a number for it, even if you aren't ready to call it yet. It might mean that you could have a plan of action involving going to the library or to a large book chain and spending a whole evening or afternoon or day skimming or reading every book on perimenopause or menopause that you can find that addresses your situation and buying as many as you can afford as a way of offering yourself bibliotherapy. It might mean calling around and finding the name and number of a well-respected psychologist for talk therapy, or a psychopharmacologist for drug therapy, or a clinical endocrinologist for other-than-estrogen hormone advice, in case you think thryoid or other hormones might be involved. Having names and numbers ready to call will give you options and keep you from feeling your back is up against the wall. Part of your contingency plan could be indulging in escape fantasies that you might act on if you really feel bad enough. It could be deciding that you will treat yourself and get away from your problems with a trip to St. Lucia for a tropically lush vacation and getting as many brochures and fliers as you can. Or it might entail having a plan to treat yourself to something you have been wanting for a long time but thought was too foolish to indulge in.

The idea is to give yourself "outs" and options and to "mother" yourself when you need extra nurturance.

Garnering Social Support for What You Are Going Through

Going through fearful or uncertain or tough times that you may not feel like openly sharing with others can exact a toll in physical and psychic stress and in health resilience as research from the field of psychoneuroimmunology has shown in recent years (particularly the work of Janice Kiecolt-Glaser). Research from the same field has shown, however, that social support can be a strong moderator of just such kinds of stresses, even extending survival in cases of advanced cancer. You might then try, when times feel tough with respect to WHMS, to reach out to others who may be going through the same thing as you as a way of easing your burden.

Dr. Fredericka Xerov, when she was tired of living with WHMS symptoms, in desperation one day looked in the telephone directory and found a doctor who ran menopause support groups. She went to one on her birthday as a present to herself. She says, "From the group I learned it wasn't just me. That there were other women experiencing what I was. We were able to let it out, what was happening to us. It was a relief to find I wasn't alone in this . . ."

Social support can mean having even just one understanding person you can talk to about what you need to when you need to. So you might plan to try to find such a person, to drop some discrete ambiguous hints about what you are experiencing to other women you feel comfortable with who are the same age, to see if they pick up on what you are talking about. WHMS is what I call a releasing topic. If you mention it first you will be surprised how many other people will feel free to talk to you about what *they* are experiencing. So plan to be a little brave if you think you might need some support in going through WHMS. The pleasure of unburdening yourself and sharing with another person the rather comical "shows" WHMS affords self-spectators can be enormous from what women have told me.

Social support these days might mean going online and chatting with other women in computer chat groups.

It might mean writing a letter to yourself to open in the future or addressed to your daughter to be opened when she turns your age.

Reassuring Yourself with Self-Talk

In my pure research days before I trained as a health psychologist I would have said that "self-talk" was "for the birds," that children could benefit from self-talk but not normal healthy adults. On the basis of experience I've come to see things differently. Self-talk is education, it's self-cuing, it's a reminder that there is a different way of looking at things. Sometimes it's just reassurance or nurturance.

What can you say to yourself that might help?

"Millions of women have lived through this and are doing so now. They endured and so will I."

"All over the country women are going through the same thing I am. We are a secret club. I'm not alone in this."

A friend of mine found a little book from a religious group left in her hallway that advised that in times of need to say to oneself "All will be well." She says she doesn't know why but she feels a tension-releasing weight lift from her shoulders when she says this to herself in times of need. She's no mystic. She has a doctorate in public health and tends to be rather rational most of the time.

Harvard cardiologist Dr. Herbert Benson, who wrote the book *The Relaxation Response,* in his later book *The Faith Factor* describes the beneficial relaxation effects in those who say the equivalent of "Father have mercy" that relates to their religious convictions. Perhaps at some level we always remain children in need of a good or kind word.

"What doesn't break me makes me stronger."

"I'll do the best I can and leave the rest alone."

Developing "Cover" Statements To Use When WHMS Glitches Occur

Some women develop anticipatory anxiety if they have had an embarrassing experience with a WHMS symtpom and spend considerable energy worrying about "what if it happens again?" One way to lessen such anxiety is to have prepared, even if you never choose to use them, "covering" statements that let you escape the situation with a less than "I'm losing my mind" confession. Statements such as:

- "I caught barely a wink last night—a car alarm (or a neighbor's blasting music) kept me up all night."
- "Let me get back to you on that. I want to be sure I'm giving you the right information."
- "I've been on information overload this week—would you please repeat that again."

Becoming Aware of Where Your Mind Is: Bringing Directed Attention to What Was Automatic

Practice tuning in and taking the equivalent of regular depth soundings to try to become more aware of what your mind feels like with respect to attention and focus during different times in the day. Do this so that you can clue yourself into how much self-prompting you need to rouse yourself out of a torpid "inattentive" state when it is important. Or to cue yourself as to when you should be taking added compensatory measures to assist you if your attention is flagging, as in tape recording a meeting you are about to go to so you can listen to it later if you are feeling foggy before the meeting. You probably know what that after–Thanksgiving dinner feeling can do to your mind as the blood drains from your brain to your digestive tract. You know what daydreaming feels like. See if you can over time distinguish different feeling tones to your state of alertness, how it varies with fatigue or sleep deprivation. In a course on sleep in infants I recall being taught that there were some six stages on a continuum of wakefulness-to-sleep in newborn infants and that infants learned best during only some of them. See if you can distinguish your own stages of attention and wakefulness and use that knowledge for your own benefit to guide your compensatory response if one is necessary. I know from using biofeedback with patients with different physical problems that it is quite possible to use your mind to tune in to many otherwise ignored sensations, i.e., the feel of a bra strap on your shoulder, or the weight of a shoe on your foot if you beam your attention there with interest and do it often enough. I suspect that by drawing your interest to your mind's stages of alertness you might become an adept spectator of yourself. You might then try to cue yourself with unspoken self-statements such as "stay focused" or "tune in" when you detect your attention is flagging or as a practice exercise. You might also use occasions when you sense your alertness is flagging to see if eating glucose or a complex carbohydrate makes a difference.

WHMS AT WORK

The good news from the evidence of my interviews is that WHMS tends to pose a challenge to a woman's personal life more often than her work life typically, which is no small comfort, however, if it's affecting *you* at work. If it is and fits the culture of your work situation, laugh off your glitches the way some women do by laughing at themselves and making a joke of an "I seem to be losing it!" statement or adopting Sherry Strumph's in-your-face "mind like a sieve" "that's the way I am now" bravado, showing confidence in your larger non-WHMS self with a "big deal, we're all fallible sometimes" attitude.

If you can't do that perhaps the falsifiable cover of most WHMS symptoms will throw people off from detecting the pattern in your symptoms. Or if you have a dramatic flair hint that your glitches are due to the added stress of "unspeakable family problems." Then use your "glitch" as a cue to heighten your resting self-monitoring vigilance and "directed attention" at work and hope for the best.

If you feel it's safe, confide as Polly Van Benthusen did and as Cheryl Calhoun has, in a boss who may become your ally in this adventure and appreciate how usually effective you are most of the time, overlooking your occasional glitches.

And remember when things get really hairy to have a contingency plan of escape, an alternative escape career fantasy—realizable—that you will pursue if things really become dire. Several very bright women I've interviewed for this book did make such WHMS-inspired career switches successfully, defining for themselves alternative satisfying careers that now give them more control over their lives and that do not necessitate minute-by-minute rigid precision with no room for biological realities. "Perhaps when one door closes . . ."—you know the rest. Aim to reframe WHMS as possibly sending you a life message you may ultimately benefit from, as possibly setting you off on a new adventure that years from now may have you saying "it was the best thing that ever happened to me." Whatever else happens don't forget that there are many ways to live a life and to be a person.

V

THE BIG PICTURE

14

WHMS Symptoms and Men

I first detected WHMS symptoms as I've noted earlier in my women patients, and in members of all-women reading groups I belong to. When I made the estrogen/brain connection in my mind, after searching the research literature on estrogen and the brain, I naively assumed that the symptoms had to be a woman's issue because of the time-linkage of WHMS symptoms with altered menstrual cycles and often in proximity to hot flashes symptoms in those who had them. I thought of estrogen then as primarily a female hormone. And even when I learned that in men some of their testosterone is converted in the body and brain to estrogen by the enzyme aromatase I still did not stop to think that men might be experiencing WHMS symptoms too. In fact when I went to advertise for and recruit possible subjects to interview through physician referrals and other means I never initially considered advertising for men or getting referrals to men from physicians.

But gradually I began to get clues from my environment that WHMS might not only be a woman's set of symptoms. My first clue came from interviewing Letty Cottin Pogrebin for the *New York* magazine article. Discussing the verbal and behavioral malapropisms and the memory and delayed retrieval symptoms she had described in her book *Getting Over Getting Older,* she told me, after we had spoken for a while, that it was her impression that most of the men she knew had these symptoms too and at similar ages. I mentally filed the information.

At an evening summer party in Woodstock just after the *New York* magazine article came out a circle of women were asking me questions about what I knew about their strange symptoms (of WHMS). Afterward two who I had never met before came up and to my surprise embraced me and thanked me for having relieved them of enormous fears. The boyfriend of one of the women who had been listening to the discussion, a man I imagine to be in his early fifties, said to me, "You know, I have a lot of those symptoms too."

After I gave a talk about WHMS at a women's professional group the leader of the group told me in private that she didn't have WHMS, but her husband who was forty-nine did. He had been putting strange things in the refrigerator for a while now, made malapropisms, and was considerably more absentminded overall than he used to be. (The refrigerator seems to be a key object of WHMS behavioral malapropisms.)

Still another time I was treated by an associate of my usual, wonderful dentist who was unavailable for a dental emergency. Dr. D., let's call him. When the receptionist popped in to mention having read my article, Dr. D. and I entered into a discussion about memory and he proceeded to tell me that his memory had changed quite noticeably over the last few years. I at first found this difficult to credit since he was only forty-two and not likely to be "perimenopausal," and my private thought was "Maybe it's from the occupational hazard of mercury-vapors poisoning or chemical toxicity from dental fumes over the years." Did he really mean "noticeably," I asked? He stuck by his intensity rating. He also said he wasn't alone, that other men he knew had told him the same thing in private.

One day I came upon a funny Steve Martin essay on men and memory at fifty, in the back page of an issue of *The New Yorker.* It's now part of a recent book of his writings. To my surprise it sounded like he was experiencing WHMS.

Then a book titled *Male Menopause* came on the scene and in early 1998 I called to arrange an interview with its author, Jed Diamond, a California psychotherapist who had been treating and writing about men for many years. I called the book's publicist to arrange the interview and was first sent a packet of press information about the book. It included a cover article in *USA Today* by staff writer Anita Manning with an intriguing title: BOOMER BRAIN MELTDOWN. Manning described not only baby boomer women but men with "brain lapses" that were "ubiquitous." In the article a forty-five-year-old male botanist, the director of the Morris Arboretum in Philadelphia, describes himself as having "senior moments." What troubled him most, he said, was not being able to remember plants. "I'll look at a plant and know perfectly well what it is, but I just can't recall its [name]." A fifty-one-year-old man who runs a data center in Wilmington, Delaware, told Manning that "it's in the nonwork part of his life that he finds his memory unreliable." (Sound familiar?) The man was quoted as saying "You just find yourself in the kitchen not knowing what you went in the kitchen for." The man describes having conversations in which neither he nor his conversational partner can recall the name of the person they are talking about. In another example in the article the fifty-one-year-old director of a social research institute describes his employees as snickering when he leaves work: "I get to the car and say, oh, I forgot . . . whatever. After my second or third time back in the room sometimes I get so embarrassed I say the hell with it. I don't need it. I'll get it tomorrow."

When I ultimately interviewed Jed Diamond he told me that about ten years ago in his private practice he began observing changes in men aged forty to fifty-five in both physical and psychological domains but didn't yet "get" what was happening. When he read a popular article about male menopause he frankly doubted that such a thing existed. He started to research the topic formally and found that there was "a lot of research in Europe on it." He said, "Contrary to what I believed, men go through real hormonal changes and a midlife crisis. I found and others found that this occurs between the ages of forty and fifty-five but can start as early as the thirties, and that some men lose as much as 30% of their testosterone while at the same time experiencing changes in their estrogen levels, while some men don't have declines in testosterone levels. There seems to be much more complexity [in what is happening to them hormonally] than we thought." And also much more variability among men in what might be happening. He also added that there was evidence that even when testosterone levels were not radically shifting "testosterone may be being metabolized in different ways."

What kinds of changes did he see in men? I asked without telling him about WHMS symptoms yet. He said, "Men can change cognitively, psychologically, and sexually." Examples? "Forgetfulness or memory loss. They'll say I'm losing my mind and getting early Alzheimer's disease. I forget where I put my keys, where I left my car. The names of good friends. The names of things. Dates. They don't, however, lose their map-reading skills," he added. "They'll say, My brain went dead for a moment, it went off-line." They also report experiencing more "irritability, a lot more anger, anxiety, aggressiveness, depression and more suicidal thoughts." They experience sexual changes, "reduced force of ejaculation, loss of erections, reduced interest and increased anxiety over this. Also increased fear of sexual encounters, and both increased and decreased masturbation. They want to know 'does it still work.' They'll say, 'I don't feel like a failure when I'm masturbating.'" Diamond went on and on, and I'll refer you to his excellent book for more comments.

I then probed, asking Diamond whether he had heard complaints of specific WHMS symptoms in men with male menopause, describing them as nonspecifically as I could. Wrong words popping out? "Yes," he said. Being at a loss for words? "Yes." As we proceeded in this prompted way he described men in their forties "who go out and forget they haven't shaved or brushed their hair. They'll say this has never happened to them before but now all of a sudden it is." Men who have blackouts of memory who say "I'll go to a movie and don't remember what I just saw." Men who can't remember faces, or where car parts go, or which person e-mailed them yesterday. Men who describe themselves as having "spaghetti brains," who say "I can't find the thread, it gets lost in the morass of feeling fuzzy-headed." Men who develop writing inaccuracies, who say "I'll start to spell a word [as I'm writing] and can't remember the next part" or who say "This doesn't look right" but then don't know how to fix it (Diamond said "No," however, when I asked him if men complain of spelling uncertainties.) He described men who "say they are not feeling at home in their body. Like their 'parts don't fit together.'" Who experience a change in coordination. Who experience a change in time spent reading: "I can't sit still and concentrate," they'll say. "I lose my train of thought." When I ask about fatigue Diamond said "Yes, that's one of the most common ones they mention, that and feeling numb—experiencing emotional flatness." Diamond also responded in the affirmative and with examples with respect to changes in computation skills and handling stress differently. He said, "A lot of midlife breakups are due to the projection of the man's changes onto their wives. They blame the wives for what's happening to them. They fear the memory loss. They are in terror of it. One man, a taxi-cab driver, told me, 'I'm losing my sexual desire, my erections, and my mind. I'm afraid my wife will lose interest in me. I've never told a soul about this. I'm afraid to tell my doctor.'"

When I looked in one of several textbooks on menopause I had by now acquired, I found two chapters on the aging male in one from 1994. One chapter titled "Andropause, Fact or Fiction?" opened with "The concept of a male equivalent to the menopause, the andropause, is still the subject of debate" and closed with "Strictly speaking, the male equivalent of the menopause, with its sudden definitive end of reproductive capacities and a sudden decrease in sex hormone levels, does not occur in males. However, in the great majority, if not all, elderly men there is clear-cut evidence for an age-associated progressive decline both in fertility and in plasma androgen [testosterone] levels, responsible for the clinical signs of decreased virility." In another chapter, however, titled "The Aging Male" it said "The term 'climacterium virile' was created in 1939 by Wermer, who described men at or beyond the fifth decade of life [forties+] who suffered from . . . a number of symptoms such as impaired memory, lack of concentration, tiredness, nervousness, and lowered resistance to stress." (Does this sound like a two-ring circus of symptoms that includes WHMS?) The article goes on to say: "The decline in testosterone levels observed in old age is gradual, and although the germinal epithelium [source of sperm production] shows age-related changes, there is great interindividual variability: functioning germ cells are found in men over eighty years. The existence of a male climacteric is therefore questionable."

To me, however, it seemed quite possible that many of the symptoms women with WHMS experienced might also apply to at least some men. These were my reasons for the switch in the name of WHMS from "The Women's Hormonal Misconnection Syndrome" to "Warga's Hormonal Misconnection Syndrome."

For the moment, however, I have provisionally concluded for myself that while some men's testes may possibly go on working proficiently for a lifetime, some men's brains don't—at least not fully—for whatever biological reasons. And that from the cognitive standpoint they may be more like women when it comes to the machinery of memory and attention and cognition at midlife. This is a body-part disconnect in men that I doubt would surprise *either* gender very much in terms of what they already know! Some may suggest that the commonality between women and men's apparent symptoms probably points to "aging" as the common factor in their symtpoms rather than hornones. However, I suggest that my association of WHMS with the perimenopausal symptoms of hormonal change in women first was propitious and instead has served as a useful cue guiding me to understand that unsuspected hormonal changes in *men* may well prove to be the basis for their symptoms rather than the cover-all concept of "aging."

It will be interesting in the years to come to see just how much overlap or difference in the symptoms of the WHM syndrome will exist between the genders, ultimately: to what degree we are "hard-wired" the same; to what degree differently; and to what degree the *X* factor, the common genetic link between XY men and XX women, is the common default mode of the generic human mind and brain.

In the meantime provocative findings keep on being reported on the pivotal role of *estrogen in males* sexually and cognitively: For example:

- In an article titled "A New Breadth to Estrogen's Bisexuality" Rockefeller University researcher Donald W. Pfaff was quoted as saying, "Estrogen appears to be 'a basic contributor to normal sexuality in both genders,'" in response to his research published in the Feb 18, 1997, Proceedings of the National Academy of Sciences. Pfaff's work with colleagues showed that mutant male mice without *estro-*

gen receptors were far less aggressive and showed less typical masculine social behavior than littermates who responded normally to the presence of estrogen. Moreover, these male mutant mice had mating problems—they were unable to sexually penetrate female mice or release sperm, despite attempts to do so. Estrogen thus appears to play a critical role in male sexual mating.

- In related research, it's been found that sperm too depend on estrogen. It was found that male mutant mice, missing an estrogen receptor—so-called estrogen receptor knockout mice (they are missing the gene for the alpha estrogen receptor, which allows cells to take up the hormone)—are rendered sterile by the loss of this gene for making use of estrogen. (The females were rendered sterile too.) In the males the ability to generate sperm was found to be reduced and their testes atrophied progressively.

- In studies of male rats estrogen improved memory of a previously learned task. Researchers found that injections of estrogen (estradiol) into the hippocampus after learning a water maze task preferentially enhanced retention of the same task in rats twenty-four hours later compared to rats given injections with salt water (not unlike the glucose facilitation effect after learning).

- In another study it was found that not only estrogen, but testosterone and another type of androgen—all steroid hormones—at some dosage levels but not others facilitated learning on a specific avoidance task in male rats. Some doses facilitated short-term memory, and other doses facilitated long-term learning. This suggests that dosing levels of all these hormones may be critical in maximizing learning effects, short-term and long-term.

- A *New York Times* headline declared on December 8, 1998: "Weak Bones Among Men Are Linked to Estrogen."

What all this tells us is that testosterone is no longer solely a male hormone, just as estrogen is no longer purely a female hormone. The intriguing question of course is what then specifically renders us female, and what makes us male besides the obvious evidence? It looks as though for a while at least things may become less clear in this regard before they become clearer again.

15

The Big Picture

After I began detecting the symptoms of WHMS I kept asking myself what could all these symptoms possibly mean? What could they possibly add up to, or tell us? What could tie them together? They were such an odd assortment. What, for example, did *spelling certainty* have to do with anything? Why should that get shaky with estrogen loss in so many women? In this chapter I describe some of the thoughts and provisional answers I came up with to these and other questions as they apply to my knowledge of *women's* changes with WHMS. (I know too little that is yet definite about the male side of this picture to factor it into my suppositions.)

ESTROGEN IN WOMEN FACILITATES THE MOTIVATION TO TALK

One of the first things that seemed fairly evident to me from having waded in the waters of estrogen/mind/brain research and from observing what happened to speech in those with WHMS symptoms of estrogen decline was that it seemed fairly clear that estrogen's presence *played some part in making women "on average" preferentially verbal and loquacious* as opposed to more "yup"/"nope" binarily efficient types (something that presumably has to do with the double XX genetic load of women as opposed to males' single X.) Perhaps over the span of history, a verbal facility tied to women's distinctive biological roles over the course of evolution as the nurturers and nearby educators of children conferred a survival advantage to those offspring who had nonterse moms. Being loquacious and verbally fluent as opposed to tongue-tied could be an advantage in promoting survival skills, in transmitting the skills of a culture via specific corrective "mastering-life" feedback to children (who, in case you haven't noticed, spend an inordinate amount of childhood saying "look, ma" for related adaptive feedback reasons, I suspect). Verbal agility could offer subtly variant forms of verbal reinforcement and motivating nurturance to the species in contrast to primitive "uh-huhs" or mute undifferentiated nods. (On the other hand, perhaps being a gabby "here-I-am" male hunter led to starvation or too-ready detection and death.)

Barbara Sherwin's estrogen and verbal memory research certainly pointed to the verbal advantage conferred by estrogen. She had found consistent *verbal* deficits in recall, learning, and fluency in many different kinds of estrogen-deprived women, verbal deficits that were consistently reversible with estrogen replacement. So too did the studies of cognitive skill changes over the course of the normal menstrual cycle with different hormone balances in healthy younger women by Elizabeth Hampson and Doreen Kimura. Estrogen-high phases were consistently associated with better scores on verbal tests while estrogen-low phases were associated with better scores on tests of spatial skills (small but reliably present differences).

So too do the studies on giving estrogen to women with Alzheimer's disease such as those of Howard Fillet and his colleagues and Sanjay Asthana's, where it was found that replacement estrogen improved verbal skills. So too do the verbal malapropisms, word reversals, "echo" intrusions, naming, and variant forms of word-finding difficulties that are characteristic of WHMS.

WHAT ESTROGEN GIVETH, ESTROGEN LOSS TAKETH?

As I asked myself what WHMS symptoms meant, one of the earliest formulations I came up with was "Perhaps what estrogen preferentially *giveth* to girls it *taketh* when it proceeds to go." I remembered that girls tended on average to excel in learning to read proficiently earlier than boys on average, that in one of her review articles estrogen/gender researcher Doreen Kimura mentioned that girls tend to be better spellers at younger ages. Maybe that's what the change in spelling certainty around menopause reflected—a taking of what had been uniquely given by the hormone to girls. Maybe that's what the change in reading proficiency in WHMS reflected in some strange turnaround. I knew that many women after menopause tended to lose the pinched waists that puberty molded via estrogen's activating influence. I even knew an older woman, a divorced former model in her sixties, who in seeking a partner through a dating service had requested a man with hair. The man she ultimately met, she later learned, had requested "a woman with a waist." Similarly, perhaps, the loss of libido in many but not all women after menopause reflected a turnaround in what had been turned "on" at puberty via estrogen's activating effects. Perhaps this "giveth-taketh" rule held for all the skills women were at a gender advantage for (that then changed to a degree in some women with estrogen loss, affording us a peak at how we humans "work").

And turning things around: perhaps all the things that "go" to a degree, with ovarian hormonal changes as reflected in WHMS symptoms, provide us with a reflective mirror of what estrogen subtly "does" that gives women specific advantages science doesn't yet appreciate as distinctive.

What is it that women or girls are now known to excel at on average? According to Barbara Sherwin and a coauthor, "Women are considered to excel on average in verbal abilities, perceptual speed and accuracy, and in fine motors skills. . . . Although the magnitude of these sex differences in specific cognitive abilities is modest they occur fairly reliably across studies of normal men and women." Sherwin and her coauthor also note that "On average men excel in spatial and quantitative abilities and in gross motor strength." In view of WHMS perhaps women also excel at other things apparently affected by estrogen, such as attention, or face recognition, or landmark recognition, or the reverse of any of the other symptoms of WHMS I cite.

Reflecting on specific symptoms, however, I thought perhaps the loss of certainty over spelling around menopause has something to do not only with changes in verbal skill—spelled words after all are symbolic representations of spoken words—but also with women's known advantage in perceptual speed and accuracy: quickly "taking in" a distinctive "landscape" of symbolic letters perceptually and recalling them with excellent accuracy as one might take a "snapshot" of a spatial configuration, a landscape diagram, of where one's six children are in relation to oneself in a momentary glance as one worked outdoors. Perhaps that was what this symptom reflected. Perhaps loss of spelling certainty reflected tremors in learned well-rehearsed coordinated routines that become "automatic" like driving and then undergo "tremors" in the manner of driving coordination. Perhaps the dyslexia-like reading changes too reflected earthquake-like tremors in the foundations of "automatic" routines learned long ago. Perhaps the well-worn grooves of old learning weren't being maintained as well with estrogen loss and were getting "overgrown" and in need of less lackadaisical maintenance.

Perhaps the WHMS symptom of more "dropsies" with estrogen loss was the flip side of the gender's excelling in fine-motor coordination. This "giveth-taketh" hypothesis of estrogen's functions is one that I hope researchers will actively pursue experimentally.

It is my belief as I've noted—provisional of course—that the WHM Syndrome leaks important clues to us about the selective "design" over the course of evolution of our baseline human inclinations, our resting predilections of mind and behavior, our "instincts" when we are "just being," our human nature when we are in default mode and are not actively striving and choosing how we want our lives and ourselves to be, in the sense that the late Rockefeller University scientist/philosopher René Dubos described in his book *Choosing to Be Human*. Namely that we *are* our biological individuality—our fingerprints, or our "default mode reflex instincts." We become who we *choose to be,* our true "selves," by the sum total of the choices we actively, directedly, assert in life, when we say "I want this kind of life, not that one," "I will do that, but not this." WHMS leaks to us information about who we are during our reproductive years when we aren't trying—what settings we have been "set" to by an unknowable designer. Though in discussions of evolution we more commonly tend to think of *body parts* as being "selected" and "shaped" for their environmental or survival advantages, nonetheless sociobiologist Edward O. Wilson, among others, believes that evolutionary biology has shaped the human mind too, and that implicit in our brains are programmed rules that define our human nature.

WHMS, I believe, leaks information to us about such rules. Writing in the book *Mindblindness,* psychologist Simon Baron-Cohen suggests in the introduction that "we experience 'instinct blindness'. . . . We have been blind," he says, "to the existence of the machinery that constitutes most of the evolved architecture of the human mind—what might reasonably be called our cognitive instincts."

It is my suspicion that the very traits of mind, speech, and behavior in WHMS that become somewhat disregulated with the shift in biological agenda represented by perimenopause and menopause—a shift away from a strict priority on skills that facilitate survival of the species—leak to us clues about the very traits of mind, speech, and behavior that "nature" particularly "values" highly and keeps tightly constrained, regulated, and "girdled" during those years when the programmed drive of reproducing the species is prime. Traits that are the opposite of WHMS *confer distinct survival advantages* in communication (speech); quick retrieval skills and access to learned past-memory; attention, concentration, fast accurate thinking, and perceptual speed and accuracy; behavioral "on-target" reflex accuracy and recall of prior mastery; accurate anticipation, planning, and navigational precision; quick prioritizing and problem solving; rapid numerical assessments; and symbolic translations and representation.

The fact that so many WHMS symptoms occur when people are

"just being"—storing something in the refrigerator, walking from one room to another, putting things down as they walk in the door, throwing laundry in the hamper—suggests to me that during our estrogen-high years of reproductive potential, we have a "default setting" with a checklist of implicit rules we are not aware of, geared to keeping us attentive, able to concentrate at will, expectantly and unconsciously, able to track important events and time, and able to stay abreast of our self's innocuous behaviors even when we aren't actively engaged in monitoring them. These rules are set to keeping us *ever mindful,* in all senses of the word, and relatively error-free when we are in "automatic-pilot behavior" mode. The rules are set so that we have quick and ready access mentally to our past experience and learning and problem-solving machinery, so that we have quick verbal access to memory "files" for precise communication and transmission of the information and experience we have within us.

To make it clear, the traits of mind and mood necessary for fulfillment of this drive for perpetuating the species include not merely successfully giving birth, but the attendant skills of attracting a mate who will make a pregnancy possible, using the advantageous lure of a non-depressed, cheerful, noncontentious "get-along" baseline mood or demeanor (not an irritable and cranky one—estrogen keeps us relatively cheerful); remembering which navigational landmarks marked a prospective hunk's cave or patch of trees; distinguishing with accuracy his perhaps bushy-bearded head and face from those of all the other bearded males around. They include the abilities of being able to attend and concentrate well so as to remain continually vigilant within one's environment to the actions and context of one's self and one's children, particularly around issues of safety.

The traits of mind include being able to keep track over time where it is safe to rest for the night, where it's safe to engage in sex without predatory attacks during vulnerable moments, where supplies of food and water exist at different times of the year over a conceivably navigationally wide terrain; being able to keep ten things in mind while holding one child and grabbing another; being able to focus in at an instant on life-and-death decisions; being able to think of the right child's name rapidly and speak precisely (i.e. "Johnny (my son), jump off that rock, there's a deadly snake right next to you" versus "er . . . whatsyourname, over, you know where. . . . look . . ."); having a baseline readiness to instinctively grasp and deftly prioritize in a second solutions needed for immediate action; being able to handle much stress well, taking in with a quick, potentially life-rescuing glance where your children are before the fire or flood engulfs them. All these conferred survival advantages on those who had them. These traits led to the survival and perpetuation of one's genes in one's self and in offspring, and led to the opportunity to have more children to perpetuate those genes. Those of us alive today are the direct descendants of those who manifested these adaptive cognitive/behavioral survival traits and are likely inheritors of those same advantages.

Consider for the moment the WHMS symptom of increased scheduling errors, of poor time-keeping or poor anticipation of events of personal relevance. *When looked at in reverse* it confers a survival advantage, according to experimental psychologist Dr. John Gibbons of the New York State Psychiatric Institute, a researcher who studies "foraging behavior in animals and how they use time when they are foraging." Gibbons in 1998 was quoted as saying in an article in the *New York Times* on time estimation and the existence in humans and animals of an interval-tracking stopwatch internal clock, the "ability to estimate . . . durations of time is critical for learning and survival and those that had the ability to remember and recall where they last got food or with what frequency of reward survived better than those that didn't have this accurate clock or barometer of past schedules of reward." (The clock's unit of chemical measurement involves dopamine, a neurotransmitter known to be affected by estrogen loss.)

ESTROGEN IS A PERFORMANCE-ENHANCING AGENT THAT APPEARS TO BOOST THE *PREPAREDNESS* TO BE INTUITIVELY INTELLIGENT

Athletes trying to enhance their athletic performance are known to use steroids to boost their strength, endurance, speed, etc., using most typically androgens such as testosterone or variants of testosterone. Estrogen too is a steroid hormone. Animal research with estrogen indicates that it can act to boost energy, activity, speed, and accuracy. In studies with women, estrogen has also been shown to be a mood elevator, an "upper." These findings suggest to me that estrogen too is a performance-enhancing drug. However, the symptoms of WHMS (when looked at in reverse) and other animal research on estrogen's roles in attention and memory, etc., suggest to me that estrogen is a drug that enhances the pre-paredness to act intelligently, bypassing centers of conscious processing, planning, and thinking, relying on more intuitively grasped outside-of-consciousness mechanisms of "thinking" and "knowing." Perhaps it is this facet of estrogen that makes women appear to be the more intuitive of the two genders.

I am not at all suggesting that estrogen loss deprives women of active intelligence. Rather my interviews with women have indicated to me that even when women are in the full throes of WHMS symptoms and feeling foggy and not "with it," they can still achieve and attain. What is necessary, however, is directed, active, conscious effort—actively choosing to engage tasks and challenges while perhaps overriding now less-engaged prior motivational instincts and inclinations of less hypervigilant second-by-second monitoring of all "relevant" fields, which may now be signaling internally "Why bother?" "It's too daunting." "What for?" I don't think native intelligence changes, but the baseline preparedness to be alert to and respond to grasping the essence of a situation in a split second may change. It's quite possible, however, that there may be unrecognized advantages in the alternative view of the world afforded by WHMS changes and that some skills may actually be sharpened by the redirection. It is also possible that longer experience with life and its lessons in how things tend to "go" may well compensate for changes in resting cognitive/behavioral "friskiness."

The Thinking, Remembering Parts of the Brain Are a Major Organ of Reproduction

Scientists long knew estrogen to be a hormone essential for reproduction and long thought of it solely in that connection. When in the eighties estrogen was first found to be a "player" in parts of the brain having to do with learning and memory, scientists wondered "What could estrogen possibly be doing there?" in parts that have virtually nothing to do with reproduction. It didn't make sense.

I believe that the thinking brain is a major "organ" of reproduction, that its functions are critical for successful reproduction—even today— and that that is why estrogen is present in the hippocampus and frontal lobes of the cortex and other brain regions involved in thinking, planning, remembering, and learning. Yes, conception and delivery may be essential to reproduction, but learning and processing and remembering that learning; planning and choosing wisely; benefiting from past experience through the exercise of memory; choosing a nonbrutal, altruistic, nonjealous mate; choosing where it's safe to "nest," where it's safe to deliver, how to protect one's children, whether to stay with a mate, whether to leave an area when food is getting scarce or stay in a flood zone, etc., possibly have as much bearing on the ultimate outcome of a child's survival and the survival of the species when viewed collectively, as do pregnancy and delivery and the state of one's other reproductive organs.

CLUES FROM CASES IN THIS BOOK: IS ESTROGEN THE VIGILANCE AND SAFETY HORMONE? THE INTIMATE CONTACT HORMONE?

In the realm of speculation, I find intriguing some of the comments of the women I interviewed in this book with respect to what they might be leaking to us about possible functions of estrogen.

Sherry Strumph, for instance, describing her experiences around WHMS, said to me: "Things I feared before [estrogen-loss changes] I could do now like drive at night." "I used to be so driven to be right. It's kind of refreshing not to have to do that." Later she said, "I'm more trusting than I used to be. I used to see traits in people and I'm no longer as suspicious of them, you know, mistrusting the looks of someone. I used to think 'I don't want to be caught in an alley with such a person.' Now I'm not as suspicious. I would give people motives that they don't have from my suspiciousness." Sherry no longer is vigilant about carrying keys, or being as compulsive as she used to be about locking up her house and setting the alarm. Are these changes simply a function of an erratic memory, or do they suggest that estrogen may keep us motivated and "tuned" to being attentive at all times—so that we aren't typically aware of it—to instinctive issues of safety in mothers: around keeping our home, i.e., nest, safe and protected (mindful of keys and locking up); sizing up others implicitly for their potential for danger; not engaging in personally risky behavior (driving at night); *caring* about things being right, in getting them "just so" right—a type of obsessive/compulsive symptom those with Tourette's syndrome sometimes manifest. These traits too conferred survival advantages in those who had them.

Yes one case is not much to go on. I readily acknowledge that. But taking seriously clues from patients and friends and subjects and then checking them out further is how I came to detect this syndrome and write this book in the first place. I hope it will prompt others to do more investigatory interviews.

I was also intrigued by the comments of Patricia Estrich in this book, the woman with WHMS who experienced a three-ring circus of perimenopausal symptoms and got lost at the mall she had once worked at. Her hormonally associated antipathy to her kind, funny, supportive husband, and her children, and the similar reactions of a friend going through a similar experience, provoked added thoughts about estrogen.

Estrich had said, "Another thing that happened was I wanted to leave my husband. For no reason. Just because of the way I was feeling. I didn't want to be around anyone. I wanted to be by myself where no one knew me. It didn't make sense logically. My husband is a wonderful guy but I just didn't want to be around him. I wanted to leave him. I was telling this to a friend at the time and she confessed she felt the same way. She wanted to leave her kids who meant everything to her. She was as crazy as I was.

"I confessed these feelings to my old doctor and he sent me to a doctor for psychotherapy and told me not to act on what I felt till I spoke to the doctor. I told my husband what I was feeling and he said, 'Fight it, fight it, fight it.' I didn't act on my feelings."

Now, were Patricia Estrich's feelings simply reactions to depression, related somehow to her loss of libido? Possibly. Did her comments suggest possibly that estrogen might have a role in making us ultimately social creatures, readily receptive to the human touch of a partner and continual engagement, making us tolerant of the tactile intimacy that is essential to both mates' attraction, the breast-feeding nurturing of children, and the bigger "default-setting goal" of assuring survival of the species? Was the tolerance for ongoing social engagement, touch by a partner, and having one's intimate space constantly intruded upon by the small-fingered whims of children something that was hormonally regulated? These thoughts intersected with my recall of an interview I had had with Yale Medical School menopause expert Dr. Phillip Sarrel. He had told me that after menopause women's sensitivities to touch sometimes changed. Fabrics, he said, women had found tolerable in the past now annoyed them. Could an added tolerance for much unpredictable touch from children and an ongoing intimate availability for contact be again an example of what estrogen giveth, it taketh? I don't know but it's provocative conjecture. Certainly women's sensory sensitivities are known to change with the hormonal alterations of pregnancy. Was this so different? Again I have no sense of certainty but I think such possible clues warrant further investigation.

My conclusions after this roundabout journey—in how I see things differently now—are that more than I suspected before, we are hormonal machines, largely unmindful of the degree to which we are "driven." However, I also believe that WHMS leaks to us clues—leaks them to me—that if we *actively* choose to, we have within us considerable power through effort and will to control and direct the reins of our lives more than we might suspect.

In my graduate school years, as I interviewed many scientists for the Swiss Government Broadcasting System for Physicians' Radio Network, for interviews for *Medical Tribune* and *OMNI* magazine, and profiles for *Psychology Today*, I made an interesting discovery about scientists: They tend to be an optimistic breed. The reason? Because their work continually exposes them to difficult problems, which they have often seen solved.

As I see it this is an exciting time in which to make the discovery of WHMS, in fact, in which to *have* WHMS. Why? Because I see the prospects for multiple solutions to WHMS being imminent, for those in need of such solutions.

- The neurosciences at the moment are "exploding" virtually daily with revolutionary discoveries fueling both curiosity and likely funding for this "hot" promising field. As I have been writing this book, it's been discovered, for example, that a bedrock assumption about the brain—that its neurons can't divide—is no longer true. DISCOVERY OF DIVIDING NEURONS IN HUMAN BRAINS EXCITES RESEARCHERS was the headline of an article in the medical journal *Lancet,* November 7, 1998. The particular discovery entailed evidence of neurons dividing in an area particularly relevant to WHMS and memory—namely, the dentate gyrus. (Thus, even more prospects of WHMS being ultimately reversible.) What all this means to me is that neuroscientists are likely to "jump" on WHMS because of all the intriguing inroads into understanding the brain that it affords, and that there will be funding for such research. WHMS, I suspect, is likely to provoke a good deal of *basic sciences* curiosity and research, which I believe will pay off in better understanding of what is going on in the brain and in better applied treatments for specific WHMS symptoms—perhaps not even necessitating specific estrogen replacement but rather more targeted treatments for the subcomponent parts that estrogen affects.
- The ability to "look" within the brain noninvasively and watch what it is doing while it is remembering, speaking, thinking, or "just being" is reaching a new level of sophistication at the moment in basic research and in medicine. So scientists are getting to the point where they will be able to do the equivalent of "mammograms" for the mind and brain of those with WHMS soon. This will facilitate the ability to understand what is happening for the goal of effective solutions. You will also I suspect be able to know soon if your "brain reserve cushion" is shrinking, or changing over time, or if you are at risk for cognitive erosion and need to act somehow now—not unlike screening for osteoporosis of the bones.

- Baby boomer women and men are in the ascendance at this moment. They constitute an enormous potential market for entrepreneurs to exploit. Finding cures for WHMS symptoms holds enormous financial potential for those smart enough to exploit it. Business is likely to rush in to fill the vacuum of a market no one has even known existed. Drugs and other substances and products that can help memory, attention, speech, and WHMS specifically are likely to be potentiated by the huge market of baby boomers in need.

- Designer estrogens—estrogens that do only good things but not bad things—are also "happening." Two are already on the market and the research technology for developing new ones are in place and ongoing. The discovery of WHMS is likely to push to the front of the line the hunt for designer estrogens that do good things for the brain.

- Fear of the public health costs of Alzheimer's on the horizon for baby boomers and the desire to head it off "at the pass" with preventive maintenance measures *now* for this generation will also promote public health drives to sponsor research that can do just that, and this too will help baby boomers now with WHMS.

So have cheer. Help is likely to be on the way if you need it.

Then too the reality of WHMS for most women is not a dreadful one, certainly not when one understands what it is and recognizes that it is "normal" and not likely a prelude to early Alzheimer's. In fact WHMS is often downright funny! I laughed and laughed as Polly Van Benthusen told me the things that happened to her and how she viewed them. When it becomes socially acceptable to acknowledge WHMS—and it will because so many otherwise sane and competent people will have it—I suspect WHMS will ultimately serve to draw people together and have them belly laughing—even openly at work—over the strange foibles of the human condition. Women, men, breast-feeding mothers. We are all in this together, I suspect. Expect a new crop of TV movies soon.

Appendix I: Possible Emotional and Physical Changes Associated with Years Surrounding Menopause

Possible (but Not Inevitable) Emotional/Mood Changes

T he symptoms below are based on my own interviews with women and with menopause experts I have confidence in. They may not reflect the views of the larger menopause research community. Many of these symptoms, for example, are not described as associated with perimenopause and menopause in a leading medical textbook on menopause: *Treatment of the Post-Menopausal Woman, Basic and Clinical Aspects,* edited by Rogerio Lobo.

These changes in emotion or mood can be *occasional,* spontaneous intrusions into an otherwise normal emotional profile—moments or intervals when an unexpected emotion, or "storm front," intrudes suddenly or leaves suddenly for no good reason. Or these changes in emotion or mood can be more *ongoing* changes that alter the "color tone" of one's previous "normal" emotional range.

Women report that sometimes their unusual emotional reactions seem entirely unrelated to the context of what is going on, and sometimes they seem somewhat appropriately triggered by what is going on, but tend to be over-the-top reactions—inappropriately intense. As you saw in chapter 4 there are now potential scientific explanations, biological explanations, for why emotional/mood changes might occur with changing ovarian/hormonal function in the years of perimenopause and menopause. For the most part emotional/mood changes have remained little studied as yet by menopause researchers.

Possible Emotional/Mood Symptoms

1. A diminished degree of control over one's negative emotions: more "moodiness"
2. "Flattened" emotion or affect without apparent cause: not full-blown depression but the sense that a pall is dimming one's resting mood level (repetitive difficulty trying to sound upbeat or cheerful while trying to tape a message on an answering machine; the inability to put a positive-sounding lilt in one's voice)
3. Depression, subclinical and clinical, for no apparent reason
4. Rapid mood shifts—mood lability—encompassing primarily negative moods
5. A lower threshold for experiencing intolerance/annoyance, which can be variously characterized as:

   • greater impatience compared with the past and/or
   • greater short-temperedness compared with the past and/or
   • greater irritability/grumpiness than in the past

6. Increased anger compared with the past
7. A lower-than-usual threshold for becoming tearful or crying: reduced control over such emotions
8. Disaffiliation: less of a desire for wanting closeness, or tolerance for letting others intrude with impunity on one's physical or psychic space, particularly in relation to those one has typically let in on these "spaces," e.g., children, a spouse or partner. (My hypothesis is that the ovarian hormones facilitate the emotional and physical closeness of mating and childrearing.)
9. Anxiety/restlessness/"vibrating with tension"
10. The new onset of panic disorder with possible agoraphobia
11. Suicidal thoughts or intentions
12. Feelings of paranoia (as in the case of Patricia Estrich)
13. Psychotic symptoms: hallucinations, delusions, psychotic obsessions, etc.

Possible (but Not Inevitable) Physical Changes

It is now well established that estrogen can affect the bones throughout the body and the cardiovascular system—the heart and the blood vessels throughout the body and brain.

In the 1990's scientists have been discovering the many, many areas in the brain, apart from blood vessels, in which estrogen plays an important role. In 1997 to the surprise of scientists, a second type of estrogen receptor, now known as the estrogen beta receptor, was discovered in addition to the previously known estrogen alpha receptor. Scientists are now actively exploring the many sites in the body in which the estrogen beta receptor supplies estrogen to organs dependent on it. Estrogen receptors have been newly discovered in the eyes, in the liver. . . . and the list is likely to go on and on in future years, since researchers now suspect that there are possibly multiple other types of estrogen receptors still awaiting discovery.

This means that the list of possible symptoms that might be associated with estrogen loss, and responsive to estrogen replacement and related treatments, is likely to not be a small one. Remember, however, again that women vary enormously. The following list is not therefore a forecast of doom and inevitability. Many, many women breeze through perimenopause and menopause without *any* untoward physical effects. So expect the best but be forewarned with knowledge about possible physical symptoms and what they might respond to:

Possible Physical Symptoms

1. The new onset of migraine headaches
2. Low-grade fatigue without an apparent cause (In animal and/or human research studies estrogen has been found to be both a physical and a mood activator or energizer and to act as an antidepressant.)
3. Chronic fatigue
4. Symptoms of rheumatoid arthritis
5. Symptoms of osteoarthritis
6. Symptoms of fibromyalgia

7. Heart palpitations
8. Restless leg
9. Atypical angina or Syndrome X (severe angina, positive EKG changes with exercise but normal coronary arteries)
10. A change in skin sensitivity to fabrics and the touch of another person
11. Diminished sexual desire (libido)
12. Vaginal dryness
13. Vaginal itchiness
14. Hot flashes or hot flushes/sensations of heat with sweating
15. Nighttime awakenings in association with hot flashes
16. Insomnia: nighttime awakenings without hot flashes and difficulty falling back to sleep
17. Decreased metabolic rate and weight gain
18. Increased deposition of fat on stomach and hips
19. Lower urinary tract symptoms:

    • Stress incontinence (incontinence with coughing, sneezing, laughing, etc.)
    • Greater urgency in urination
    • Urge incontinence (inability to resist urination after one experiences the urge to)
    • Greater frequency of urination during the day
    • Greater frequency of urination at night

20. More frequent bladder and vaginal infections
21. Increased risks of osteoporosis
22. Increased risks of developing heart disease
23. Increased tooth loss
24. Increased risk of colon cancer

AND NOW FOR SOME GOOD NEWS:
25. The end of a prior pattern of migraine headaches
26. The shrinking of estrogen-dependent fibroids
27. Decline in the symptoms of endometriosis, an estrogen-dependent condition

Soy Products with Genistein

Soy Products	Isoflavone Content	Soy Protein Content
White Wave Tempeh (3 oz cake)	47 mg	18 grams
Soyboy Not dogs (1.5 oz hot dog)	34 mg	10 grams
Edensoy Original drink (8 oz)	43 mg	10 grams
White Wave Fruit Silk Dairyless drink (8 oz)	41 mg	8 grams
1 oz Take Care Soy Protein Powder	57 mg	20 grams (to be mixed in a drink of your choice)
Nature's Plus Ultra Isoflavone (one pill)	50 mg	(No protein)
Nature's Way Soy Isoflavones pills (two pills)	25 mg	(No protein)
Rainboy Light Soy Supercomplex pills (two pills)	24 mg	(No protein)

Source: Bonnie Liebman, "The Soy Story," *Nutrition Action Newsletter,* September 1998. Published by Science in the Public Interest.

Appendix II:

IF YOU WANT TO SHARE YOUR WHMS STORY OR OBTAIN INFORMATION ABOUT WHMS

- If you would like to share your WHMS "story" or your examples of verbal or behavioral "slips" with me please send them to me via (1) written, or preferably typed or computer-disk form, or (2) on an au- diotape cassette, (3) via e-mail, or write and tell me where and when you can be contacted to set up a later interview. Be sure to indicate in writing that I have permission to use this information in future published material. Please indicate if you would like your name to be used if your material is published or if you would like your name not to be used if your material is published. Send this material to:

Dr. Claire Landsberg Warga
P.O. Box 943
Stone Ridge, NY 12484-0943
e-mail: gL/1or@is3.nyu.edu

For more information, see also my Web site: menopause101.com

- To obtain the fifty-page booklet titled *Your Memory: What Changes and What You Can Do about It,* written by Dr. Margie Lachman, send $4.00 to:

The National Center on Women & Aging
Heller School, MS 035
Brandeis University
Waltham, MA 02254-9110
800-929-1995 or 617-736-3866

You can request information about their newsletter *Women & Aging Letter,* $5.00 for six issues/year, and other booklets:

Estrogen Replacement: Interpreting Media Reports about New Research Estrogen Replacement: Is It Right for You? (both are available as a set for $3.00)

- To order copies of the *WHMS Screening Instrument* (the *Short Form* in this book is for individual use over different intervals, or for use in physicians' offices; the *Longer Form* is available for personal or research use). Send requests for information to:

Dr. Claire Landsberg Warga
Human Services Development Associates
P.O. Box 3380
Brooklyn, NY 11202

- To attempt to improve memory by decreasing associated stress, order Dr. Claire Warga's *Behavioral Medicine/Relaxation Techniques Audiotape.* Send check or money order for $15.95 made payable to **Human Services Development Associates** to:

Dr. Claire Landsberg Warga
Human Services Development Associates
P.O. Box 3380
Brooklyn, NY 11202

TO REQUEST THAT RESEARCH ON WHMS BE DONE

- Write a letter requesting that research be done on the causes and treatment of Warga's Hormonal Misconnection Syndrome, mention your awareness of the existence of WHMS in some of those you know, and mention the name of this book. Send your letter to:

Dr. Richard Hodes, Director
National Institute on Aging (NIA)
9000 Rockville Pike
Bethesda, MD 20892
800-222-2225

and to:

National Women's Health Network
Office of the Director
514 10th Street NW, Suite 400
Washington, DC 20024
202-347-1140

("an advocacy organization giving women a greater voice in the U.S. healthcare system")

MEMORY-ASSISTING DEVICES

- The Day-Timer Appointment Reminder Multi Alarm system is a low-cost, low-tech, highly useful, inconspicuous 5" x 1½" gadget that lets you schedule up to thirty-one alarms at half-hour intervals from morning till night by moving a little switch from left to right; it beeps you discreetly at the right time or times. It costs at this writing $14.99 with batteries included if you order it from Day-Timer by phone directly. Or you may be able to find it in some Staples stores. To order Day-Timer: 800-805-2615, product number 50120 "Day-Timer Appointment Reminder Multi Alarm." You might also order the free Day-Timer's catalog.
- RadioShack has several useful devices: A new digital voice-memory recording-alarm device lets you prerecord reminders to yourself at up to four preset times with up to four messages. It can fit in your palm (4" x 2½" x ½"), has up to 116 seconds of recording time, costs $29.99, and comes with a battery. You can remind yourself before an appointment what to bring with you, before leaving work what you need to take with you, before getting home what you need to pick up. It also has a built-in talking clock function. It also tells you how much remaining memory you have left. To order: 800-THE-SHACK or go to a store near you, product number 63-948.
- RadioShack also sells a four-minute tapeless digital personal recorder that's some 4½" tall with a clip and stand that requires three AAA batteries. It costs $39.99. It lets you skip messages or play only the last

message. To order: 800-THE-SHACK or go to a store near you, product number 14-1114.

- To order the *Memory Catalog,* a directory of gadgets, books, products, and electronic and mechanical devices for assisting your own memory, send a check or money order for $9.95 payable to HSDA to the *Memory Catalog,* HSDA, P.O. Box 3380, Brooklyn, NY 11202.
- I suggest for days when you are not feeling entirely yourself you purchase a small lightweight microcassette tape recorder to tape meetings as a backup to memory, or to tape what follow-up things you need to do right after a meeting. RadioShack offers an inexpensive microcassette tape recorder with fast playback that lets you record on one ninety-minute tape up to three hours of information. It requires two AA batteries or a power adapter and costs $39.99. To order: 800-THE-SHACK or go to a store near you, product number 14-1163.

FILOFAX INFO

For a Filofax catalog of personal organizers and calendars or to order a specific product or refill: 800-635-4321.

INFORMATION ABOUT SOY ISOFLAVONE CONTENT

For information about soy products and the amounts of isoflavones and proteins they reputedly contain obtain the September 1998 issue of the *Nutrition Action Healthletter* published by the Center for Science in the Public Interest (vol. 25, no. 7, pp. 3–7, $2.50). Ask your librarian for a copy of this issue or order it directly: Nutrition Action Healthletter, 1875 Connecticut Avenue NW, Suite 300, Washington, DC 20009-5728, Fax 202-265-4954.

MENOPAUSE AND WOMEN'S HEALTH NEWSLETTERS

Menopause News
Bimonthly: $25/year
2074 Union Street
San Francisco, CA 94123
415-567-2368 or 800-241-MENO

A Friend Indeed (Menopause)
10 issues: $30/year
A Friend Indeed Publications, Inc.
Box 1710
Champlain, NY 12919-1710
514-843-5730

Harvard Women's Health Watch
Monthly: $24/year
164 Longwood Avenue
Boston, MA 02115
800-829-5921

Women & Aging Letter
6 issues: $5.00/year
The National Center on Women & Aging
Heller School, MS 035
Brandeis University
Waltham, MA 02254-9110
800-929-1995 or 617-736-3866

HEALTH AFTER 50
$28/year
P.O. Box 420179
Palm Coast, FL 32142
940-446-4675

Hot Flash: Newsletter for Midlife & Older Women
Quarterly: $25/year
Box 816
Stony Brook, NY 11790-0609

Menopause Management
Bimonthly: $65/year
Carrington Communications, Inc.
P.O. Box 658
Flanders, NJ 07836
201-584-3040

Midlife Woman
Bimonthly: $25/year
Midlife Women's Network
5129 Logan Avenue South
Minneapolis, MN 55419-1019
612-925-0020/800-886-4354

Via: A Guide Through Menopause and Beyond
Quarterly: $19.97/year
Carrington Communications, Inc.
P.O. Box 658
Flanders, NJ 07836
201-584-3040

Health Forum for Midlife Women
Published by the Oregon Menopause Network
Quarterly: $20/year
Greenwood Center for Women
2607 SE Hawthorn Boulevard, Suite B
Portland, OR 97214

Connections
Women's Health Connection
Bimonthly: $12/year
P.O. Box 6338
Madison, WI 53716-338
800-366-6632

The Crone Chronicles
Quarterly: $18/year
Crones
P.O. Box 81
Kelly, WY 83011
307-733-1726

The Felix Letters
P.O. Box 7094
Berkeley, CA 94707

Health Wisdom for Women
Monthly: $67.95/year
Christiane Northrup
Phillips Publishing, Inc.
7811 Montrose Road
Potomac, MD 20854
301-424-3338

Oregon Menopause Information Network
Quarterly: $15/year
OMIN Newsletter
1253 SE 32nd Place
Portland, OR 97214

Women's Health Access
Bimonthly: $18/year
Women's Health America, Inc.
P.O. Box 9690
Madison, WI 53715
608-833-9012

RELATED ORGANIZATIONS

North America Menopause Society (NAMS)
P.O. Box 94527
Cleveland, OH 44101-4527
800-774-5342
216-844-8748
Fax: 216-844-8708

To obtain Menopack information booklets, send $5.00 for shipping and handling. Request the list of menopause clinicians, clinics, and information on how to start a support group. Allow two weeks for delivery. Credit cards accepted.

American Menopause Foundation
Marie Lugano, Director
350 Fifth Avenue, Suite 2822
New York, NY 10018
212-714-2398

Contact for referrals to support groups throughout the United States, directory of physician members, newsletter, and other information.

American College of Obstetrics and Gynecology
(ACOG)
409 12th Street SW
Washington, DC 20024
202-638-5577

National Women's Health Network
514 10th Street NW, Suite 400
Washington, DC 20024
202-347-1140

National Women's Health Network offers "Taking Hormones and Women's Health: Choices, Risks and Benefits," a thirty-seven-page position paper by the National Women's Health Network, an advocacy organization giving women a greater voice in the U.S. healthcare system.

National Institute on Aging (NIA)
9000 Rockville Pike
Bethesda, MD 20892
800-222-2225

National Women's Health Resource Center (NWHRC)
2440 M Street NW
Suite 201
Washington, DC 20037
202-293-6045

Alliance for Aging Research
2021 K Street NW, Suite 305
Washington, DC 20006
202-293-2856

Female Cancer

American Cancer Society
90 Park Avenue
New York, NY 10016
212-736-3030

Y Me National Organization for Breast Cancer & Support
212 West Van Buren Street
Chicago, IL 60607
800-221-2141

National Cancer Institute Cancer Information Service
9000 Rockville Pike
Bethesda, MD 20892
800-4CANCER (800-422-6237)

American Cancer Society National Headquarters
1599 Clifton Road NE
Atlanta, GA 30329
800-ACS-2345 (800-227-2345)

Mental Health

American Psychological Association
1200 17th Street NW
Washington, DC 20036
800-964-2000

American Psychiatric Association
14 K Street NW
Washington, DC 20005
202-682-6000

DEPRESSION (Awareness, Recognition, and Treatment Program
National Institute of Mental Health)
D/ART Public Inquiries
5600 Fishers Lane
Room 15C-05
Rockville, MD 20857
301-443-4513

National Mental Health Association (NMHA) Information
Center
1021 Prince Street
Alexandria, VA 22314-2971
703-684-7722/800-969-6642

Heart Disease

American Heart Association
7320 Greenville Avenue
Dallas, TX 75231
214-373-6300

American Lung Association
1740 Broadway
New York, NY 10019
212-315-8700

Hysterectomy Education

HERS (Hysterectomy Educational Resource and Service)
422 Bryn Mawr Avenue
Bala Cynwyd, PA 19004
215-667-7757 or 387-6700

Sexuality in Midlife and Beyond

Sexuality Information-Educanon
Council of the U.S. (SIECUS)
130 West 42nd Street, Suite 350
New York, NY 10036
212-819-9770

The Jacobs Institute of Women's Health
409 12th Street SW
Washington, DC 20024-2188
202-863-4900

Birth Control in Midlife

Planned Parenthood Federation of America
810 Seventh Avenue
New York, NY 10019
212-541-7800

Alan Guttmacher Institute
120 Wall Street
New York, NY 10005
212-248-1111

The Institute for Reproductive Health
Georgetown University School of Medicine
Washington, DC 20007
202-687-1392

Premature Ovarian Failure
Premature Ovarian Failure Support Group
703-913-4787

Osteoporosis

National Osteoporosis Foundation
1150 17th Street NW, Suite 500
Washington, DC 20036
800-223-9994

To find out where you can get a *bone density test,* call the *NOF,* 800-464-6700.

Urogenital Health

Help for Incontinent People (HIP)
P.O. Box 544
Union, SC 29379
800-BLADDER

National Vulvodynia Association
P.O. Box 19288
Sarasota, FL 34276

Simon Foundation for Continence
P.O. Box 815
Wilmette, IL 60091
800-23SIMON

Wider Opportunities for Women (WOW) National Commission
on Working Women
1325 G Street NW
Lower Level
Washington, DC 20005
202-638-3143

American Dietetic Association (ADA)
216 West Jackson Boulevard
Suite 800
Chicago, IL 60606
312-899-0040

National Heart, Lung, and Blood Institute (NHLBI)
9000 Rockville Pike
Bethesda, MD 20892
301-496-4236

National Arthritis and Musculoskeletal and Skin Diseases
Information Clearinghouse
Box AMS
9000 Rockville Pike
Bethesda, MD 20892
301-495-4484

Hypnosis Referrals

Society for Clinical and Experimental Hypnosis: 509-332-7555
American Society of Clinical Hypnosis: 847-297-3317

Pharmacies

For information about different estrogen/progesterone formulations you are considering taking speak to a pharmacist. Or to order micronized progesterone via a doctor's prescription:

Women's International Pharmacy: 800-279-5708

Madison Pharmacy Associates (the only women-owned pharmacy in America): 800-558-7046

Bajamur Women's HealthCare Pharmacy: 800-255-8025

College Pharmacy: 800-888-9358 ext. 116 (ask for Pete)

Jaye Pharmacy: 818-789-8111 (prescription compounding, natural hormone specialist)
13322 Riverside Drive
Sherman Oaks, CA 91423

Hazle Pharmacy: (Bill Spears) compounding pharmacy
800-439-2026
http://www.hazledrugs.com

Menopause Clinics

List available through North American Menopause Foundation (See above.)

All Saints Health System Place: Health Enhancement and Renewal for Women
1400 Eighth Avenue
Ft. Worth, TX 76104
817-922-7470

Cleveland Menopause Clinic: 216-442-4747

Menopause Institute of Northern California (Male and Female Sex Hormone Disorders)
700 West Parr Avenue, Suite D
Los Gatos, CA 95030
408-370-1833

Women's Medical and Diagnostic Center and Climacteric Clinic
Gainesville, FL
904-372-5600

Books

Listening to Your Hormones
Gillian Ford
Prima Books
1997

Menopause and Madness
Marcia Lawrence
Andrews McNeel Publishing (Kansas)
1998

The Silent Passage
Gail Sheehy
PocketBooks (New York)
1998

Women and Doctors
John Smith, M.D.
The Atlantic Monthly Press
1992

Male Menopause
Jed Diamond
Sourcebooks (Naperville, Ill.)
1997

The Testosterone Syndrome
Eugene Shippen, M.D. and William Fryer
M. Evans & Co. (New York)
1998

Declining to Decline
Margaret Morganroth Gullette
University of Virginia Press (Charlottesville, VA)
1997

Potatoes not Prozac
Kathleen DesMaisons, Ph.D.
Simon & Schuster (New York)
1998

Notes

Chapter 1

Page

4 *thirties, forties or fifties:* Note: *My research method*: After detecting the initial symptoms of this syndrome through observation and insight and confirming their existence in menopausal and/or perimenopausal women I knew from several settings or read about (i.e., Letty Cottin Pogrebin's book *Getting Over Getting Older*), my method in uncovering the remaining symptoms was to ask women of menopausal age what symptoms they personally associated with menopause. I learned for example about "spelling uncertainty" in this way thanks to L.G., a teacher then in her mid-fifties who was a formerly great speller. Typically, at the end of an open-ended interview of each woman about what symptoms she associated with menopause, I would engage in a "probing" query. In this section I would ask her about specific symptoms I was investigating, i.e., if she experienced any changes in "spelling, for the better or worse," or other symptoms I had been led to in prior interviews or which I detected *de novo*. In this probing part of the interview, women often acknowledged the existence of new symptoms, which they had not at all associated with menopause on their own. Adequate redundancy of confirmation of a symptom in women led to my inclusion of this symptom question in later interviews at the probing end stage. The process of probing often led women to bring up other "strange" symptoms that they had no explanation for but which fit the "new" bill. I would then include these in later probings with new women, to see if they met with redundant confirmation. (I have not included all symptoms that may ultimately pertain to this syndrome for lack as yet of sufficient redundancy in my sample.) Eventually I expanded my search to perimenopausal women and discovered that *as a group* they equaled menopausal women in familiarity with the symptoms. Thus, not all of the women I have interviewed have been asked about *all* the symptoms I eventually enumerated. The process of discovery was an emergent one. My research method can best be described as that of a "*bricoleur*" as described in the *Handbook of Qualitative Research:* "A *bricoleur* is a 'Jack of all

trades or a kind of professional do-it-yourself person' (Levi-Strauss, 1966, 17). The *bricoleur* produces a . . . pieced together close-knit set of practices that provide solutions to a problem in a concrete situation. 'The solution . . . is an [emergent] construction' . . . that changes and takes new forms as different tools, methods, and techniques are added to the puzzle." *Handbook of Qualitative Research,* ed. Norman Denzin, Yvonna S. Lincoln. Sage Publications, Thousand Oaks, California, 1994: 2.

4 *often be reversed:* Ingrid Wickelgren, "Estrogen stakes claim to cognition," *Science,* 276(5313)2; 1997: 675-8.

5 *in a woman's life:* M. Lock, P. Kaufert, and P. Gilbert, Cultural construction of the menopausal syndrome: the Japanese case, *Maturitas,* 10(4); 1988: 317–32; M. Lock, Ambiguities of aging: Japanese experience and perceptions of menopause. *Cult. Med. Psychiatry:* (10)1986: 23–46.

11 *after their discoverers.":* Edward O. Wilson, *Sociobiology: The New Synthesis.* The Belknap Press of Harvard University Press, Cambridge, Mass. and London, 1975: 154.

12 *listed in Table 1:* Gail Sheehy's 1991 book *Silent Passage,* to her credit, does mention in greater detail memory and concentration problems without specifying in detail the many specific and broad range of symptoms of the WHM Syndrome. But for reasons that are not clear, this aspect of her message in 1991 has not carried over into our culture's overall grasp or understanding of what menopause and perimenopause can consist of for many women. Janine O'Leary Cobb, editor of the menopause newsletter *A Friend Indeed,* has mentioned the symptom of not recognizing faces and menopausal forgetfulness in her newsletter, and in an interview with me.

26 *this tentative diagnosis:* Barry Gordon, *Memory.* Mastermedia Ltd., 1995: 196–200, the case of fifty-five-year-old Dr. S.

29 *thinking and speaking:* Interview with psychiatrist/thyroid expert, Dr. Peter Whybrow, UCLA.

29 *on thyroid changes:* Interview with thyroid/mind expert Dr. Peter Whybrow, UCLA.

29 *not an uncommon finding:* Interview with menopause expert Dr. Maurice Cohen.

Chapter 2

Page

36 *about normal women:* NIHs SWAN Study press release.

37 *eight women!:* Interview with Dr. Leon Speroff; B. M. Sherman, J.H, West, and S. Korenman, The Menopausal Transition: Analysis of LH, FSH, estradiol, and progesterone concentrations during menstrual cycles of women. *J. Clin. Endocrinol. Metab.* 42(4); 1976: 629–36; S. G. Korenman, B. M. Sherman, Hormonal regulation in normal and abnormal menstrual cycles, in *The Endocrine Function of the Human Ovary,* V. H. James et al., eds. London: Academic Press, 1976: 359–72.

37 *attention deficits:* Victoria Liune, M. Rodriguez, Effects of estradiol on radial arm maze performance of young and aged rats. *Behav. & Neurol. Biol.* 62; 1994: 230–236; J. Simpkins, P. Green, K. Gridely, and J. Shi, Estrogen and memory protection. *J. Society of Obstet. and Gynec. of Canada:* Supplement 1997: 14–19. (Memory deficits). M. Voytko, J. Hinshaw, Consequences of estrogen loss and replacement on cognitive function of surgically menopausal monkeys (Abstract), Society for Neuroscience: 22; 1966: 1387; M. Voytko, Cognitive function of the basal forebrain cholinergic system in monkeys: memory or attention? *Behav. & Brain Res.* 75; 1996: 13–25; interviews with Voytko, Simpkins, and Liune (attention deficits).

37 *associated with depression:* M. Rehavi, H. Sepcuti, and A. Weizman, Upregulation of imipramine binding and serotonin uptake by estradiol in female rat brain, *Brain Res.* 410(1); 1987: 135–9; S. Maswood, G. Stewart, and L. Uphouse, Gender and estrous cycle effects of the 5-HT1A agonist, 8-OH-DPAT, on hypothalamic serotonin, *Pharmacol., Biochem. & Behav.,* 51 (4); 1995: 807–13; B. B. Sherwin and B. E. Suryani-Cadotte, Up-regulatory effect of estrogen on platelet 3H-imipramine binding sites in surgically menopausal women, *Biological Psychiatry* 28 (4); 1990: 339–48; Johanna S. Archer, Relationship between estrogen, serotonin and depression, 1998, in press.

38 *uncover the symptoms":* Interview with Dr. William Andrews.

38 *psychological tests":* Interview with Dr. William Andrews.

42 *severe brain damage:* Interviews with Drs. Sonia Lupien, Jimmy Golumb, Elkhanon Goldberg, Donna Korol.

43 *the WHM Syndrome:* Interview with Dr. Robert Sapolsky.

43 *estrogen administration:* S. Campbell and M. Whitehead, Estrogen therapy and the menopausal syndrome, *Clinics in Obstet. Gynecol.,* 4; (1)1977: 31–47.

43 *women's own assessments:* In this case, noting on what is called a "visual analog scale" to indicate their self-observed degree of improvement.

43 *actively complaining about:* Interview with Barbara Sherwin.

45 *on the topic:* Interview with Dr. Michele Warren, Director of Columbia-Presbyterian Center for Menopause, Hormonal Disorders and Women's Health.

54 *on average at age 51.7:* Different sources vary around this general mean.

55 *not simply my fertility":* New York Times, Apr. 1997.

56 *related to menopause":* J. Coope, Hormonal and non-hormonal interventions for menopausal symptoms. *Maturitas,* 23 (2); Mar. 1996: Abstract 159–68.

56 *"presenting symptom":* A continuing medical education program for total healthcare of the mature woman. *The Postmenopausal Health Curriculum 101;* 1997: 11.

56 *climacteric* [menopause]." [Emphasis added.] ibid., 11.

61 *spatial memory skills:* Eric Poehlman, Michael J. Toth et al., Changes in energy balance and body composition at menopause: a controlled longitudinal study. *Annals of Internal Med.,* 123(9); Nov. 1, 1995: 673–5; Susan Resnick, J. Metter, and Alan Zonderman, Estrogen replacement therapy and longitudinal decline in visual memory. A possible protective effect? *Neurol.,* 49(6); Dec. 1997: 1491–7.

Chapter 3

Page

67 *sensitive to estrogen"*: Dr. Frederick Naftolin, address at 1997 meeting of American College of Obstetrics and Gynecology, Las Vegas.

68 *Yale University School of Medicine:* Interview with Phillip Sarrel; P. M. Sarrel, E. G. Lufkin, M. J. Oursler, and D. Keefe, Estrogen actions in arteries, bone and brain. *Sci. Am. Med.,* 1(44); 1994.

68 *capacity to function."* [Emphasis added.]: Interview with the author Phillip Sarrel, Estrogen changes during menopause; cellular actions and reactions. *The Female Patient,* Supplement; Feb. 1995: 6–9.

68 *past later childhood.* Note; The work of E. H. Lenneberg.

71 *news analysis article:* Ingrid Wickelgren, Estrogen stakes claim to cognition, *Science,* 276(5313); May 2, 1997: 675–8.

71 *Gynecologists of Canada in October of 1997.* Guest editor Barbara Sherwin, Estrogen and the brain. *J. Society of Obstet. and Gynec. of Canada,* Supplement (four articles). Oct. 1997.

71 *in the medical textbook:* Rogerio Lobo, ed., *Treatment of the Postmenopausal Woman.* Philadelphia: Lippincott-Raven, 1996.

72 *hormone deficiency states"*: Interviews with Dr. Dominique Toran-Allerand.

72 *the [brain's] neurons"*: Natalie Angier, How estrogen may work to protect against Alzheimer's, *New York Times,* Mar. 8, 1994: C3.

74 *McEwen, and others:* H. Fillet, H. Weinreb, I. Cholst, V. Liune, B. McEwen et al., Observations in a preliminary open trial of estradiol therapy for senile dementia—Alzheimer's type, *Psychoneuroendocrinol.,* 11(3); 1986: 337–45.

74 *within forty-eight hours:* C. S. Wooley, B. S. McEwen, Estradiol mediates fluctuation in hippocampal synapse density during the estrus cycle in the adult rat, *J. Neurosci.* 12; 1992: 2549–54.

75 *run around frantically.):* Interview with Dr. Sheryl Smith.

75 *says Dr. Victoria Liune:* Ingrid Wickelgren, Estrogen stakes claim to cognition, *Science,* 276; May 2, 1997: 675–8.

77 *to the hippocampus"*: Interview with Dr. Mary Lou Voytko regarding her research on attention in ovariectomized cynomolgus monkeys, presented in 1997 at Society for Neuroscience annual meeting.
  P.S. Green, K. Gordon, and J.W. Simpkins, Phenolic A ring requirement for the neuroprotective effects of steriods, *J. Steroid Biochem. & Mol. Biol.,* 63(4–6); 1997: 229–35.

80 *in recent years:* B. Smith, Activating effects of estradiol on brain activity; B. S. McEwen, Ovarian steroids have diverse effects on brain structure and function; S. Smith, Hormones, mood and neurobiology—a summary, in *The Modern Management of Menopause,* G. Berg and M. Hammar, eds., Parthenon Publishing, New York, 1994.

80 *acetylcholine:* V. N. Liune et al., Immuno-chemical demonstration of increased choline acetyltranferase concentration in rat prepoptic area after estradiol ad-

ministration, *Brain Res.* 191(1); 1980: 273–7; dopamine: T. Di Paolo, Modulation of brain dopamine transmission by sex steroids. *Rev. Neurosci.,* (5); 1994: 27–41

82 *after stroke and brain injury:* Work of Mark Matson cited by Dr. Robert Sapolsky in interview. A. J. Bruce, Y. Goodman, Mattson, Estrogen attenuates and corticosterone exacerbates excitotoxin oxidative injury and amyloid beta-peptide toxicity in hippocampal neuron, *J. of Neurochem.* 66(5); 1996: 1836–44.

82 *neurons in Alzheimer's disease:* Annlia Paganini-Hill, Alzheimer's disease in women, *The Female Patient,* 23; Mar. 1998: 10–20.

82 *in different ways:* D. Wagner et al., The effects of hormone replacement therapy on carbohydrate metabolism and cardiovascular risk factors in surgically post-menopausal cynomolgus monkeys, *Metabolism,* 45(10); 1996: 1254–62; J. Simpkins, Chronic weight loss in lean and obese rats with a brain-enhanced chemical delivery system for estradiol, *Physiol. & Behav.* 44, 1988: 573–80.

82 *(blood deficiency) damage:* Kristine Yaffe, George Sawaya, Ivan Lieberburg, and Deborah Grady, Estrogen therapy in postmenopausal women: effects on cognitive function and dementia, *JAMA,* 279(9); Mar. 4, 1998: 688–95 (Quote 690).

82 *blood, oxygen, nutrients:* Philip Sarrel, Ovarian hormones: Recent findings of cardiological significance, *Cardiology in Practice,* Mar.–Apr. 1991: 14–17.

82 *metabolism in women:* Eric Poehlman, Michael Toth, and Gardner, Changes in energy balance and body composition at menopause: a controlled longitudinal study, *Annals of Internal Med.,* 123(9); Nov. 1995: 673–5; P. J. Arciero, M. Goran, and E. T. Poehlman, Resting metabolic rate is lower in women than in men, *J. Applied Physiol.,* 75; 1993: 2514–20.

83 *tasks as driving:* Interview with Uriel Halbreich.

84 *cognitive changes:* Kristine Yaffe, George Sawaya, Ivan Lieberburg, and Deborah Grady, Estrogen therapy in postmenopausal women: effects on cognitive function and dementia, *JAMA,* 279(9); Mar. 4, 1998: 688–95; R. A. Srivastava, N. Bhasin, and N. Srivastava, Apolipoprotein E gene expression in various tissues of mouse and regulation by estrogen, *Biochem. Mol. Biol. Int.,* 38; 1996: 91–101; K. Yaffe, J. Cauley, L. Sands, and W. Browner, Apolipoprotein E phenotype and cognitive decline in a prospective study of elderly community women, *Arch. Neurol.* 54; 1998: 1110–4.

84 *"nature's psychoprotectant":* G. Fink and B. E. Sumner, Estrogen control of central neurotransmission: effect on mood, mental state, and memory, *Cellular & Mol. Neurobiol,* 16(3); 1996: 325–44.

84 *disorder schizophrenia:* G. Fink, B. E. Sumner, R. Rosie, O. Grace, and J. P. Quinn, Estrogen control of central neurotransmission: Effect on mood, mental state and memory. *Cellular & Mol. Neurobiol.,* 16(3); 1996: 325–44.

84 *depression—serotonin:* Archer, Relationship between estrogen, serotonin, and depression, in press; Uriel Halbreich, Role of estrogen in postmenopausal depression, *Neurol.* 48(5) Supplement 7; 1997: 516.

85 *serotonin in women:* Johanna Archer, Relationship between estrogen, serotonin, and depression, in press; P. Guicheney, D. Leger, J. Barat et al., Platelet sero-

tonin content and plasma tryptophan in peri and postmenopausal women: Variations within plasma oestrogen levels and depressive symptoms, *Europ. Clinic. Invest.*, 18; 1988: 297–304; Uriel Halbreich, Role of estrogen in postmenopausal depression, *Neurol.*, 48 (Supplement 7); 1997: 516.

85 *mental state, cognition:* B. E. Sumner, G. Fink, Estrogen increases the density of 5-hydroxy tryptamine 2A receptors in cerebral cortex and nucleus accumbens in the female rat, *J. Steroid Biochem. Mol. Biol.*, 54; 1995: 15–20.

85 *to placebo treatment:* E. L. Klaiber, D. M. Broverman, W. Vogel et al., Estrogen therapy for severe persistent depressions in women, *Arch. Gen. Psychiatry,* 36; 1979: 550–54.

85 *evoked by stress:* Annlia Paganini-Hill, Alzheimer's disease in women, *The Female Patient,* 23; Mar. 1998: 10–20.

85 *of stress hormones:* M. F. Kritzer, S. G. Kohama, Ovarian homones influence the morphology, distribution, and density of tyrosine hydroxylase immunoreactive axons in the dorsolateral prefrontal cortex of adult rhesus monkeys, *J. Comp. Neurol.*, 395(1); May 25, 1998: 1–17; B.S. McEwen, Protective and damaging effects of Stress Mediatiors. *New Eng. J. Med.*, 338(3); 1998: 171–79; M. G. Meaney, S. Lupien, Individual differences in hypothalamic-pituitary-adrenal activity in later life and hippocampal aging, *Experiment. Gerontol.*, 30(3–4); 1995: 229–51.

85 *receptors for stress hormones:* Interview with Dr. Robert Sapolsky.

85 *atrophy, or die":* Natalie Angier, How estrogen may work to protect against Alzheimer's, *New York Times,* Mar. 8, 1994: C3.

86 *as Alzheimer's disease":* Stanley Birge, The role of estrogen deficiency in the aging CNS." *Treatment of the Post-Menopausal Woman,* ed. Rogerio Lobo, Lippincott-Raven, 1996: 154.

87 *and Alzheimer's disease":* J. Simpkins, P. Green, K. Gridely, and J. Shi, Estrogen and memory protection. *J. Society of Obstet. and Gynec. of Canada:* Supplement; 1997: 14–9.

87 *other cognitive decline":* Kristine Yaffe, George Sawaya, Ivan Lieburburg, and Deborah Grady, Estrogen therapy in postmenopausal women: effects on cognitive function and dementia, *JAMA,* 279(9); Mar. 4, 1998: 688–95 (Quote 689).

88 *or surgical menopause":* Bruce McEwen, Ovarian steroids have diverse effects on brain structure and function, *The Modern Management of Menopause,* Parthenon Publishing Co., New York, 1994: 269–78.

88 *the most important:* J. Simpkins, P. Green, K. Gridely, and J. Shi, Estrogen and memory protection, *J. Society of Obstet. & Gynec. of Canada:* Supplement; 1997: 14–19.

90 *normal acetylcholine activity:* D. Aarsland, J. P. Larsen, I. Reinvang, and A. V. Aasland, Effects of cholinergic blockade on language in healthy young women. Implications for the cholinergic hypothesis in dementia of the Alzheimer type. *Brain,* 117 (pt. 6); Dec. 1994: 1377–84; Y. Tanaka, Masao Miyazaki, and M. Albert, Effects of increased cholinergic activity on naming in aphasia, *Lancet,* 350(9071); July 12, 1997: 116–17; S. Sorbi, P. Antuono, and L. Amaducci,

Choline acetyltransferase and acetylcholinesterase abnormalities in senile dementia: importance of biochemical measurements in human post-mortem brain specimens, *Ital. J. Neurol. Sci.,* 11(2); Mar. 1980: 75–8.

90 *namely, this one!:* H. M. Bryson, P. Benfield, Donepezil, *Drugs Aging,* 10(3); Mar. 1997: 234–39.

90 *neurotransmitter dopamine:* Russell A. Barkley, Attention-deficit hyperactivity disorder. *Scient. Am.,* Sept. 1998: 66–71; G. J. Lahoste et al., Dopamine D4 receptor gene polymorphism is associated with attention deficit hyperactivity disorder, *Molecular Psychiatry,* 1(2); May 1996: 121–4.

91 *daily activities:* Russel A. Barkley, Attention-deficit hyperactivity disorder, *Scient. Am.* 279(3); 1998: 66–71.

91 *research gets going:* Sandra Blakeslee, Running late?: researchers blame aging brain, *New York Times Science Times,* Tuesday, Mar. 24, 1998. The article points to research by Dr. Warren Meck and Matthew Matell on time estimation; Dr. Peter Mangan on time estimation; Dr. Hudson Hoagland on temperature regulation and time estimation; Dr. Sean Hinton, brain-imaging studies of time-estimating subjects; the research of Dr. John Gibbon with time estimation difficulties of dopamine-deficient Parkinson's disease patients; Dr. Guinever Eden's research with the time-keeping problems of dyslexics, and theories suggesting that time-estimation and internal interval "clock" can be "off" due to changed dopamine levels and by alterations in normal temperature regulation.

91 *express a thought:* T. Di Paolo, Modulation of brain dopamine transmission by sex steroids, *Rev. Neurosci.,* 5; 1994: 27–41. G. V. Williams, P. S. Goldman-Rakic, Modulation of memory fields by dopamine D1 receptors in prefrontal cortex, *Nature,* 376(6541); 1995: 572–5.

92 *in younger women?:* M. Sano et al., A controlled trial of selegiline, alpha-tocopherol [vitamin E] or both as treatment for Alzheimer's disease, *New Eng. J. Med.,* 336(17); 1997: 1216–22; Roberta Diaz Brinton and Rose Yamazaki, Advances and challenges in the prevention and treatment of Alzheimer's disease, *Pharmaceut. Res.,* 15(3); 1998: 386–98.

92 *in women experiencing estrogen loss:* M. Odawara, A. Tamaoka, and K. Yamashita, Ginkgo biloba. *Neurol.,* 48(3); 1997: 789–90.

Chapter 4

Page

93 *at elevated risk:* PBS art of women's health: Post-menopausal women. Life after menopause, aired Oct. 24, 1998, New York City.

94 *have the disease:* M. Larkin, Alzheimer's disease prevalence may quadruple, *Lancet,* 352; Sept. 19, 1998, referring to study in *Am. J. Public Health,* 88; 1998: 1337–42, by Ron Brookmeyer.

94 *Institute of Aging:* M. Larkin, Alzheimer's disease prevalence may quadruple, *Lancet,* 352; Sept. 19, 1998.

94 *says Dr. Richard Mayeux:* Interview with Richard Mayeux.

94 *strong association:* A. Paganini-Hill, Does estrogen replacement therapy protect against Alzheimer's disease? *Osteoporosis Int.,* Supplement 1; 1997: S12–17.

95 *sixteen years:* A. Morrison et al., A prospective study of ERT and the risk of developing Alzheimer's disease in the Baltimore longitudinal study of aging, abstract, *Neurol.,* 46; 1996: A 435–6.

96 *had the lowest risk:* M. Tang, D. Jacobs, Y. Stern, and Richard Mayeux, Effect of oestrogen during menopause on risk and age at onset of Alzheimer's disease, *Lancet,* 348(9025); 1996: 429–32.

96 *developing Alzheimer's:* A. Paganini-Hill, V. W. Henderson, Estrogen replacement therapy and risk of Alzheimer's disease, *Arch. Intern. Med.,* 156(19); 1996: 2213–7.

97 *pairs of words:* Interview with Dr. Howard Fillet.

97 *were assessed on:* Victor Henderson, Estrogen replacement therapy for the prevention and treatment of Alzheimer's disease, *CNS Drugs,* 5; Nov. 8 1997: 343–51.

98 *placebo patch:* Interview with Asthana; also, S. Asthana, S. Craft, L. D. Baker et al., Transdermal estrogen improves memory in women with Alzheimer's disease (abstract), *Neurosci. Abstr.,* 22; 1996: 200.

99 *in the WHM Syndrome:* Victor Henderson, Estrogen replacement therapy for the prevention and treatment of Alzheimer's disease, *CNS Drugs,* 5; Nov. 8, 1997: 343–351.

99 *involve naming skills:* Victor Henderson, Leanne Watt, and J. Galen Buckwalter, Cognitive skills associated with estrogen replacement in women with Alzheimer's disease, *Psychoneuroendocrinol.,* 21(4); 1996: 421–30.

99 *and, likely, brains:* Barbara Sherwin, Presentation at the Society for Behavioral Neuroendocrinology, Baltimore, May 1997.

99 *taken into account:* James Simpkins, Pattie Green et al., Role of estrogen replacement therapy in memory enhancement and the prevention of neuronal loss associated with Alzheimer's disease, *Am. J. Med.,* 103(3A); Sept. 22, 1997: 19S–25S.

99 *mild cognitive deficits* [Emphasis added]": Victor Henderson, Estrogen replacement therapy for the prevention and treatment of Alzheimer's disease, *CNS Drugs,* (5); Nov. 8, 1997: 343–351 (quote 345).

100 *a professional audience, says:* Victor Henderson, Estrogen replacement therapy for the prevention and treatment of Alzheimer's disease, *CNS Drugs,* (5); Nov. 8, 1997: 343–51.

100 *I interviewed him.):* Interview with Richard Mayeux.

101 *onset of menopause]":* Interview with Howard Fillet.

101 *Stanley Birge wrote:* S. Birge, Is there a role for ERT in the prevention and treatment of dementia? *J. Am. Geriatr. Soc.,* 44(7); July 1996: 865–70.

102 *AD. [Alzheimer's Disease]:* James Simpkins, Pattie Green et al., Role of estrogen replacement therapy in memory enhancement and the prevention of neuronal loss associated with Alzheimer's disease, *Am. J. Med.,* 103(3A); Sept. 22, 1997: 19S–25S.

102 *duration-related manner:* Note: the studies involved women who had in the past used only estrogen replacement therapy, and women who in more recent years have used estrogen/progesterone replacement regimens.

Chapter 5

Page

105 *with estrogen therapy:* B. M. Caldwell, R. I. Watson, An evaluation of psychologic effects of sex hormone administration in aged women: Results of therapy after six months, *J. Gerontol.,* 7; 1952: 228–44, cited in Barbara Sherwin, Estrogen and cognitive functioning in women. *Proc. Soc. Exp. Biol. Med.,* 217(1); Jan. 1998: 17–22.

106 *same time interval:* H. I. Kantor, C. M. Michael, and H. Shore, Estrogen for older women, *Am. J. Obstet. Gynecol.,* 116; 1973: 1115–1118; cited in Barbara Sherwin, Estrogen and cognitive functioning in women. *Proc. Soc. Exp. Biol. Med.,* 217(1); Jan. 1998: 17–22.

107 *due to fibroids:* B. B. Sherwin, T. Tulandi, Add-back estrogen reverses cognitive deficits induced by a gonadotropin-releasing hormone agonist in women with leiomyoma uteri, *J. Clin. Endocrinol. & Metab.* 81(7); Jul. 1996: 2545–9.

108 *kinds of women:* B. B. Sherwin, M. M. Gelfand, A prospective one-year study of estrogen and progestin in postmenopausal women: Effects on clinical symptoms and lipoprotein lipids, *Obstet. Gynecol.,* 73(5 Pt1); 759–66.

109 *adult brain":* Interview with Barbara Sherwin.

109 *women on ERT:* D. Robinson, L. Friendman, R. Marcus, J. Tinklenberg, and J. Yesavage, Estrogen replacement therapy and memory in older women, *J. Am. Geriatr. Soc.,* 42; 1994: 919–22.

109 *who had not:* D. M. Jacobs, M. Tang, Y. Stern, M. Sano, K. Marder, K. L. Bell, P. Schofield, G. Dooneief, B. Burland, and R. Mayeux, Cognitive function in non-demented older women who took estrogen after menopause, *Neurol.,* 50; Feb. 1998: 368–73.

109 *areas of function:* Barbara Sherwin, Linda Carlson, Estrogen and memory in women, *J. Society of Obstet. & Gynec. of Canada,* Supplement; Oct. 1997: 7–13.

110 *in that paper:* Doreen Kimura, Estrogen replacement therapy may protect against intellectual decline in postmenopausal women, *Hormones & Behavior,* 29; 1995: 312–321.

110 *she speculated:* Ibid., 319.

110 *speed-of-processing factor":* Ibid., 319.

110 *Visual Retention Test:* Susan Resnick, J. Metter, and Alan Zonderman, Estrogen replacement therapy and longitudinal decline in visual memory. A possible protective effect?, *Neurol.,* 49; Dec. 1997: 1494–7.

111 *replacement treatment:* Uriel Halbreich et al., Possible acceleration of age effects on cognition following menopause, *J. Psychiat. Res.,* 29; 1995: 153–63; U. Halbreich, et. al., Effect of estrogen antagonist on mood and cognition, Presentation at Annual meeting of the Society of Biol. Psychiatry, San Francisco, Calif., 1993.

113 *in this field":* Interview with Doreen Kimura.

113 *"smarter-than-normal"):* M. Singh, E. Meyer, W. Millard, and J. Simpkins, Ovarian steroid deprivation results in a reversible learning impairment and compromised cholinergic function in female Sprague-Dawley rats, *Brain Res.,* 644; 1994: 305–12.

113 *learning/memory behavior:* J. W. Simpkins, P. S. Green, K. E. Gridley, M. Singh, N. C. de Fiebre, and G. Rajakumar, *Am. J. Med.,* 103(3A); Sept. 22, 1997: 19S–25S.

113 *improved working memory:* P. Dohanich et al., Estrogen regulation of learning and memory, *Society for Behavioral Neuroendocrinology,* May 28–31, 1997, Baltimore Md., 47.

114 *"reversible" findings:* Victoria Liune, M. Rodriguez, Effects of estradiol on radial arm maze performance of young and aged rats, *Behav. & Neurol. Biol.,* 62; 1994: 230–236; also the research of Mark Packard.

114 *of working memory":* Christina Williams, Gillian Einstein, Organizational and activational effects of estradiol on spatial ability and hippocampal morphology across the lifespan program. *Society for Behavioral Neuroendocrinology,* May 28–31, 1997: Baltimore, Maryland, 45.

114 *with memory improvement:* R. B. Gibbs, Effects of estrogen on basal forebrain cholinergic neurons vary as a function of dose and duration of treatment, *Brain Res.,* 757(1); May 16, 1997: 10–6.

116 *was being applied:* Interviews with neuroscientist Dr. Sonia Lupien, neuropsychologist and Alzheimer's researcher Dr. Allan Kluger.

Chapter 6

Page

130 *estrogen loss alone:* B. B. Sherwin, B. E. Suryani-Cadotte, Up-regulatory effect of estrogen on platelet 3H-imipramine binding sites in surgically menopausal women, *Biol. Psychiatry,* 28; 1990: 339–48; M. Rehavi, H. Sepcuti, and A. Weisman, Upregulation of imipramine and serotonin uptake by estradiol in female rat brain, *Brain Res,* 410; 1987: 130–135; S. Maswood, G. Stewart, and L. Uphouse, Gender and estrous cycle effects of the 5-HT1A agonist, 8-OH-DPAT, on hypothalamic serotonin, *Pharmacol. Biochem. Behav.,* 51; 1995: 807–13; Johanna S. Archer, Relationship between estrogen, serotonin and depression, 1998, in press.

133 *at the same age.* [emphasis added.]" [Ref: From an article in press: Relationship beweeen estrogen, serotonin and depression, 1998 by Johanna S. Archer, V.M.D., M.S., M.D. (pages not numbered). The investigators referred to are E. L. Vliet, V. L. H. Davis, New perspectives on the relationship of hormone changes to affective disorders in the perimenopause, *NAACOG's Clin. Is.,* 2; 1991: 453–71.]

141 *their blood test or hormone test numbers:* Interviews with Dr. John Arpels, Dr. Maurice Cohen, Dr. Robert Greene.

142 *ovarian/hormonal changes):* Dr. Susan Love informed me that this is called "chemo brain." Interview with Dr. Susan Love.

142 *(the luteal phase):* Sarah Berga, Understanding premenstrual syndrome, *Lancet,* 351; 1998: 465–66.

142 *postpartum depression:* John C. Arpels, The female brain: Hypoestrogenic continuum from the premenstrual syndrome to menopause. *J. Reprod. Med.,* 41(9); Sept. 1996: 633–39.

142 *WHM symptoms:* John Arpels, ibid.

143 *and physical estrogen loss symptoms:* Ibid.

143 *varies among women:* Interview with Dr. Galen Buckwalter, University of Southern California; Manual of La Leche League.

143 *make of the fact:* Interview with Dr. John Arpels.

143 *to again "kick in":* Note: A number of these same women have told me they experienced some of the same WHMS symptoms during certain phases of pregnancy. This too warrants further investigation.

144 *to be researched:* Note: So too does the question of whether women who have breast-fed for many years—experienced estrogen loss during breast-feeding cumulatively for conceivably many years—are at a cognitive disadvantage later in life, at greater risk for later cognitive decline. Indeed, research whether women with Alzheimer's disease have breast-fed more children or longer than women without Alzheimer's disease would help cast light on the potential cost, if any, of estrogen deprivation on cognitive function in women over the long term.

144 *What was that about?":* Lisa Belkin, Now accepting applications for my baby. *New York Times Magazine* Apr. 5, 1998, 56.

144 *non-supplemented breast-feeding:* Note: I have interviewed seven other women with not dissimilar symptoms.

Chapter 7

Page

152 *unexpectedly pregnant:* Interview with Marie Lugano, president American Menopause Foundation.

156 *would know about":* Note: Virginia psychiatrist Dr. Susan Trachtman, who works with perimenopausal and menopausal women, told me that the "fogginess" symptom is what women with PMS not infrequently report—a symptom that she says tends to go away when they get their period.

158 *simply my fertility."* Anna Quindlen *New York Times Health Supplement,* 1997.

163 *but also bizarre":* Note: These are referred to as "paraphasias" by neuropsychologists. New York University Medical Center neuropsychologist Dr. Allan Kluger notes that the use of these phrases in patients with traumatic brain injuries is associated with changes in the left temporal cortex.

164 *Changes in the "Beam":* Note: Without further research it is difficult to distinguish "problems in attending" from "problems in encoding or registering short-

term memories," i.e., to know if someone wasn't paying attention as the basis for not remembering something, or *was* paying attention but failed to "register" or "encode" in memory what was being attended to. Research will be needed to distinguish between these two possibilities.

170 *shores of memory":* Letty Cottin Pogrebin, *Getting Over Getting Older: An Intimate Journey.* Boston: Little, Brown, 1996, p. 99.

177 *stress differently:* My thanks to ob/gyn Dr. Maurice Cohen for alerting me to this complex symptom. From my interviews with women I too believe it is a distinct symptom.

177 *in the recent past:* S. Lindheim, R.S. Legro, and L. Bernstein et al., Behavioral stress responses in premenopausal and postmenopausal women and the effects of estrogen, *Am. J. Obstet. Gynecol,* 167; 1992: 1831–6.

178 *hormonal change:* Note: This symptom of not handling stress in the same way may reflect:

(1) a decreased tolerance for the same *outward* amount of stress possibly because the body during perimenopause and menopause is already adapting to many more subtle new *interior* biological shifts and changes (stressors) that are reflected in other WHM Syndrome symptoms. The load of added internal changes may reduce the overall tolerance for outward stress that the body can handle. I am referring here to one possible definition of stress that has been used in health psychology: "having to adjust to change."

(2) This symptom may also reflect on the integrity of the "stress handling" emergency coping system that Hans Selye described—the General Adaptation Syndrome. It's now known that prolonged intense stress, by elevating the levels of such stress hormones as cortisol, can damage neurons in the hippocampus—sometimes reversibly (see McEwen below). But research suggests that estrogen-replacement therapy, i.e., estrogen, can buffer the effects of stress, reducing the negative physiological consequences of such stress in postmenopausal women. S. Lindheim, R. S. Legro, L. Bernstein et al., Behavioral stress responses in premenopausal and postmenopausal women and the effects of estrogen, *Am. J. Obstet. Gynecol,* 167; 1992: 1831–6.

(3) Furthermore, estrogen loss has been associated with both architectural and chemical changes in the hippocampus—the major memory coding organ of the brain, processing incoming information. And the hippocampus has been found "to regulate the stress response" and to "inhibit the response of the HPA to stress." [The HPA is the hypothalamic-pituitary axis—a hormone-based interactive signaling system that responds to stress with a cascade of events.] Thus, by altering the functioning of the hippocampus, estrogen may alter the integrity of the stress-response system under the control of the hippocampus. B. McEwen, Protective and damaging effects of stress mediators, *New England J. Med.,* 338(3); Jan. 15, 1998: L. Jacobson, R. Sapolsky, The role of the hippocampus in feedback regulation of the hypothalamic-pituitary adrenocortical axis, *Endocrin. Rev.,* 12(2); 1991: 118–34; J. Herman, W. E. Cullinan, Neurocircuitry of stress: Central control of the HMA axis, *Trends Neurosci,* 20; 1997: 78–84. Thus, declining estrogen levels may act in some to compromise the ability to handle stress to a noticeable degree. It would make sense that being alert and highly responsive to danger and handling high loads of stress would be an important trait advanta-

geous to assure the survival of the species during the years of fertility and be tied to ovarian/hormonal functioning. It would make sense too that this "handling high loads of stress" would possibly assume lesser relative importance when the goal of assuring the propogation of the next generation of the species becomes irrelevant—after fertility is over.

(4) Or this symptom may be just a temporary change in response to factors we are not yet aware of. Research will have to disentangle the basis for this observed symptom.

185 *feel ourselves disappear":* Letty Cottin Pogrebin, *Getting Over Getting Older,* p. 99.

Chapter 8

Page

205 In the Notes you will find a number you can call to find out where these are available: Wilson Sports 800-622-7955, Golf-Score Caddy W327.

Chapter 9

Page

215 *needs of patients":* Interview with Pam Boggs.
216 *Listening to Your Hormones:* Gillian Ford, *Listening to Your Hormones,* Prima Publishing, 1997: 303.
216 *of menopausal issues:* Interview with Dr. Michelle Warren, director of Columbia-Presbyterian Medical Center's Center for Menopause and Hormonal Disorders.
217 *Our Health, Our Lives:* Eileen Hoffman, *Our Health, Our Lives, A Revolutionay Approach to Total Health Care for Women,* Pocket Books, 1995.
218 *Dr. Nachtigall said:* Interview with Dr. Lila Nachtigall.
218 *and HMO picture:* Interview with Dr. Maurice Cohen.
218 *unlike Quiana Mortier:* Interviews with Dr. Frederick Naftolin, Dr. William Andrews, Dr. Bruce McEwen, Dr. Jim Morrison.

Chapter 10

Page

224 *hormone replacement therapy (See below.):* Richard J. Santen, M.D., Treatment of menopausal symptoms when estrogen is not acceptable or is contraindicated. North American Menopause Society, Eighth Annual Meeting, Sept. 4–6, 1997; Learning objectives narrative outlines.
225 *another step forward:* ACOG Educational Bulletin (247); May 1998, Hormone Replacement Therapy; replaces number 166, April 1992.

226 *headaches:* Note: Here they cited a 1977 placebo-controlled study of an English researcher, S. Campbell, in which women reported on an evaluative visual analog scale subjective ratings of improvement in their prior memory problems after use of estrogen alone: S. Campbell, M. Whitehead, Estrogen therapy and the menopausal syndrome. *Clin. Obstet. Gynecol.,* 4; 1977: 31–47.

226 *and improve function.* Studies by Barbara Sherwin were cited: 2, ACOG Educational Bulletin (247); May 1998, Hormone Replacement Therapy, 1–10. It is implicit in this educational directive that progesterone will also be given together with estrogen in women with a uterus.

226 *and adult tooth loss:* ACOG Educational Bulletin No. 247, May 1998, Hormone replacement therapy, 1–10.

227 *New York at Buffalo:* Interview with Dr. Uriel Halbreich.

229 *the following conditions:* North American Menopause Society, Menopause treatments, 1997; RA-10794-10019028.

229 *Replacement Therapy:* ACOG Educational Bulletin (247); May 1998, Hormone Replacement Therapy, 1–10.

231 *2.5 milligrams daily:* Richard J. Santen, M.D., Treatment of menopausal symptoms when estrogen is not acceptable or is contraindicated, The North American Menopause Society, Eighth Annual Meeting, Sept. 4–6, 1997, Learning objectives narrative outlines.

231 *onset after age fifty-five:* Jane Brody, Weighing the pros and cons of hormone therapy, *New York Times,* Sept. 8, 1998: F7.

231 *writing in Scientific American:* Nancy Davidson, Is hormone replacement therapy a risk. *Scientific American,* Sept. 1996: 101.

232 *smart (I think . . .)":* Letters to the editor in response to Claire Landsberg Warga's Estrogen and the brain, *New York* magazine, Sept. 8, 1997: 16.

233 *pharmaceutical houses:* Robin Marantz Henig, Behind the buzz on designer estrogens, questions linger. *New York Times,* June 21, 1998, women's health section.

234 *does in the brain:* V. Craig Jordan, Designer estrogens. *Scientific American,* Oct. 1998: 60–67. They are raloxifene (marketed as Evista) for the prevention of osteoporosis, and tamoxifen (marketed as Nolvadex), for preventing breast cancer.

234 *alpha and beta":* Interview with Dr. James Simpkins.

235 *to understand this.):* Pattie S. Green, Katherine Gordon, and James W. Simpkins, Phenolic A ring requirement for the neuroprotective effects of steroids. *J. Steroid Biochem. Molec. Biol.,* 63(4–6); 1997: 229–235.

235 *neuronal outgrowths":* Roberta Diaz Brinton, Julie Tran, Pam Proffitt, and Maria Montoya, 17 B-estradiol enhances the outgrowth and survival of neocortical neurons in culture. *Neurochemic. Res.,* 22(11); 1997: 1339–1351; Roberta Diaz Brinton, Pan Proffitt, Julie Tran, and Richarde Luu, Equilin, a principal component of the estrogen replacement therapy Premarin, increases the growth of cortical neurons via an NMDA receptor-dependent mechanism. *Exp. Neurology,* 147; 1997: 211–220; R. Diaz Brinton and Rose Yamazaki, Advances and challenges in the prevention and treatment of Alzheimer's disease. *Pharm Res,* 15(3); 1998: 386–98.

236 *we now know of":* Interview with Dr. James Simpkins.

237 *Women's lives today:* Interview with Dr. Roberta Brinton.

237 *all their life":* Interview with Dr. Susan Love.

237 *functioning of women.]":* Interview with Dr. Robert Butler.

247 *you are taking:* Interview with Barbara Sherwin.

252 *menopause and beyond:* Claire Landsberg Warga, "Estrogen and the brain. *New York* magazine, August 11, 1997.

Chapter 11

Page

260 *postsurgical complications: Lancet,* 1994.

263 *and behavioral measures . . .":* P. E. Gold, Role of glucose in regulating the brain and cognition. *Am. J. Clin. Nutr.,* 61 (4 Suppl); Apr. 1995: 987S–995S.

263 *in [such] patients . . .":* S. Craft, J. Newcomer, S. Kanne, Jack S. Dagogo, et al., Memory improvement following induced hyperinsulinemia in Alzheimer's disease. *Neurobiol. Aging,* 17(1); Jan.-Feb. 1996: 123–30.

264 *and fluency performance":* J. B. Allen, A. M. Gross, M. S. Aloia, C. Billingsly, The effects of glucose on nonmemory cognitive functioning in the elderly. *Neuropsychologia,* 34(5); May 1966: 459–65.

265 *previously observed object:* C. Messier, Object recognition in mice: Improvement of memory by glucose. *Neurobiol. Learning & Memory,* 67(2); Mar. 1997: 12–5.

265 *following estrogen treatment":* Jiong Shi and James W. Simpkins, 17 B-estradiol modulation of glucose transporter 1 expression in blood-brain barrier. *Am. J. Physiol.* (endocrinol. Metab. 35) 1997: E1016–E1022.

266 *a glucose transporter 1:* Jiong Shi, Yu Zhang, James W. Simpkins, Effects of 17 b-estradiol on glucose transporter 1 expression and endothelial cell survival following focal ischemia in the rats [sic], *Exp. Brain Res.,* 117; 1997: 200–206.

266 *of flushing episodes:* J. W. Simpkins, and M. J. Katovich, Relationship between blood glucose and hot flushes in women and an animal model. In: *Thermoregulation: Research and clinical application.* P. Lomax and E. Schonbaum, eds. Basel: Karger, 95–100.

266 *glucose supplies:* James W. Simpkins and Michael J. Katovich, Hypoglycemia causes hot flashes in animal models. *Multidisciplinary Perspectives on Menopause,* vol. 592 of the *Annals of the New York Academy of Sciences,* June 13, 1990.

267 *via diet:* Interview with nutritionist Lea Anztis; Kathleen DesMaisons, *Potatoes not Prozac,* Simon & Schuster, 1998.

268 *Genistein:* Source: Bonnie Liebman, The soy story. *Nutrition Action Healthletter,* (Center for Science in the Public Interest), 25(7); Sept. 1998: 3–7.

268 *protein:* Note: Isoflavone estimates are the ones published by the companies involved and reported by Bonnie Liebman, The soy story. *Nutrition Action Healthletter,* (Center for Science in the Public Interest), 25(7); Sept. 1998: 3–7. The isoflavone and protein figures may only be rough estimates according to this source.

268 *in the Public Interest: Nutrition Action Healthletter,* 25(7); 3–7. Ask your librarian for a copy of this issue or check the appendix for an address or fax to order it directly: *Nutrition Action Healthletter,* 1875 Connecticut Avenue NW, Suite 300, Washington, DC 20009–5728. Fax: 202-265-4954. $2.50.

269 *women's arteries:* P. J. Nestel et al., Soy isoflavones improve systemic arterial compliance but not plasma lipids in menopausal and perimenopausal women, *Arteriosclerosis, Thrombosis & Vascular Biology* 17(12); 1997: 3392–8.

269 *density in the spine: Amer. J. Clin. Nutr.,* in press.

269 *individual starting factors: Circulation,* 97; 1998: 816.

269 *So go figure!:* T. Clarkson, S. Anthony, and C. Hughes, Estrogenic soybean isoflavones and chronic disease. *TEM,* 6(1); 1995: 11–16.

270 *in Alzheimer's patients:* James Simpkins, Pattie Green, et al., Role of estrogen replacement therapy in memory enhancement and the prevention of neuronal loss associated with Alzheimer's disease. *Am. J. Med.,* 103 (3A), Sept. 22, 1997: 19S–25S.

270 *native repair mechanisms:* Ibid.

271 *of Alzheimer's disease":* M. C. Morris, L. A. Beckett, P. A. Scherr, et al., Vitamin E and vitamin C supplement use and risk of incident Alzheimer's disease. *Alzheimer's Disease Assoc. Disord.,* 12(3); Sept. 1998: 121–6.

271 *The Alternative Medicine Handbook:* Barrie Cassileth, *The Alternative Medicine Handbook,* New York, W. W. Norton, 1998.

271 *800 IU daily:* Ibid., 71.

271 *uncommon" she says:* Ibid., 74.

"antioxidant cocktail": Sarah Fremerman, Clearing the fog: How to sharpen your mind. *Natural Health,* March/April 1998: 99–181.

274 *through different routes:* Uriel Halbreich, Role of estrogen in postmenopausal depression, *Neurology,* 48 (supplement 7); 1997.

275 *by Kathleen DesMaisons:* Kathleen DesMaisons, *Potatoes not Prozac,* Simon & Schuster, New York, 1998.

275 *in the middle:* David J. Morrow, Lusting after Prozac. *New York Times,* October 11, 1998.

Chapter 12

Page

280 *sprouting neuronal connections:* I. J. Weiler, N. Hawrylak, W. T. Greenough, Morphogenesis in memory formation: Synaptic and cellular mechanisms. *Behav. Brain Res.,* 66 (1–2): Jan. 23, 1995; J. E. Black 1–6, K. R. Isaacs, W. T. Greenough, Usual vs. successful aging: Some notes on experiential factors. *Neurobiol. Aging,* 12 (4); 1991: 325–8.

282 *and abnormal aging":* P. S. Timiras, Education, homeostatsis, and longevity. *Experim. Geront.,* 30 (3–4); May-Aug. 1995: 189–98.

282 *among other factors:* J. E. Black, K. R. Isaacs, W. T. Greenough, Usual vs. successful aging: Some notes on experiential factors. *Neurobiol. Aging,* 12 (4); 1991: 325–8.

282 *declare in their work:* J. E. Black, K. R. Isaacs, W. T. Greenough, Usual vs. successful aging: Some notes on experiential factors. *Neurobiol. of Aging,* 12 (4); 1991: 325–8.

283 *unresponsive to change]":* Marcia Barinaga, The brain remaps its own contours. *Science,* 258; October 9, 1992: 216–18.

283 *supply routes to the brain:* K. R. Isaacs, B. J. Anderson, A. A. Alcantara, J. E. Black, W. T. Greenough, Exercise and the brain: Angiogenesis in the adult rat cerebellum after vigorous physical activity and motor skill learning. *J. Cerebral Blood Flow & Metab.,* 12 (1); Jan. 1992: 110–9; J. E. Black, K. R. Isaacs, B. J. Anderson, A. A. Alcantara, W. T. Greenough, Learning causes synaptogenesis, whereas activity causes angiogenesis in cerebellar cortex of adult rats. *Proceed. Nat. Acad. Sci. U.S.A.,* 87(14); July 1990: 5568–72.

284 *branching in the brain."* Interview with the author.

284 *new brain cells:* John Rowe and Robert L. Kahn, *Successful Aging,* Pantheon Books, New York; 1998.

284 *mental performance:* Dr. J. Michael Murphy, *Arch. Ped. & Adol. Med.,* September 1998.

284 *are hurt by hunger:* Jane Brody, People who skip breaskfast pay a high price. *New York Times,* October 6, 1998: F7.

285 *the stress hormone: Science News,* 153; April 25, 1998: 263.

288 *forget, you often do":* Interview with Dr. Margie Lachman.

288 *her colleagues write:* Margie E. Lachman, Suzanne L. Weaver, Mary Bandura, Elaine Elliott, and Corinne J. Lewkowicz, Improving memory and control beliefs through cognitive restructuring and self-generated strategies. *J. Geront.: Psych. Sci.,* 47(5); 1992: 293–2.

288 *show poorer performance.*(Berry, West & Dennehy, 1989; Hertzog et al., 1990; Lachman, Steinberg & Trotter, 1987): Ibid., 293–99.

289 *problem solving":* Interview with the author.

289 *used for recall":* O. Burack, M. E. Lachman, The effects of list-making on recall in young and elderly adults. *J. Geront.: Psych. Sci.,* 51B; 1996: 226–233.

290 *through glucose disregulation:* M. Vanhanen, K. Koivisto, et al., Risk for non-insulin-dependent diabetes in the normoglycaemic elderly is associated with impaired cognitive function. *Neuroreport,* 8(6); Apr. 14, 1997: 1527–30; J. Dey, A. Misra, N. G. Desai, et al., Cognitive function in younger type II diabetes. *Diabetes Care,* (1); Jan. 2, 1997: 32–5.

Chapter 13

Page

302 *and synthesize better.* Interview with Dr. Donna Korol.

Chapter 14

Page

313 *men for many years:* Jed Diamond, *Male Menopause,* Sourcebooks, Inc., Naperville, Ill., 1997.

313 *brain meltdown:* Anita Manning, Boomer brain meltdown. *USA Today,* January 6, 1998.

315 *resistance to stress":* A. Vermeulen, Andropause, fact or fiction? In *The Modern Management of the Menopause,* G. Berg and M. Hammar, eds., Parthenon Publishing Group, New York, 1994, pp. 567–77.

316 *is therefore questionable:* W. B. Schill, F. M. Kohn, G. Haidl, The aging male. In *The Modern Manaagement of the Menopause,* G. Berg and M. Hammar, eds., Parthenon Publishing Group, New York, 1994: 552.

317 *male sexual mating:* J. Raloff, A new breadth to estrogen's bisexuality. *Science News,* vol. 151, Feb. 22, 1997: 116.

317 *testes atrophied progressively:* J. Raloff, Estrogen's emerging manly alter ego. *Sci. News,* 152; Dec. 6, 1997: 356.

317 *injections with salt water:* M. G. Packard, J. R. Kohlmaier, G. M. Alexander, Post-training intrahippocampal estradiol injections enhanced spatial memory in male rats: Interaction with cholinergic systems. *Behav. Neurosci.,* 110(3); June 1996: 626–32.

317 *short-term and long-term:* F. Vazquez-Pereyra, S. Rivas-Arancibia, Castillo A. Loaeza-Del, S. Schneider-Rivas, Modulation of short term and long term memory by steroid sexual hormones. *Life Sci.,* 56(14); 1995: P1255–60.

Chapter 15

Page

321 *normal men and women":* Barbara Sherwin and Linda Carlson, Estrogen and memory in women. *J. Soc. Obstet. and Gynec. of Canada,* Oct. 1997: 7.

322 *do that, but not this":* René Dubos, Choosing to be human. Interview with Dubos by Warga in *OMNI,* 1979.

322 *shaped the human mind too:* E. O. Wilson, *Consilience,* Alfred Knopf, New York, 1998.

324 *schedules of reward":* Interview with Dr. John Gibbons, "Running late? Researchers blame aging brain. *New York Times,* March 24, 1998: E1.

326 *It didn't make sense:* Interview with Dr. Bruce McEwen.

327 *those who had them:* Note: It's my suspicion that obsessive/compulsive traits may possibly reflect on the existence in humans of adaptive built-in "default-mode" or innate rules—as do WHMS symptoms—that we all have within us to lesser "normal" degrees but that somehow go "awry" and are overboard in execution in those with Tourette's and other obsessive/compulsive disorders. Or stated somewhat differently, that obsessive/compulsive traits leak to us clues about some of the implicit default mode "rules" that drive "just being human" behavior.

329 *Lancet*, November 7, 1998: Marilynn Larkin, Discovery of dividing neurons in human brains excites researchers. *Lancet*, 352, November 7, 1998.

Appendix I

Page

331 *textbook on menopause: Treatment of the Post-Menopausal Woman, Basic and Clinical Aspects*, Rogerio A. Lobo, ed., Lippincott-Raven, Philadelphia, 1996.

332 *menopause researchers:* For the most part emotional/mood changes have remained little studied by menopause researchers. Menopause researchers in recent years have been focusing on whether depression is at all a feature associated with menopause and perimenopause. As noted earlier a dominant view at present (wrong in my opinion) is that depression is not commonplace in women during perimenopause and menopause, and when present is not the likely result of the biological events surrounding menopause, but when present is more likely a secondary reaction to sleep disruption and fatigue and/or the life-cycle psychosocial factors that occur in women at this stage of life.

332 *delusions, psychotic obsessions, etc.:* I have not had direct experience with women who have expressed such feelings, but in the recent book *Menopause and Madness*, author Marcia Lawrence describes her own and others' experience with psychotic symptoms, in relation to perimenopause. She provides research evidence that helps explain the plausible basis for such reactions in some women. *Menopause and Madness*, Marcia Lawrence, Andrews McMeel Publishing, Kansas City, 1998.

333 *migraine headaches:* "Continuous treatment with exogenous estrogens has been demonstrated to prevent migraine attacks," Philip Sarrel, Blood Flow. *Treatment of the Post-Menopausal Woman*, ed. Rogerio Lobo, Lippincott-Raven Publishers, Philadelphia, 1997: 259; and to act as an antidepressant, Ibid., 257–68. S. S. Smith, Hormones, mood, and neurobiology—a summary. *The Modern Management of Menopause*, ed. G. Berg and M. Hammar, Parthenon Publishing Group, New York, 1994.

333 *Chronic fatigue:* Note: In one study, twenty-two of twenty-eight patients with chronic fatigue syndrome improved with the use of estrogen patches used together with cyclical progestins, J. W. W. Studd, and N. Panay, Chronic fatigue syndrome. *Lancet*, 1996: 348, 384. Also, *Progress in the Management of the Menopause*, ed. Barry G. Wren, Parthenon Publishing Group, New York, 1997: 391.

333 *Symptoms of rheumatoid arthritis:* G.H.M. George and T. D. Spector, Arthritis, menopause and estrogens. *Progress in the Management of the Menopause*, ed. Barry G. Wren, the Parthenon Publishing Group, New York, 1997: 323.

333 *Symptoms of osteoarthritis:* Ibid., 324.

333 *Symptoms of fibromyalgia:* Ibid., 325.

334 *Atypical angina or Syndrome X (severe angina, positive EKG changes with exercise but normal coronary arteries):* Sarrel et al. "have reported an association between

Syndrome X and estradiol [a form of estrogen] deficiency. . . . The findings suggest that coronary symptoms in some women may be due to estrogen deficiency effects on coronary blood flow and that estrogen replacement may serve to stabilize coronary blood flow and vasodilator reserve capacity," Philip Sarrel, Blood Flow. *Treatment of the Post-Menopausal Woman*, ed. Rogerio Lobo, Lippincott-Raven Publishers, Philadelphia, 1997: 259–60.

334 *touch of another person:* Interview with Dr. Philip Sarrel.

334 *Diminished sexual desire (libido):* A. Graziottin, Hormones and libido. *Progress in the Management of the Menopause,* ed. Barry G. Wren, Parthenon Publishing Group, New York, 1997: 393–400.

334 *Vaginal dryness:* Ibid.

334 *Decreased metabolic rate and weight gain:* Eric Poehlman, Michael J. Toth et al., Change in energy balance and body composition at menopause. A controlled longitudinal study. *Annals Internal Med.,* 123(9); Nov. 1, 1995: 673–75.

334 *deposition of fat on stomach and hips:* Ibid.

334 *urinary tract symptoms:* M. Formosa, M. Brincat, L. Cardozo, J. Studd, The significance in skin, bones and bladder. *Treatment of the Post-Menopausal Woman,* ed. Rogerio Lobo, Lippincott-Raven Publishers, Philadelphia, 1997: 143–151.

334 *stress incontinence:* Ibid., 149.

INDEX